Paclitaxel in Cancer Treatment

BASIC AND CLINICAL ONCOLOGY

Editor

Bruce D. Cheson, M.D.

National Cancer Institute
National Institutes of Health
Bethesda, Maryland

1. Chronic Lymphocytic Leukemia: Scientific Advances and Clinical Developments, *edited by Bruce D. Cheson*
2. Therapeutic Applications of Interleukin-2, *edited by Michael B. Atkins and James W. Mier*
3. Cancer of the Prostate, *edited by Sakti Das and E. David Crawford*
4. Retinoids in Oncology, *edited by Waun Ki Hong and Reuben Lotan*
5. Filgrastim (r-metHuG-CSF) in Clinical Practice, *edited by George Morstyn and T. Michael Dexter*
6. Cancer Prevention and Control, *edited by Peter Greenwald, Barnett S. Kramer, and Douglas L. Weed*
7. Handbook of Supportive Care in Cancer, *edited by Jean Klastersky, Stephen C. Schimpff, and Hans-Jörg Senn*
8. Paclitaxel in Cancer Treatment, *edited by William P. McGuire and Eric K. Rowinsky*

ADDITIONAL VOLUMES IN PREPARATION

Paclitaxel in Cancer Treatment

edited by

William P. McGuire
Emory University
Atlanta, Georgia

Eric K. Rowinsky
Johns Hopkins Oncology Center
and Johns Hopkins Hospital
Johns Hopkins University School of Medicine
Baltimore, Maryland

Marcel Dekker, Inc.   New York • Basel • Hong Kong

ISBN: 0-8247-9307-2

The publisher offers discounts on this book when ordered in bulk quantities. For more information, write to Special Sales/Professional Marketing at the address below.

This book is printed on acid-free paper.

Marcel Dekker, Inc.
270 Madison Avenue, New York, New York 10016

Current printing (last digit):
10 9 8 7 6 5 4 3 2 1

Printed in the United States of America

Series Introduction

The current volume, *Paclitaxel in Cancer Treatment*, is the eighth in the Basic and Clinical Oncology series.

Many of the advances in oncology have resulted from close interaction between the basic scientist and the clinical researcher. This volume follows and expands on these aims to illustrate the success of this relationship as demonstrated by new insights into the development and use of a new class of anticancer drugs, the taxanes.

As editor of the series, my goal is to recruit volume editors who have not only established reputations based on their outstanding contributions to oncology, but also an appreciation for the dynamic interface between the laboratory and the clinic. To date, the series has consisted of monographs on topics that are of a high level of current interest; *Paclitaxel in Cancer Treatment* certainly fits into that category as a most important addition to the series.

Volumes in progress focus on supportive care of the cancer patient, the use of purine analogs in cancer therapy, gene therapy in cancer, and controversies in breast cancer, consultations in gynecologic cancer, principles of anticancer drug development, and cancer drug resistance. I anticipate that these volumes will provide a valuable contribution to the oncology literature.

BRUCE D. CHESON

Preface

In the past 50 years, since the initial discoveries that the alkylating agent nitrogen mustard and the antimetabolites methotrexate and 5-fluorouracil possessed cytotoxic activity against several human malignancies, fewer than 100 compounds have been licensed for the treatment of cancer, and many of these have rare indications. Additionally, many of these compounds are congeners of each other, with little difference in therapeutic index. The process of developing novel anticancer drugs with unique mechanisms of action and broad clinical activity has been arduous and partly serendipitous; however, this process has led to tremendous successes in identifying several classes of agents capable of curing and palliating a broad range of human tumors.

In the 1960s, the taxanes, a structurally and mechanistically unique class of antineoplastic agents, was identified. This book is dedicated to the journey taken by the first of this class of compounds, paclitaxel. Despite the elucidation of its broad activity and its unique structure by Wall and Wani in the late 1960s, developmental efforts with paclitaxel ceased for nearly a decade until Horwitz discovered that paclitaxel induced novel biological effects and had a unique mechanism of action. Solubility problems and a limited drug supply from the natural resource, *Taxus brevifolia*, slowed the initiation of clinical trials. Early clinical trials were also hampered by significant toxicity, such as hypersensitivity reactions.

An alternative and renewable natural resource for paclitaxel has been identified and clinical toxicities have been successfully ameliorated through the tenacity of clinical investigators. Thirty years after its original identification, paclitaxel was approved by the Food and Drug Administration for treatment of refractory ovarian cancer, and more recently for refractory breast cancer. In fact, paclitaxel may be one of the most broadly active compounds available to treat human malignancy, with activity demonstrated in cancer of the ovary, breast, lung, head and neck, esophagus, bladder, testis, endometrium, and possibly some hematological and pediatric malignancies. However, it is in primary therapy of human cancer that any new agent may have its greatest impact, and the role of paclitaxel in the primary therapy of many human tumors has only recently been explored. The first such trial performed in advanced ovarian cancer indicates that paclitaxel is at least as active as cisplatin was when evaluated in similar patients in the 1980s and should now become part of the standard treatment of this disease. Its activity in breast cancer is also significant, as paclitaxel is the first major new drug in this disease since the introduction of doxorubicin in the 1960s. Currently, prospective, randomized trials are evaluating the utility of paclitaxel-based therapies in the treatment of metastatic breast cancer or in the high-risk adjuvant setting. Similar studies are being conducted in cancers of the lung, head and neck, esophagus, testis, and bladder.

The success with paclitaxel has also stimulated significant interest in the microtubule as a target for new therapeutics. In addition, it has also generated enthusiasm for the development of taxane analogs that may have improved therapeutic indices. One such analog, docetaxel, is already undergoing clinical evaluation and has shown exciting activity.

This book outlines the current state of knowledge about paclitaxel from both preclinical and clinical standpoints. It is not hyperbole to state that the 1990s will be the decade of the taxanes, much as the 1980s were for the platinum coordination complexes and the 1970s were for the anthracyclines. It is our intention that this book will serve as a foundation for those interested in this exciting new arena of cancer research.

WILLIAM P. McGUIRE
ERIC K. ROWINSKY

Contents

Contributors

Susan G. Arbuck, M.D. Clinical Research Scientist, Developmental Chemotherapy Section, Investigational Drug Branch, Cancer Therapy Evaluation Program, Division of Cancer Treatment, National Cancer Institute, National Institutes of Health, Bethesda, Maryland

Barbara A. Blaylock, Ph.D. ADP/National BioSystems, Inc., Rockville, Maryland

James Burroughs, M.S. Manager, Scientific Information Systems Department, Pharmaceutical Research Institute, Bristol-Myers Squibb Company, Wallingford, Connecticut

Renzo Canetta, M.D. Vice President, Clinical Cancer Department, Pharmaceutical Research Institute, Bristol-Myers Squibb Company, Wallingford, Connecticut

Alex Y. Chang, M.D. Associate Professor, Oncology in Medicine, Department of Medicine, University of Rochester School of Medicine and Dentistry, Rochester, New York

Bruce D. Cheson, M.D. Head, Medicine Section, Cancer Therapy Evaluation Program, Division of Cancer Treatment, National Cancer Institute, National Institutes of Health, Bethesda, Maryland

Marcia Dougan, M.P.H.   Clinical Scientist, Clinical Cancer Department, Pharmaceutical Research Institute, Bristol-Myers Squibb Company, Wallingford, Connecticut

Avi I. Einzig, M.D.   Associate Professor, Division of Oncology, Department of Medicine, Montefiore Medical Center and Albert Einstein Cancer Center, Albert Einstein College of Medicine, Bronx, New York

David S. Ettinger, M.D., F.A.C.P.   Professor of Oncology and Medicine, Division of Medical Oncology, Department of Oncology, Johns Hopkins Oncology Center, Johns Hopkins University School of Medicine, Baltimore, Maryland

Craig R. Fairchild, Ph.D.   Senior Research Investigator, Department of Experimental Therapeutics, Pharmaceutical Research Institute, Bristol-Myers Squibb Company, Princeton, New Jersey

Alexander Florczyk   Manager, Clinical Cancer Department, Pharmaceutical Research Institute, Bristol-Myers Squibb Company, Wallingford, Connecticut

Arlene A. Forastiere, M.D.   Associate Professor, Division of Medical Oncology, Department of Oncology, Johns Hopkins Oncology Center, Johns Hopkins University School of Medicine, Baltimore, Maryland

Charles R. Geard, Ph.D.   Professor, Center for Radiological Research, Department of Radiation Oncology, College of Physicians & Surgeons of Columbia University, New York, New York

Barry R. Goldspiel, Pharm.D.   Oncology Clinical Pharmacy Specialist, Pharmacy Department, National Institutes of Health Clinical Center, Bethesda, Maryland

Ruth Gubits, Ph.D.   Research Scientist, Department of Radiation Oncology, College of Physicians & Surgeons of Columbia University, New York, New York

Nancy Gustafson, M.S.   Senior Research Biostatistician, Biostatistics/Data Management Department, Pharmaceutical Research Institute, Bristol-Myers Squibb Company, Wallingford, Connecticut

Susan Hellmann, M.D., M.P.H.   Associate Director, Clinical Cancer Department, Pharmaceutical Research Institute, Bristol-Myers Squibb Company, Wallingford, Connecticut

Frankie Ann Holmes, M.D.   Associate Professor of Medicine, Department of Breast and Gynecologic Medical Oncology, University of Texas M. D. Anderson Cancer Center, Houston, Texas

Susan Band Horwitz, Ph.D.   Falkenstein Professor of Cancer Research, Department of Molecular Pharmacology, Albert Einstein College of Medicine, Bronx, New York

Craig A. Hurwitz, M.D.   Medical Director, Division of Pediatric Hematology–Oncology, Department of Pediatrics, Maine Medical Center, Portland, Maine, and Clinical Associate Professor, Department of Pediatrics, University of Vermont College of Medicine, Burlington, Vermont

Sharafadeen Kashimawo   Research Worker, Department of Radiation Oncology, College of Physicians & Surgeons of Columbia University, New York, New York

David George Ian Kingston, M.A., Ph.D.   Professor, Department of Chemistry, Virginia Polytechnic Institute and State University, Blacksburg, Virginia

William P. McGuire, M.D.   Professor of Medicine, Division of Hematology/Oncology, Department of Medicine, Emory University, Atlanta, Georgia

Franco M. Muggia, M.D., F.A.C.P.   Professor, University of Southern California School of Medicine, and Director, Clinical Investigations and Medical Oncology, USC/Norris Comprehensive Cancer Center, Los Angeles, California

Nicole Onetto, M.D.   Director, Clinical Cancer Department, Pharmaceutical Research Institute, Bristol-Myers Squibb Company, Wallingford, Connecticut

George A. Orr, Ph.D.   Professor, Department of Molecular Pharmacology, Albert Einstein College of Medicine, Bronx, New York

Srinivasa Rao, Ph.D.   Research Associate, Department of Molecular Pharmacology, Albert Einstein College of Medicine, Bronx, New York

Mary V. Relling, Pharm.D.   Assistant Member, St. Jude Children's Research Hospital, and Associate Professor, College of Pharmacy, University of Tennessee, Memphis, Tennessee

Israel Ringel, Ph.D.   Department of Pharmacology, The Hebrew University, Jerusalem, Israel

William C. Rose, Ph.D.   Senior Research Fellow, Department of Experimental Therapeutics, Pharmaceutical Research Institute, Bristol-Myers Squibb Company, Princeton, New Jersey

Eric K. Rowinsky, M.D.   Associate Professor, Division of Pharmacology and Experimental Therapeutics, Department of Oncology, Johns Hopkins Oncology Center, Johns Hopkins University School of Medicine, and Oncologist, Johns Hopkins Hospital, Baltimore, Maryland

Marcel Rozencweig, M.D.   Executive Vice President, Clinical Cancer Department, Pharmaceutical Research Institute, Bristol-Myers Squibb Company, Wallingford, Connecticut

Susan E. Sartorius, B.S., R.N.   Clinical Trials Research Nurse, Division of Medical Oncology, Department of Oncology Nursing, Johns Hopkins Oncology Center, Johns Hopkins University School of Medicine, Baltimore, Maryland

Peter B. Schiff, M.D., Ph.D.   Professor and Chairman, Department of Radiation Oncology, College of Physicians & Surgeons of Columbia University, New York, New York

Vicente Valero, M.D.   Assistant Professor of Medicine, Department of Breast and Gynecologic Medical Oncology, University of Texas M. D. Anderson Cancer Center, Houston, Texas

Janet Ruth Walczak, M.S.N., R.N.   Clinical Nurse Specialist, Division of Medical Oncology, Department of Oncology Nursing, Johns Hopkins Oncology Center, Johns Hopkins University School of Medicine, Baltimore, Maryland

Steven D. Weitman, M.D., Ph.D.   Associate Professor, Department of Pediatric Hematology–Oncology, Medical College of Wisconsin, Milwaukee, Wisconsin

Peter H. Wiernik, M.D.   Professor of Medicine, Clinical Oncology Program, Montefiore Medical Center and Albert Einstein Cancer Center, Albert Einstein College of Medicine, Bronx, New York

Wyndham H. Wilson, M.D., Ph.D.   Special Assistant to the Director, Division of Cancer Treatment, National Cancer Institute, National Institutes of Health, Bethesda, Maryland

Chia-Ping Huang Yang, Ph.D.   Instructor, Department of Molecular Pharmacology, Albert Einstein College of Medicine, Bronx, New York

1

History and Chemistry

DAVID GEORGE IAN KINGSTON
Virginia Polytechnic Institute and State University
Blacksburg, Virginia

I. INTRODUCTION

A. Scope

This chapter covers the chemistry of paclitaxel in a book that is aimed primarily at a medical audience. For this reason, and also because of page limitations imposed by the editors, the coverage of the chemistry of paclitaxel is selective rather than complete. Attention has been focused on those aspects of the chemistry which have led to useful structure-activity relationships or which are likely to prove important in a clinical situation. Those readers interested in a more detailed approach are referred to two recent reviews (1,2).

B. Discovery of Paclitaxel

Paclitaxel was first discovered in the bark of the western yew, *Taxus brevifolia* (3), but it was not the first taxane diterpenoid (or taxoid) to be isolated. That honor goes to the toxic constituents of the yew and to their chemical derivatives. The toxic properties of yew have been known for over two thousand years; it is thus understandable that the earliest chemical and pharmacological studies on the active constituents of yew were concerned with its toxic constituents. These early studies indicated that the major toxicity was due to an alkaloid "taxine," which was later shown to be a mixture of alkaloids with taxine A and taxine B (**1.1** and **1.2**

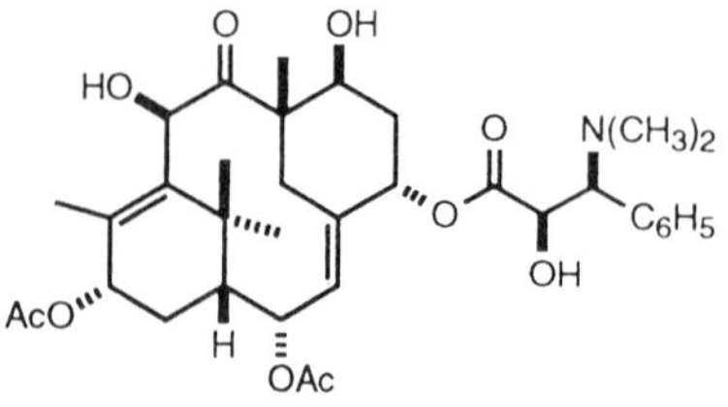

Figure 1 The structures of taxine A (**1.1**) and taxine B (**1.2**).

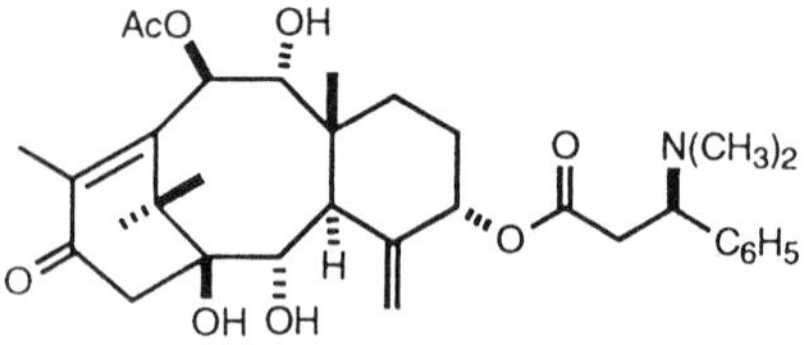

in Fig. 1) as the major components (4,5). The toxicity of yew is primarily due to taxine B, which shows cardiotoxic activity (6); this finding may yet prove to be important in view of the report that paclitaxel causes cardiac disturbances in some patients (7) and of the related structures of taxine B and paclitaxel.

Paclitaxel itself was isolated as a result of a systematic search for naturally occurring anticancer agents. This search was begun under the guidance of the late Dr. Jonathan Hartwell at the National Cancer Institute, and it initially focused on agents from higher plants and from microbial sources. Plant collections were carried out by a team from the U.S. Department of Agriculture under Dr. Robert Perdue, Jr., and fractionation work was carried out by research teams under contract with the National Cancer Institute, including a team under Dr. Monroe Wall at the Research Triangle Institute in North Carolina.

The western yew, *Taxus brevifolia*, is a small tree that grows primarily as an understory tree in the old-growth forests of the Pacific Northwest. A collection of the bark and other parts of this tree was first made in 1962, and the bark in particular was shown to have very good activity in the KB (Eagle's carcinoma of the nasopharynx) cytotoxicity assay. A large recollection was then made and assigned to Dr. Wall for fractionation in 1965. Isolation of paclitaxel proved to be a challenging task because it was present only in very small amounts in the bark. It was not until 1969 that adequate amounts were prepared for structure elucidation. The structure was solved by some careful chemical studies, including a key reaction that succeeded in cleaving paclitaxel into two pieces, which could be crystallized after derivatization. The x-ray structures of these two pieces were determined, and this work enabled the structure of paclitaxel itself to be deduced as shown by **2** in Figure 2 (3). Paclitaxel was originally named taxol, and all studies until 1993 used this chemical name.

C. Development of Paclitaxel

The biological activity of paclitaxel was not particularly impressive in comparison to that of other known and novel anticancer agents. It showed clear but modest activity in both P-388 and L-1210 leukemia and excellent cytotoxicity in the KB in

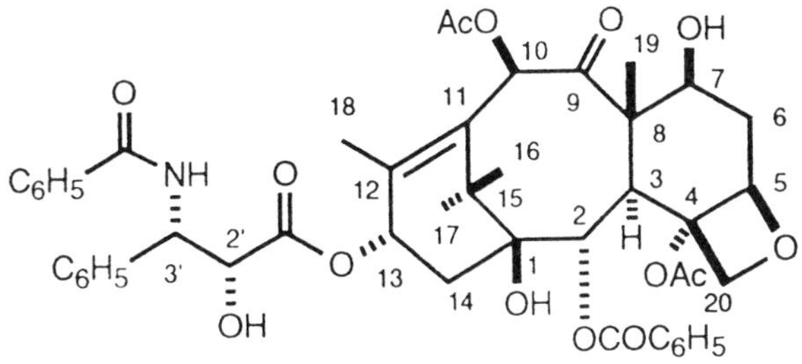

Figure 2 The structure and numbering of paclitaxel (**2**).

vitro assay. In addition, it was a costly compound to develop as a drug, both because of its lack of aqueous solubility and its very difficult isolation from a limited biological source. For these reasons, there were some questions about whether it should be considered for development, and the lack of interest is reflected in the fact that a composition-of-matter patent was never filed.

Fortunately for cancer patients, the decision was made to continue testing paclitaxel in additional animal models for various tumors as they became available, and modest additional quantities of paclitaxel material were prepared for this purpose. During the early 1970s, paclitaxel was tested in several new tumor systems, including B16 melanoma and various xenografts in nude mice. The results of this testing are summarized in Table 1, wherein it can be seen that paclitaxel shows excellent activity against the B16 melanoma, P1534 leukemia, and the MX-1 mammary xenograft (8,9). Based on this encouraging activity, the decision was made by the National Cancer Institute in 1977 to proceed with full-scale preclinical development and clinical trials of paclitaxel.

An important discovery in 1979 provided further impetus to the development of paclitaxel. In that year Dr. Susan Horwitz discovered that paclitaxel promoted the assembly of tubulin into stable microtubules (10), thus explaining the basis for paclitaxel's known action as an antimitotic drug. Although other anticancer agents, including the vinca alkaloids and the epipodophyllotoxins, are known to operate as antimitotic agents and tubulin binders, these agents acted by preventing the polymerization of tubulin into microtubules. Paclitaxel was (and still is) the only naturally occurring drug that acts by promoting the assembly of tubulin, and this discovery thus created great interest in it from a mechanistic point of view.

The period 1978–1982 saw the completion of preclinical studies on paclitaxel. The solubility problem was solved by the development of an emulsion formulation in polyoxyethylated castor oil, and toxicity studies showed that paclitaxel was relatively nontoxic to rats and beagle dogs. Phase I clinical trials were initiated in 1983; these were accompanied by some severe allergic responses that proved fatal

4

Kingston

Table 1 Selected Antitumor Activity Data for Paclitaxel

Tumor system	Route tumor/drug[a]	Regimen	Optimal dose (mg/kg/inj)	T/C (%) at optimal dose	Evaluation[b]
B16 melanoma	IP/IP	Daily × 9	5	283	++
P1534 leukemia	IP/IP	Daily × 10	3.75	300	++
P388 leukemia	IP/IP	q4d × 3	43	170	+
L1210 leukemia	IP/IP	Daily × 15	20	131	+
Colon 26	IP/IP	q4d × 2	30	161	+
MX-1 mammary xenograft	src/sc	Daily × 10	200	(−67)	++
LX-1 lung xenograft	src/sc	Daily × 10	200	(13)	+
CX-1 colon xenograft	src/sc	Daily × 10	400	(12)	+

[a]*Abbreviations*: IP, intraperitoneal; src, subrenal capsule; sc, subcutaneous
[b]++, highly active; +, active
Source: Ref. 9.

in at least one case (11). Happily, these problems did not end the trials (in part because of the interest in paclitaxel's unique mechanism of action), and the allergic reactions were minimized by the adoption of a protocol that includes premedication with glucocorticoids and antihistamines and a long infusion period.

Following the completion of phase I trials, phase II clinical trials began in 1985, and these began to show spectacular results. Full details of the clinical results with paclitaxel form a major part of this volume and thus are not discussed here, but the first published phase II clinical result showing a response rate of 30% in refractory ovarian cancer (12) should be noted, since it marked the beginning of a growing awareness among the medical community and the general public of the unusual properties of this exciting new drug.

The development of paclitaxel as an anticancer drug has recently been reviewed (13), with a particular emphasis on the supply problems and the methods used to overcome them.

II. THE CHEMISTRY OF PACLITAXEL

A. Introduction

Chemically paclitaxel is classified as a taxane diterpenoid, or taxoid. Diterpenoids are natural products with a C-20 carbon skeleton derived biogenetically from geranylgeraniol pyrophosphate, and the taxoids are a subclass of the diterpenoids with the unique tricyclo[9.3.1.0.^{3,8}]pentadecane or taxane ring system as the core structure. All known taxoids to date with one exception, discussed later, have been isolated from plants of the Taxaceae family, and most from various *Taxus* species. A few related compounds—such as taxine A (**1.1** in Fig. 1), which are obviously biogenetically related to the taxoids although they do not have the taxane ring system—are also included in the class of taxoids.

Over one hundred taxoids have been isolated to date. It is not the purpose of this chapter to review the structures of all these compounds; the interested reader is referred to a recently published comprehensive review (1) and to the current literature for information on other taxoids.

Paclitaxel differs from most other taxoids in two key respects. In the first place, its taxane skeleton is esterified at C-13 with a complex *N*-benzoylphenylisoserine ester group; in the second place, it has an unusual fourth ring in the form of an oxetane ring attached at the C-4,5 positions. Both these features are necessary for its biological activity, as will be discussed later.

Although the conventional chemical representations of paclitaxel (such as **2** in Fig. 2) make it appear to be a planar molecule, this is far from the case. Paclitaxel does, in fact, have a shape somewhat like that of an inverted cup, in which the C-13 ester side chain is free to position itself under the mouth of the cup (Fig. 3). Some of the chemistry described later depends on this juxtaposition in space of seemingly remote functional groups.

B. Nuclear Magnetic Resonance Spectroscopy

Nuclear magnetic resonance (NMR) spectroscopy is a powerful technique that has played a key role in the structure elucidation and subsequent studies of the conformation of paclitaxel. Although it is by no means the only physical technique that has been applied to paclitaxel, it is the only one to date that has yielded significant three-dimensional structural information, since an x-ray crystallographic structure of paclitaxel has not yet been published, presumably because suitable crystals could not be obtained.

Although several NMR studies of paclitaxel and related compounds have been made (14–18), two of these (17,18) are particularly interesting in that they deduce the conformation of paclitaxel both in nonaqueous solvents and in mixed aqueous-organic solvents. One study (17) also compares the conformation deduced from NMR measurements with that obtained by molecular modeling calculations using the MacroModel Program. Both groups reach the conclusion that the dominant paclitaxel conformation in chloroform solution differs from that in aqueous dimethyl sulfoxide (DMSO) mainly in the C-13 ester side chain. In organic solvents, this side chain is oriented so that the 3′-phenyl ring is exposed to the solvent, while in aqueous DMSO this ring is spatially proximate to the acetate

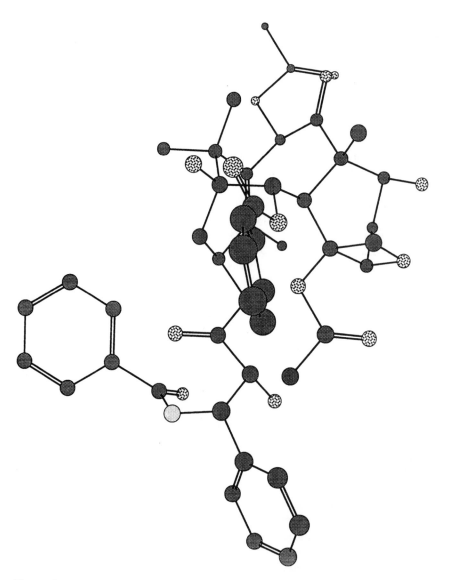

Figure 3   A perspective representation of the paclitaxel structure.

group at the 4 position and to the 2-benzoate to form a hydrophobic cluster. This work has obvious implication for the binding of paclitaxel to microtubules; indeed, a related paper on the conformation of the paclitaxel analog docetaxel (16) suggests that the taxane core of paclitaxel is first recognized and that this is then followed by orientation of the side chain on the basis of hydrophobic interactions, so that the side chain can interact with tubulin residues to give a stable drug-receptor complex.

C. Acylation and Related Chemistry

Although paclitaxel has three free hydroxyl groups, these are readily distinguished on the basis of their chemical nature. The 1-OH group is tertiary and is thus unreactive to all but the most vigorous acylation conditions. The 7-OH group is secondary but is sterically hindered by the adjacent 8-CH_3 group; thus the secondary and unhindered 2'-OH group is the most reactive. Mild acylation of paclitaxel with acetic anhydride thus yields the 2'-acetate selectively, while more vigorous conditions yield the 2',7-diacetate (19). This same order of reactivity applies to other protective groups; thus the 2'-triethylsilyl ether of paclitaxel can be prepared under mild conditions and the 2',7-di(triethylsilyl) ether can be prepared under more vigorous conditions.

D. Hydrolysis and Epimerization

Hydrolysis of paclitaxel occurs readily, but the products obtained depend very much on the conditions.

Under aqueous or alcoholic conditions, hydrolysis or methanolysis tends to yield a complex mixture of products. This is exemplified by the methanolysis of cephalomannine, a naturally occurring paclitaxel analog that differs from paclitaxel only in having an N-tigloyl group in place of the N-benzoyl group of paclitaxel. Under mild methanolysis conditions, five taxoid products were obtained (Fig. 4) and identified as 10-deacetylcephalomannine (**4.2** in Fig. 4), baccatin III (**4.3**), 10-deacetylbaccatin III (**4.4**), 7-*epi*-baccatin III (**4.5**), and 10-deacetyl-7-*epi*-baccatin III (**4.6**) (20). The formation of the C-7 epimers **4.5** and **4.6** is discussed below, but this result clearly demonstrates the lability of the side chain and the C-10 acetate to hydrolysis under aqueous conditions as well as the lability of the configuration of the C-7 hydroxyl group.

Although paclitaxel has several groups that are labile to hydrolysis under aqueous conditions, it is still possible to carry out selective hydrolysis at the 2'-position under very mild conditions. As an example of this, 2',7-diacetylpaclitaxel can be hydrolyzed in reasonable yield to 7-acetylpaclitaxel in the presence of aqueous bicarbonate (19). This chemistry forms the basis of various prodrug derivatives of paclitaxel, which are discussed in the next section.

Selective cleavage of the side-chain of paclitaxel can be accomplished under

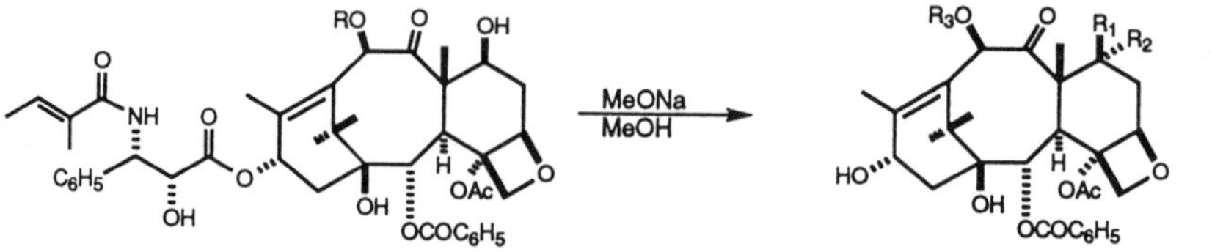

	R			R₁	R₂	R₃
Cephalomannine	**4.1**	Ac	Baccatin III	**4.3**	OH	H	Ac
10-Deacetyl cephalomannine	**4.2**	H	10-Deacetyl baccatin III	**4.4**	OH	H	H
			7-epi baccatin III	**4.5**	H	OH	Ac
			10-Deacetyl-7-epi-baccatin III	**4.6**	H	OH	H

Figure 4   Methanolysis of cephalomannine (**4.1**).

two different sets of conditions. The first method is not strictly speaking a hydrolysis, since it uses tetrabutylammonium borohydride to remove the side chain in a reductive step (21). This reaction is very clean and has become the preferred method of preparing baccatin III from paclitaxel and from mixtures of paclitaxel and cephalomannine and other related taxoids. It depends for its effectiveness on the presence of a free 2′-hydroxyl group, which complexes with the borohydride anion to deliver the hydride selectively to the side-chain carbonyl group. An alternate method using lithium iodide in methanol gives good yields only when the 7-hydroxyl group is protected as its triethylsilyl ether (22).

Cleavage of the 10-acetoxy group of paclitaxel can be achieved by treatment with zinc bromide to give 10-deacetylpaclitaxel, but this reaction is always accompanied in part by epimerization at C-7, and the yield of 10-deacetylpaclitaxel is thus not very good (23).

Selective cleavage of the C-2 benzoate has recently been achieved (24). Treatment of 2′,7-di(triethylsilyl)paclitaxel (**5.1** in Fig. 5) with base under phase-transfer conditions yielded the 2-debenzoyl derivative **5.2**, which could be reacylated under carefully controlled conditions and deprotected to yield the 2-debenzoyl-2-acylpaclitaxel analog **5.3**. If reacylation was carried out under uncontrolled conditions, an intramolecular displacement reaction gave the iso-paclitaxel derivative **5.4** as the major product.

Selective hydrolysis of the paclitaxel derivative baccatin III has been studied by several groups. Methanolysis of hexahydrobaccatin III (protected as its 7-triethyl-silyl ether) yielded the 10-deacetyl and the 4,10-dideacetyl derivatives before deacylation at C-2 took place (25). Further treatment with base led to an oxetane ring-opening reaction to give a product analogous to **5.4**. A similar product was also formed on treatment of 7,13-diacetylbaccatin III with tributyltin methoxide in the presence of lithium chloride (26), and hydrolysis of 10-deacetyl-7-triethylsilylbaccatin III also yielded an analogous product (27).

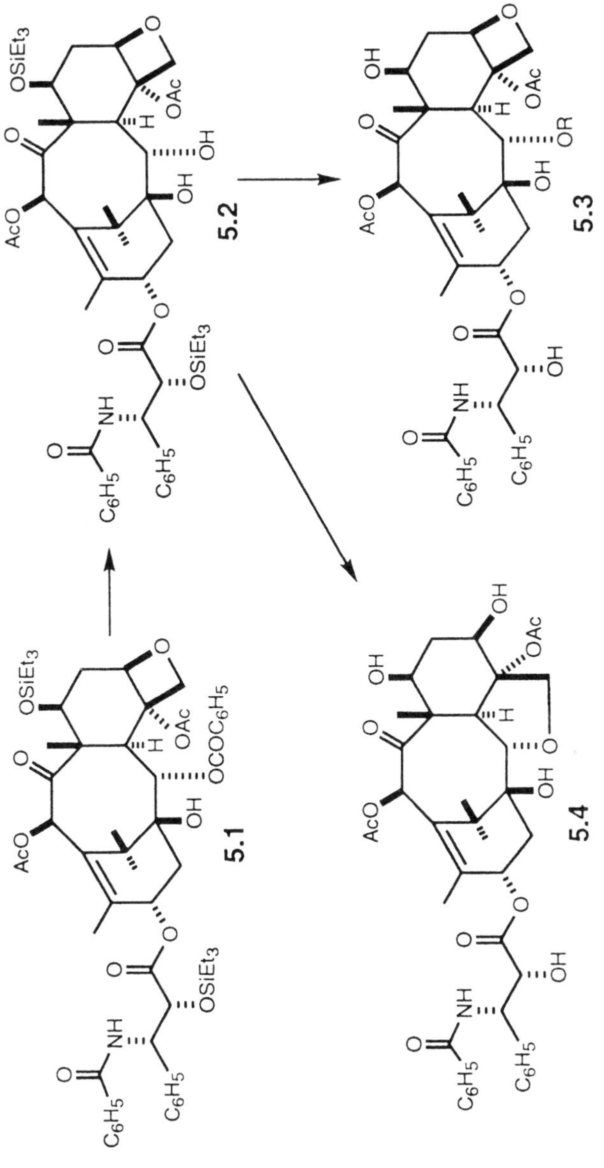

Figure 5 Preparation of 2-debenzoylpaclitaxel analogs.

As noted earlier, paclitaxel and its analogs readily undergo epimerization at C-7 in the presence of mild base. This reaction is believed to proceed through a base-promoted retro-aldol condensation to give the enolate (**6.2** in Fig. 6), which can then cyclize back to the natural configuration **6.1** or to the epimeric configuration **6.3**. The epimer **6.3** appears to be the more stable isomer, since treatment of paclitaxel with sodium hydride in an inert solvent leads to complete epimerization to 7-*epi*-paclitaxel (28). The reason for the greater stability of the epimer is probably associated with hydrogen bonding of the 7-*epi*-hydroxyl group to the 4-acetate group; this bonding can be seen in the x-ray structure of baccatin V (7-*epi*-baccatin III) (29). In hydroxylic solvents, intramolecular hydrogen bonding competes with intermolecular bonding, and an equilibrium mixture of epimers is formed. Epimerization is particularly facile in the 10-deacetyl series, and 10-deacetylpaclitaxel is converted to a mixture of epimers simply on standing in aqueous methanol (30).

The conversion of 7-*epi*-paclitaxel to paclitaxel can be accomplished in good yield by a four-step process that relies on the fact that the 7-*epi* position is even more sterically crowded than the 7 position. Formation of a xanthate ester under equilibrating conditions thus yields the normal ester regardless of whether the starting material is in the normal or the *epi* series, and hydrolysis of this ester yields the normal alcohol (28).

E. Prodrugs

The low solubility of paclitaxel in water (0.7 mg/mL) (31), coupled with its relatively low potency and thus with the need for large clinical doses, proved to be a major stumbling block in the development of paclitaxel as an anticancer agent. Although the immediate problem was solved by the polyoxyethylated castor oil emulsion mentioned earlier, a water-soluble and active paclitaxel analog would be highly desirable to avoid the difficulties associated with the use of polyoxyethylated castor oil. A prodrug approach is ideal for this situation, since cleavage of the prodrug by hydrolysis or by other means would convert it back to paclitaxel and would thus retain all the activity associated with paclitaxel.

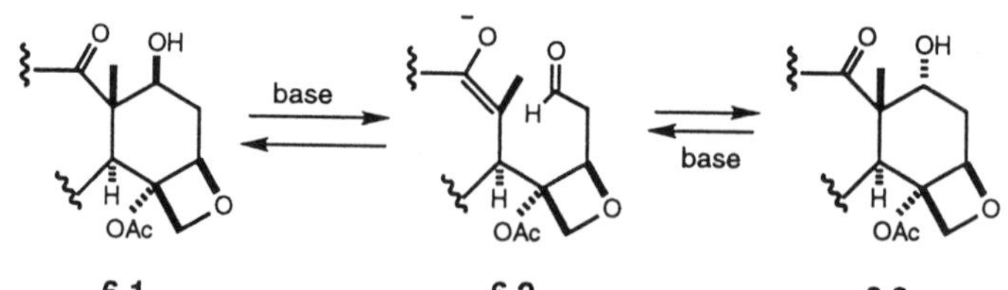

6.1   **6.2**   **6.3**

Figure 6 Proposed epimerization mechanism of paclitaxel.

The design of a successful prodrug requires that the prodrug be converted to the parent drug reasonably quickly after injection or infusion but that it be chemically stable prior to administration. In the case of paclitaxel, chemical derivatization at either the 2' or the 7 position appeared to offer the best prospects for achieving these goals, and both approaches have been tried.

Various succinate and glutarate half esters at the 2' position were prepared by ourselves (32) and by Deutsch et al. (33). The salts of these acids (such as **7.2**, **7.3**, **7.5**, and **7.6** in Fig. 7), were found to have improved activity as compared with the free acids **7.1** and **7.4** (33), and the ammonium salt **7.7** was found to show excellent activity in the B16 melanoma system and the MX-1 breast xenograft system (33). Various sulfonic acid derivatives such as **7.8** were also prepared, but these turned out to have a diminished activity as compared with paclitaxel (34). However, a recent paper reports that half esters containing sulfone groups or heteroatoms in the diacid portion do show comparable cytotoxicity to paclitaxel (35).

A number of amino acid derivatives at the 2'-position have been prepared by our group (32) and, in particular, the Stella group (31). Of these derivatives, the most promising ones were the 3-(N, N-diethylamino)propionyl derivative **7.9** and the N, N-dimethylglycyl derivative **7.10**, both of which showed good solubility and good bioactivity, with **7.9** showing better activity than **7.10** (31).

Several chemical derivatives at the 7 position have also been prepared (31–33, 35,36), but these turn out to be much more stable than esters at the 2'-position and thus do not undergo hydrolysis to paclitaxel at a suitable rate; they are thus not appropriate for use as prodrugs.

F. Oxidation

Paclitaxel has two secondary hydroxyl groups, but the 2'-hydroxyl group is α to a carbonyl group and is less readily oxidized than the 7-hydroxyl group. Oxidation of paclitaxel with normal oxidants such as Jones's reagent thus gives the 7-oxo derivative selectively; more vigorous conditions are required to give the 2',7-dioxo derivative (37).

The C-11 (12) double bond of paclitaxel is very hindered and is thus not readily oxidized. Paclitaxel is thus resistant to oxidation with osmium tetroxide, ozone, and similar reagents specific for carbon-carbon double bonds.

G. Reduction

Just as the double bond of paclitaxel is resistant to oxidation, so also is it resistant to reduction. As an example of this, baccatin III can be hydrogenated over platinum in acetic acid to yield a hexahydro derivative, with the benzoyl group reduced to a cyclohexylcarbonyl group and the C-11 (12) double bond unaffected (24).

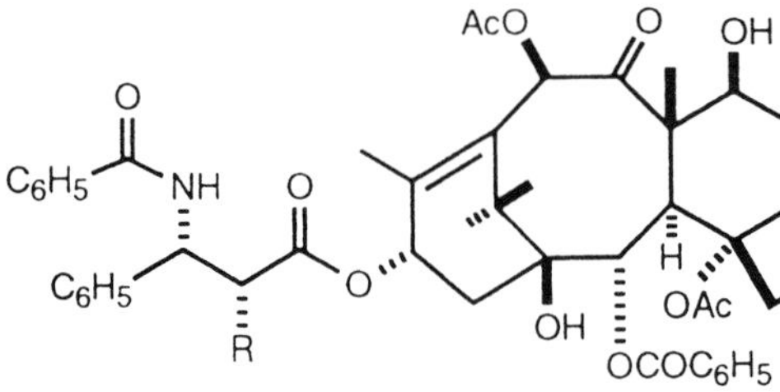

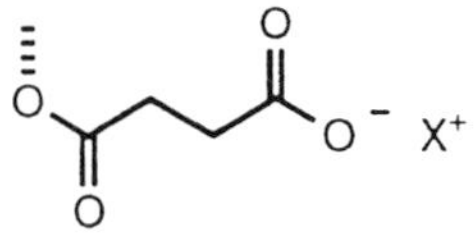

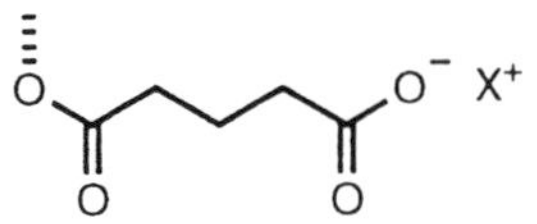

7.1 X = H
7.2 X = Na
7.3 X = (HOCH$_2$CH$_2$)$_3$NH

7.4 X = H
7.5 X = Na
7.6 X = (HOCH$_2$CH$_2$)$_3$NH

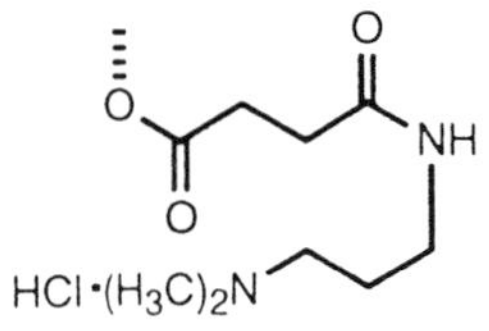

7.7

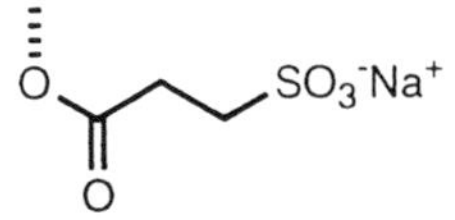

7.8

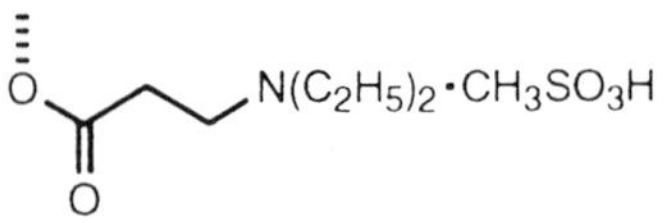

7.9

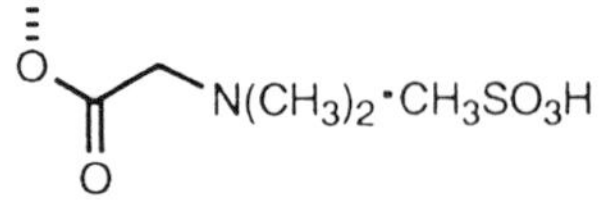

7.10

Figure 7 Prodrugs of paclitaxel with substitution at the 2'-position.

Deoxygenation of paclitaxel can be accomplished most readily by the Barton procedure, although an alternate and unexpected reaction with Yarovenko's reagent has also been used for this purpose (38). In the Barton procedure, conversion of paclitaxel to 7-deoxypaclitaxel (**8.2** in Fig. 8) was accomplished through the 7-S-methylxanthate (**8.1**) (28,39). 10-Deacetoxylpaclitaxel (**8.3**) has been prepared both by the route cited earlier (38) and also by deoxygenation of 10-deacetylbacca-

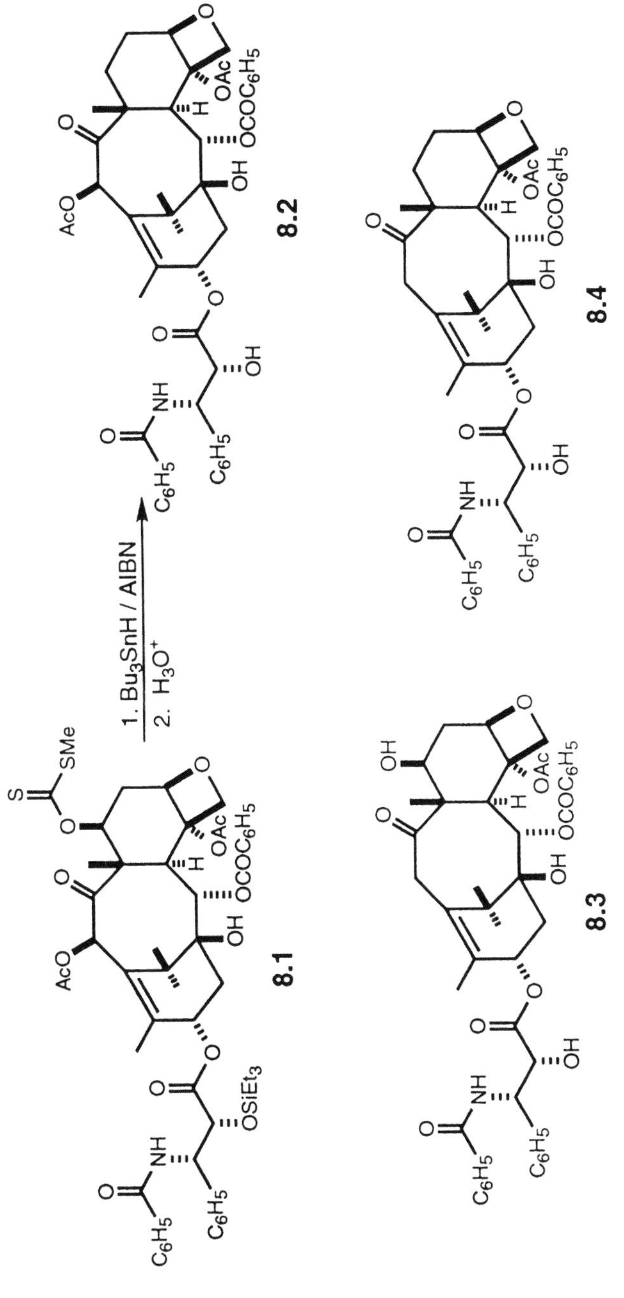

Figure 8 Deoxygenation of paclitaxel.

the Barton procedure, with subsequent introduction of the C-13 side chain (40). Recently, a direct reduction of paclitaxel to 10-deacetoxypaclitaxel with samarium diiodide has been disclosed (41). 7,10-Di-deoxypaclitaxel (**8.4**) has also been prepared by two different applications of the Barton procedure (39). In one case the 10-acetoxy group could be reduced without conversion to its xanthate derivative in the presence of excess tributyltin hydride (42), while in a second case an interesting rearrangement accompanied radical deoxygenation of 10-deacetoxy-paclitaxel (39). Deoxygenation at C-2 has also been achieved by the Barton procedure (43).

Reduction of paclitaxel with complex metal hydrides is an alternate to hydro-lysis for the selective removal of various acyl groups. Reduction of paclitaxel itself with tetrabutylammonium borohydride leads to selective cleavage of the side chain, as noted earlier, to give baccatin III (21). Reaction of protected baccatin III derivatives with lithium aluminum hydride at low temperature leads to selective or complete deacylation, depending on the conditions (27).

H. Oxetane Chemistry

The oxetane ring is one of the more unusual structural elements of paclitaxel, since this is a relatively rare feature of natural products. The oxetane ring is much more stable and less reactive than its three-membered analog the oxirane ring, but it can nonetheless undergo ring opening under various conditions.

The first ring-opening reaction was observed on treatment of 7-oxopaclitaxel with mild base; under these conditions, the oxetane ring opened in a β-elimination reaction to give **9.1** in Figure 9 (37). A ring-opening reaction with concomitant formation of a tetrahydrofuran ring has also been noted earlier (Fig. 5), and a similar reaction has been observed in the baccatin III series (26,27).

Ring opening also occurs under acidic conditions. Thus treatment of paclitaxel with Meerwein's reagent (triethyloxonium tetrafluoroborate) yields the ring-opened derivative **9.2** in a surprisingly selective reaction, which is believed to proceed with intramolecular assistance by the C-4 acetate (23). Similar reactions have been observed on treatment of a 2'-protected paclitaxel with a variety of Lewis acids such as $SnCl_4$, $TiCl_4$, or BF_3OEt_2 (22), and analogous products were obtained on treatment of baccatin III derivatives with $SnCl_4$ (22). An unusual oxido-bridged paclitaxel derivative, **9.3**, was formed when 2'-benzyloxycarbonyl-paclitaxel was treated with $SnCl_4$ at 0°; this product is probably formed by attack of the C-7 hydroxyl group on one of the cationic intermediates of the ring-opening reaction (22).

I. Rearrangement Reactions

Paclitaxel is relatively stable toward molecular rearrangement reactions, but it does undergo selective rearrangement under appropriate conditions. A ring-A

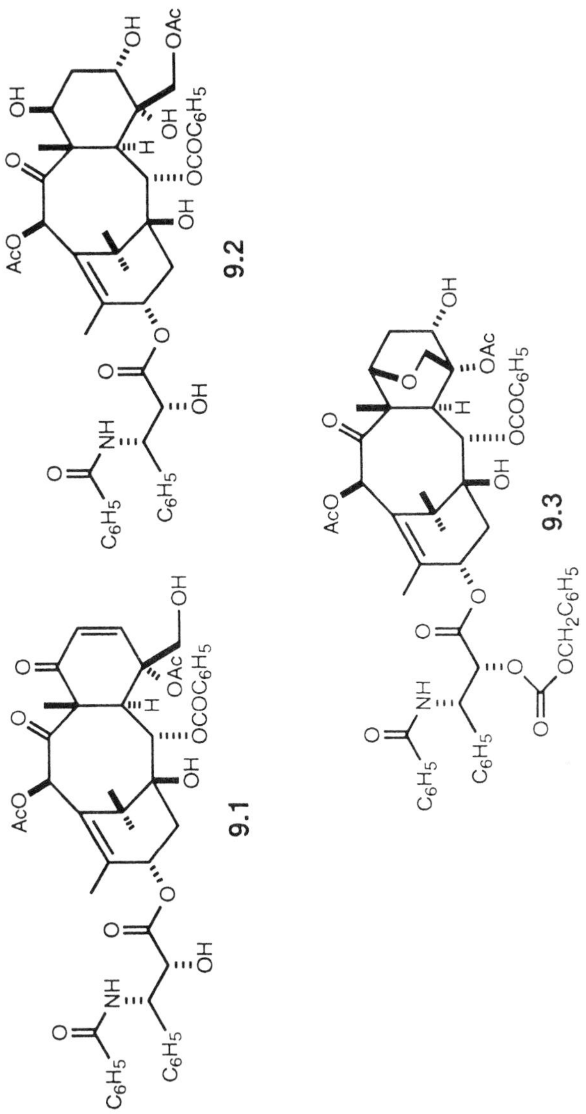

Figure 9 Oxetane ring-opened derivatives of paclitaxel.

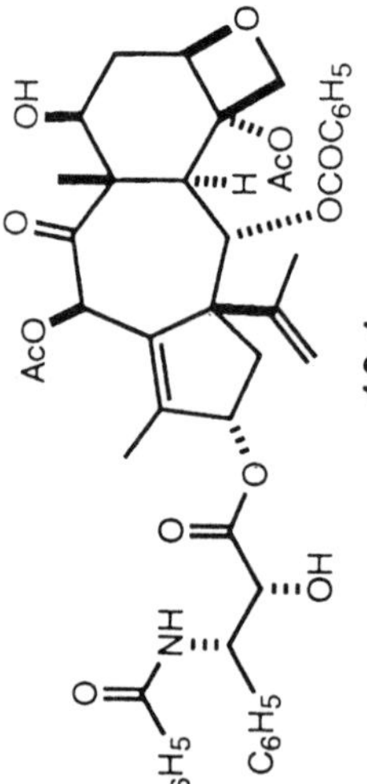

Figure 10 Rearranged paclitaxels.

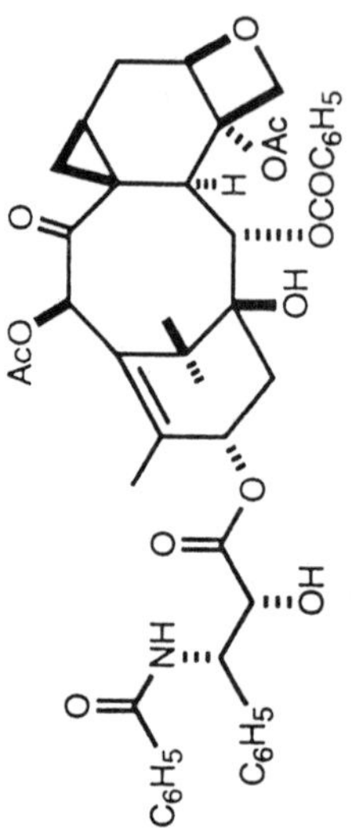

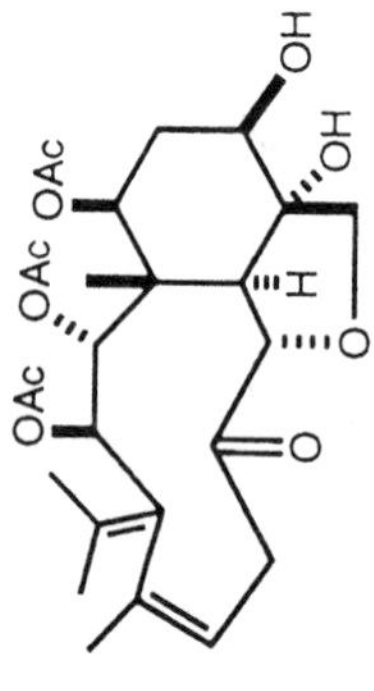

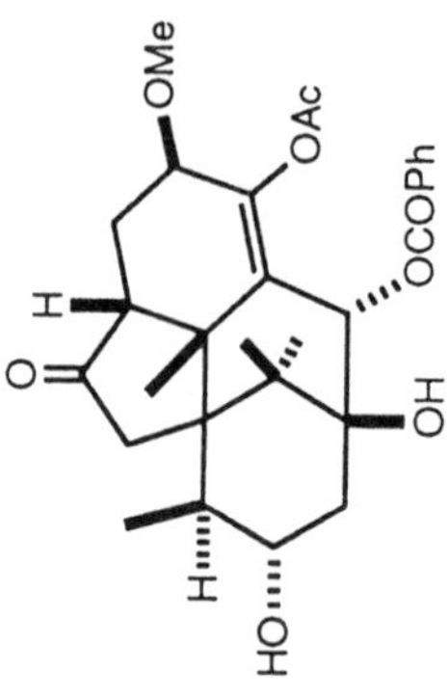

contraction of paclitaxel to yield an A-norpaclitaxel derivative was first noted when paclitaxel was treated with acetyl chloride under vigorous conditions, but these conditions also led to oxetane ring opening (23). The ring-A contraction alone could be achieved by preparation of the unstable C-1 mesylate of paclitaxel to give the A-norpaclitaxel derivative **10.1** in Figure 10 (23). A similar product is formed when docetaxel is treated with trifluoroacetic acid (27).

An interesting rearrangement of paclitaxel to the cyclopropane-containing derivative **10.2** occurs on treatment of a 2'-protected 7-*epi*-paclitaxel with the fluorinating agent DAST (44). The ring-A contraction described above also occurred readily under these conditions, but careful control of conditions led to the isolation of **10.2** in modest yield.

Numerous rearrangement reactions have also been observed in the baccatin series and on other taxoids (1). Although most of these are beyond the scope of this review, it is of interest to note that treatment of 2-debenzoyl-4,13-dideacetyl baccatin VI with acid gave the ring-opened product **10.3**, in which the A-ring has cleaved to give a 10-membered ring (45). Another unusual rearrangement occurred on attempted deoxygenation of 10-deacetoxybaccatin III; the reaction gave the tetracyclic product **10.4** in addition to the expected 7,10-dideoxy baccatin III (39). Recently, the preparation of various ring-B rearranged taxane analogs from 9-dihydrobaccatin III has been described (46).

J. Photochemistry

Paclitaxel is stable to ultraviolet irradiation under ambient light conditions, and no particular precautions are needed to protect it from light. However, irradiation with Pyrex-filtered light from a mercury lamp does lead to the formation of the C-3 (11) bridged product **11.1** in Figure 11 (47).

Irradiation of radiolabeled paclitaxel in the presence of polymerized tubulin leads to covalent bond formation between paclitaxel and the α-form of tubulin (48). It is not known at this time whether the photochemical reaction of paclitaxel with tubulin is related to the reactions leading to the formation of **11.1**.

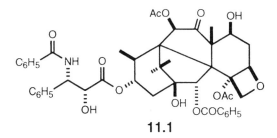

11.1

Figure 11   Photochemical product of paclitaxel.

III. SOURCES OF PACLITAXEL

A. Introduction

One of the major reasons that it took over ten years from the isolation of paclitaxel to its first clinical trial is that it is very difficult to isolate paclitaxel in large quantities. The earliest isolation from *Taxus brevifolia* bark was carried out with a 0.02% yield (3), and all the paclitaxel used in the clinical trials and initial clinical use of paclitaxel was isolated from this same source. An intensive effort to uncover better sources of paclitaxel has been carried out over the last few years, and the supply picture is now much brighter than it was as recently as 1991. This section will summarize the various approaches to obtaining paclitaxel on a large scale for clinical use.

B. Isolation

As noted above, paclitaxel was originally isolated from the bark of *T. brevifolia* in 0.02% yield (3). This source of paclitaxel was initially considered to be unsuitable for long-term use, because *T. brevifolia* grows in the ecologically threatened old-growth forests of the Pacific Northwest. Since the isolation of paclitaxel neces-sarily involves destruction of the tree and since the tree is small and slow-growing and does not occur in large stands, it was thought that it could never serve as more than a temporary source of paclitaxel. Recent surveys, however, have indicated that there are more *T. brevifolia* tress growing in the United States and Canada than previously supposed, and it is possible that this source could continue to be an important one for years to come. Thus, under one proposal, approximately 4 million lb of bark could be collected per year from federal lands alone, yielding enough paclitaxel to treat up to 150,000 patients per year (49). However, as noted below, some of the newer sources may have cost or other advantages over *T. brevifolia* bark; it is thus likely that the bark source will diminish in importance. An indication of this is the fact that the only U.S. pharmaceutical company currently marketing paclitaxel, Bristol-Myers Squibb, has announced that it will not renew its supply contract with Hauser Chemical Research when it expires in 1994. Hauser Chemical Research was the contractor used by Bristol-Myers Squibb to obtain paclitaxel from *T. brevifolia* bark, but Bristol-Myers Squibb has since developed an alternate supply strategy, described below.

   In addition to the isolation of paclitaxel from *T. brevifolia* bark, it can also be obtained from the leaves (or needles) of *T. brevifolia* and various other *Taxus* species. Although the amount of paclitaxel varies widely from plant to plant and from species to species, yields of 0.025% from needles appear to be reproducible (50). This compares well with the 0.013% reported for large-scale extraction from *T. brevifolia* bark (51). The use of needles has an obvious advantage in that they represent a renewable resource; in one scenario, a plantation of *Taxus* could be trimmed annually to yield a regular supply of needles. The isolation of paclitaxel from needles is more complicated than its isolation from bark, since needles contain large amounts of lipid material which interferes with the separation if it is not removed, but methods have been developed to do this using hexane (52) and supercritical fluid (53). Proper drying and storage of the needles is also necessary, since the paclitaxel content declines rapidly if they are stored without an initial drying (54). Given proper management of the unique problems associated with working with needles, it seems probable that needles will replace bark as the preferred source for those situations where paclitaxel itself is the desired product.

In addition to being a source of paclitaxel, *Taxus* species contain other taxoids. The most important such compound is 10-deacetylbaccatin III or 10-DAB (**12.1** in Fig. 12), which is essentially paclitaxel without the C-13 ester side chain and the C-10 acetate. Since both these groups can be introduced synthetically, as described below, 10-DAB becomes almost as valuable a taxoid as paclitaxel. It has been reported that 10-DAB can be obtained in yields of 0.1% w/w from fresh needles of *T. baccata* (55), and the large-scale isolation of 10-DAB is being carried out on a commercial scale by at least two companies, Indena S.A. in Italy and Dhabur, Ltd., in India.

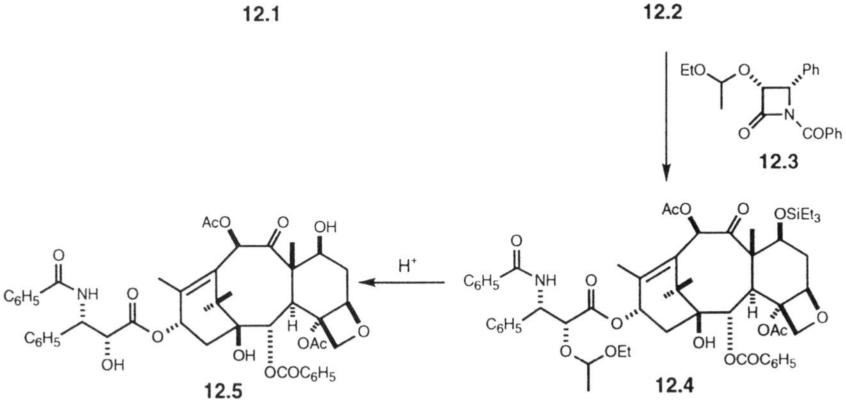

Figure 12 Semisynthesis of paclitaxel by Holton's route.

C. Plant Tissue Culture

Several workers have investigated plant tissue culture methods for producing paclitaxel. The first published report in this area was in 1989 (56), but reports from other workers have also appeared (57,58). From these reports it appears that tissue culture will certainly become a viable method for production of paclitaxel, and only time will tell whether it will be cost-effective as compared with isolation from bark and needles.

D. Fungal Production

An exciting recent development has been the report that paclitaxel is produced by the fungus *Taxomyces andreanae* (59). This fungus was found growing on one particular specimen of *T. brevifolia*, and it produces paclitaxel only in the amount of 24 to 50 ng/L. However, since strain improvement and genetic engineering techniques can be applied much more readily to fungi than to higher plants, it is very likely that this fungus could be developed as a paclitaxel producer. If this were to transpire, it would raise the attractive option of a fermentation route to paclitaxel, with production by well-developed techniques in large fermenters.

E. Semisynthesis

10-Deacetylbaccatin III (10-DAB) (**12.1**) is probably the most readily available of all the taxoids, as noted earlier. Its conversion to paclitaxel is thus an attractive option, and several methods have been devised to accomplish this.

The first requirement of a paclitaxel synthesis from 10-DAB is the preparation of the *N*-benzoyl-β-phenylisoserine side chain. A detailed discussion of the methods that have been developed to do this is beyond the scope of this review, but since at least a dozen methods have been reported in the literature, there is no shortage of available approaches. The interested reader is referred to two recent reviews which summarize those syntheses published before late 1993 (1,2).

The second requirement is that an efficient coupling mechanism be used. Although the esterification of a secondary alcohol is not normally a challenging task, the 13-hydroxyl group of baccatin III is in a hindered environment and is hydrogen-bonded to the C-4 acetate, both features which reduce its reactivity. The first group to overcome this problem used a protected side chain and forcing conditions to convert baccatin III to paclitaxel in 38% overall yield without recycling (55). Other workers have used this process or a variation of it, including one efficient method whereby the side chain is protected as a oxazolidine before coupling; in this case the coupling proceeds in excellent yield and so do the subsequent deprotection and reacylation steps necessary to make paclitaxel (60,61).

An alternate approach to the coupling problem is by the use of a β-lactam as the key reagent. This approach, which was first developed by Holton et al. (62), is illustrated in Figure 12. The coupling reaction and subsequent deprotection steps occur in high yield, and this method has been used by others in the preparation of paclitaxel analogs (63). Two enantioselective syntheses of the key β-lactam synthon have also appeared (64,65).

An important advantage of the semisynthetic route is that various paclitaxel analogs as well as paclitaxel can be prepared. Although published details are sketchy, various paclitaxel analogs have been prepared by this route, as exemplified by the synthesis of an N-debenzoyl-N-(p-chlorobenzoyl) analog (63) and a p-methoxyphenyl analog (66). It is very probable that some of these derivatives will have improved bioactivity as compared with paclitaxel and will thus serve as "second-generation" paclitaxels for clinical use. Even absent these considerations, the semisynthetic route is inherently efficient because of the relatively easy availability of 10-DAB, and—as noted earlier—Bristol-Myers Squibb will cease to purchase paclitaxel as of mid-1994 and will instead produce all its paclitaxel by this semisynthetic route.

F. Total Synthesis

A discussion of the total synthesis of paclitaxel is beyond the scope of this review; the subject has been reviewed elsewhere, and interested readers are referred to these articles for more information (1,2).

The total synthesis of paclitaxel has recently been achieved by two different research groups (67–69). Both syntheses represent towering achievements in synthetic organic chemistry, but they are unlikely to have an immediate impact on the paclitaxel supply problem. The major impact of both syntheses is that they open the doors to the preparation of additional analogs of paclitaxel, and will thus accelerate the development of improved versions of the drug.

Although the prospects for an economical total synthesis of paclitaxel itself are bleak, this does not mean that the synthetic efforts are of no value. It is very possible that an active analog of paclitaxel will be developed, either through total synthesis or by structure modification of paclitaxel itself, that will lack some of the functionality of paclitaxel and will be as active as or more active than paclitaxel. Such an analog could well be an attractive synthetic target, and its preparation by total synthesis could well be more efficient than its preparation by chemical manipulation of paclitaxel itself.

IV. STRUCTURE-ACTIVITY RELATIONSHIPS OF PACLITAXEL ANALOGS

A. Introduction

Extensive studies on the synthesis of paclitaxel analogs and the development of structure-activity relationships have been carried out over the last several years, and some important general structure-activity relationships have emerged. While these relationships will clearly be refined in the years to come, current knowledge is potentially adequate for the design of improved analogs of paclitaxel. This current knowledge is summarized rather than treated exhaustively in the following sections: fuller treatments are available in an earlier review (70) and in a forth-coming book chapter (71). For purposes of discussion, the structure of paclitaxel is divided into four regions: the northern hemisphere of the diterpenoid ring, encompassing carbons 6–12; the southern hemisphere, consisting of carbons 14 and 1–5, including the oxetane ring; the diterpenoid ring system itself; and finally the C-13 side chain. Each of these regions is discussed in turn.

B. The Northern Hemisphere

Modifications along the northern hemisphere of paclitaxel have been focused primarily at positions 7, 9, and 10. In early studies on the effect of acetylation at C-7 on the activity of paclitaxel, it was shown that 7-acetyl paclitaxel (**13.1** in Fig. 13) does not significantly reduce the tubulin-assembly activity of paclitaxel (19,72), and various other derivatives at this position have been prepared (70). Most importantly, it has been shown recently that deoxygenation of paclitaxel at C-7 to desoxypaclitaxel (**13.2**) results either in an increase in cytotoxicity (28) or in no decrease in cytotoxicity (39), depending on the assay used. In addition, the cyclopropane derivative **13.3** was almost as cytotoxic as paclitaxel in the HCT116 cell line (44). 9-Dihydropaclitaxel (**13.4**), prepared by attachment of the C-13 side

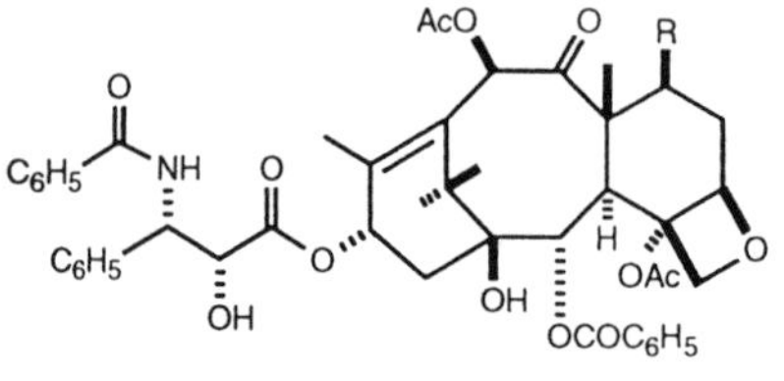

13.1 R = OAc
13.2 R = H

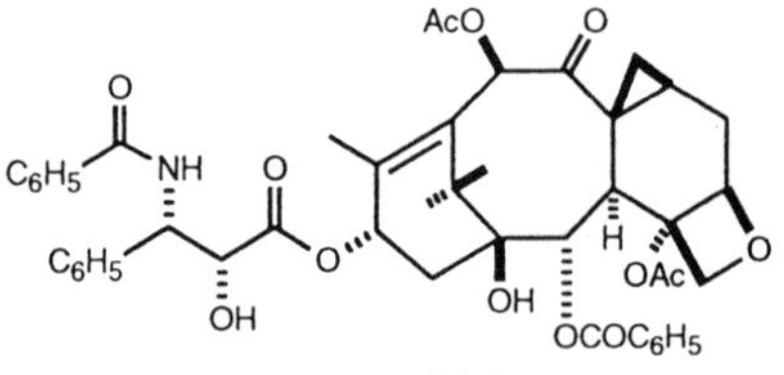

13.3

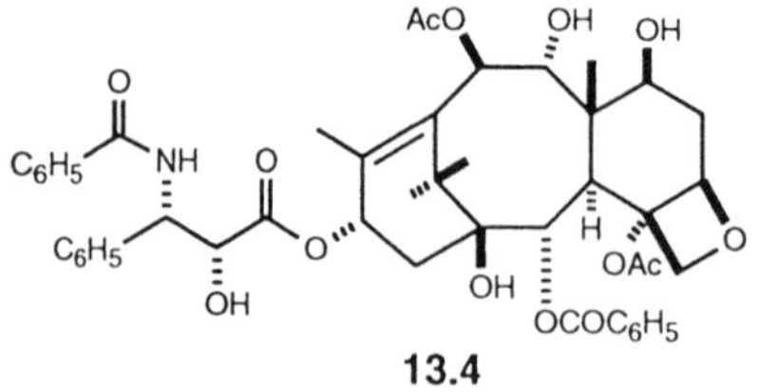

13.4

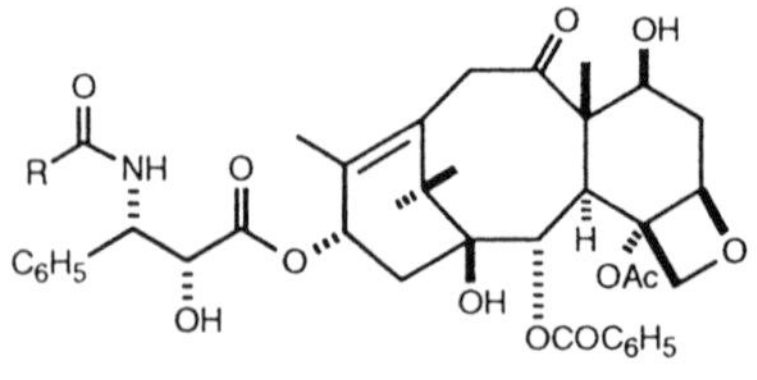

13.5 R = Ph
13.6 R = (CH₃)₃CO

Figure 13   Paclitaxel analogs modified in the northern hemisphere.

chain to a 9-dihydrobaccatin derivative, is slightly more active than paclitaxel in a tubulin-assembly assay (73).

The synthesis of 10-deacetoxypaclitaxel (**13.5**) has been achieved by three groups (38–41); the product is slightly less active than paclitaxel in two different cytotoxicity assays. Interestingly, 7-deoxydocetaxel (**13.6**) is significantly more active than paclitaxel in the P-388 assay (38).

Taken together, these results indicate that the northern hemisphere of paclitaxel is not intimately associated with its tubulin polymerization and cytotoxic activities. Results that appear to contradict this conclusion, such as the lack of activity of 7-oxopaclitaxel in KB cell culture (37), can be explained by the instability of this compound under cell culture conditions.

C. The Southern Hemisphere

In contrast to modifications in the northern hemisphere, structural changes in the southern hemisphere produce dramatic and usually deleterious effects on paclitaxel's activity.

The first modifications in the southern hemisphere were associated with the oxetane ring. Opening of this ring, either after oxidation to give the derivative **14.1** in Figure 14 (37) or on treatment with electrophilic reagents to give the derivative **14.2** (23), gave products which were essentially inactive in cytotoxicity assays. Similar results have been reported by others (22).

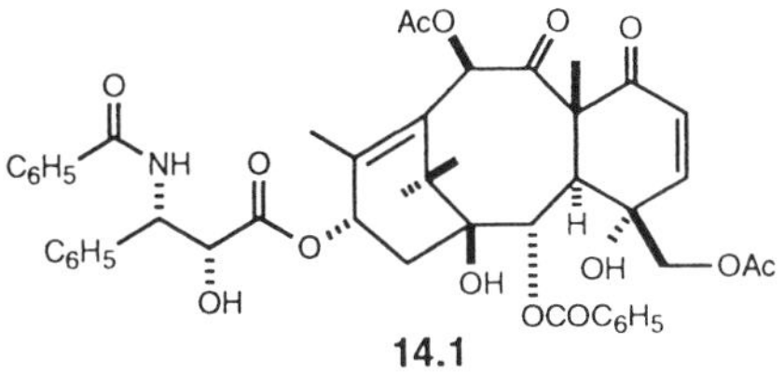

14.1

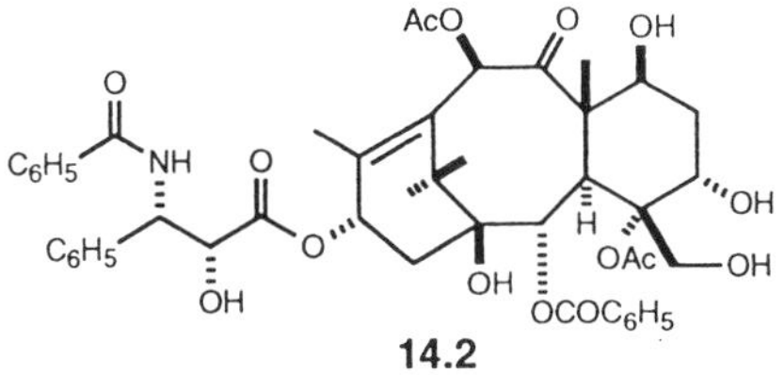

14.2

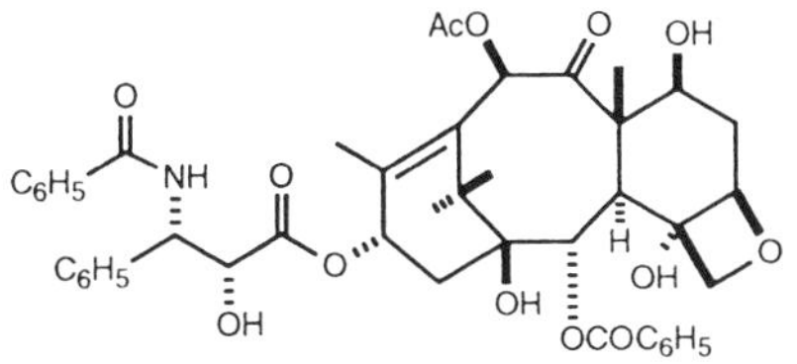

14.3

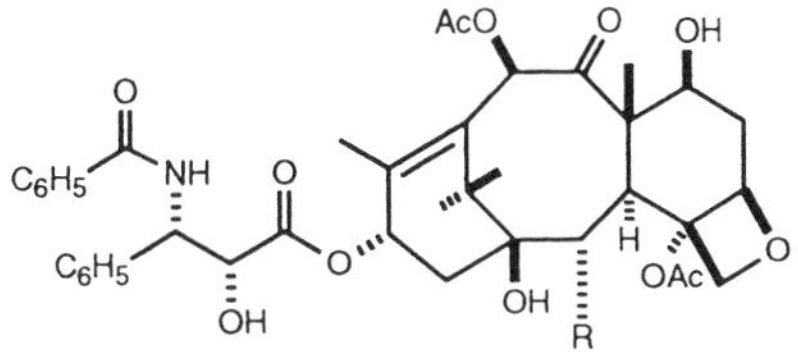

14.4 R = H
14.5 R = $OCO_6H_4N_3$ (*m*)
14.6 R = $OCO_6H_4N_3$ (*p*)

Figure 14 Paclitaxel analogs modified in the southern hemisphere.

The 4-acetyl group appears to have a significant effect on the activity of paclitaxel, since it can be removed to give 4-deacetylpaclitaxel (**14.3**) with large changes in cytotoxicity and tubulin-assembly activity (74).

The C-2 benzoyl group is essential for the activity of paclitaxel. Not only is 2-debenzoyloxypaclitaxel (**14.4**) inactive (43), but so are many of the 2-debenzoyl-2-acylpaclitaxel analogs that we have prepared (24). Some analogs, however, show very good activity; the difference is well illustrated by the *meta* and *para*-azido-benzoyl derivatives **14.5** and **14.6**. 2-Debenzoyl-2-(*m*-azidobenzoyl)paclitaxel (**14.5**) shows strikingly better tubulin-assembly activity and cytotoxicity than paclitaxel, with activities as high as 500-fold better than paclitaxel's in some assays. The isomeric *para*-azido derivative **14.6**, however, is significantly less active than paclitaxel in these same assays (24).

Taken together, these results indicate that the southern hemisphere of paclitaxel is intimately associated with its tubulin assembly and cytotoxic activities. The importance of the oxetane ring is at first sight surprising, since it is chemically inert and has only an oxygen atom as its "functional group." It is probable, however, that the oxetane ring serves to maintain the conformation of the diterpenoid ring system of paclitaxel (23), and a recent NMR and molecular modeling study of the ring-opened analog **14.2** indicates that the A ring of paclitaxel is flattened in **14.2** to bring the C-13 side chain closer to the diterpenoid ring system (71). The importance of the benzoyl group at C-2 may be associated with a π-stacking interaction that has been proposed between the C-2 benzoyl group and the phenyl group of the side chain (17), although the difference in activity of **14.5** and **14.6** shows that steric effects must also play a major role.

D. The Ring System

Paclitaxel can be converted to the ring-A contracted analog **15.1** in Figure 15 by mesylation (23), and docetaxel can similarly be converted to the analog **15.2** by reaction with electrophilic reagents (27). Both these derivatives have tubulin-assembly activity comparable to that of paclitaxel, but **15.1** was found to be much less cytotoxic to KB cells than paclitaxel, suggesting that differential absorption or metabolism may play a role in this lack of cytotoxicity. Interestingly, some of the ring B contracted analogs recently prepared (46) show comparable cytotoxicities to paclitaxel.

The nor-secopaclitaxel analog **15.3**, prepared by oxidation of 10-deacetyl-baccatin III, was found to be 20 times less active than paclitaxel against several cancer cell lines (75).

E. The C-13 Side Chain

The C-13 (2'*R*, 3'*S*)-*N*-benzoyl-3'-phenylisoserine side chain of paclitaxel is the easiest part of the molecule to manipulate synthetically; consequently, a large number of modifications have been made to it.

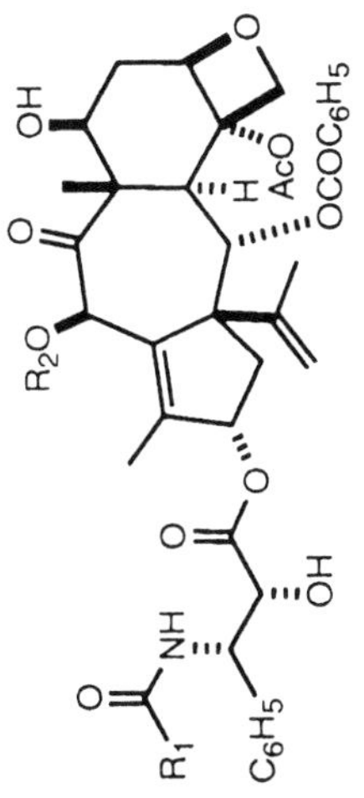

Figure 15 Paclitaxel analogs with modified ring systems.

15.1 R_1 = PhCO, R_2 = Ac
15.2 R_1 = $(CH_3)_3COCO$, R_2 = H

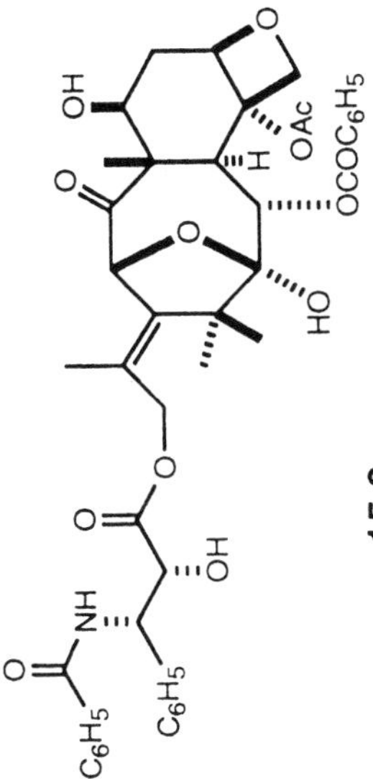

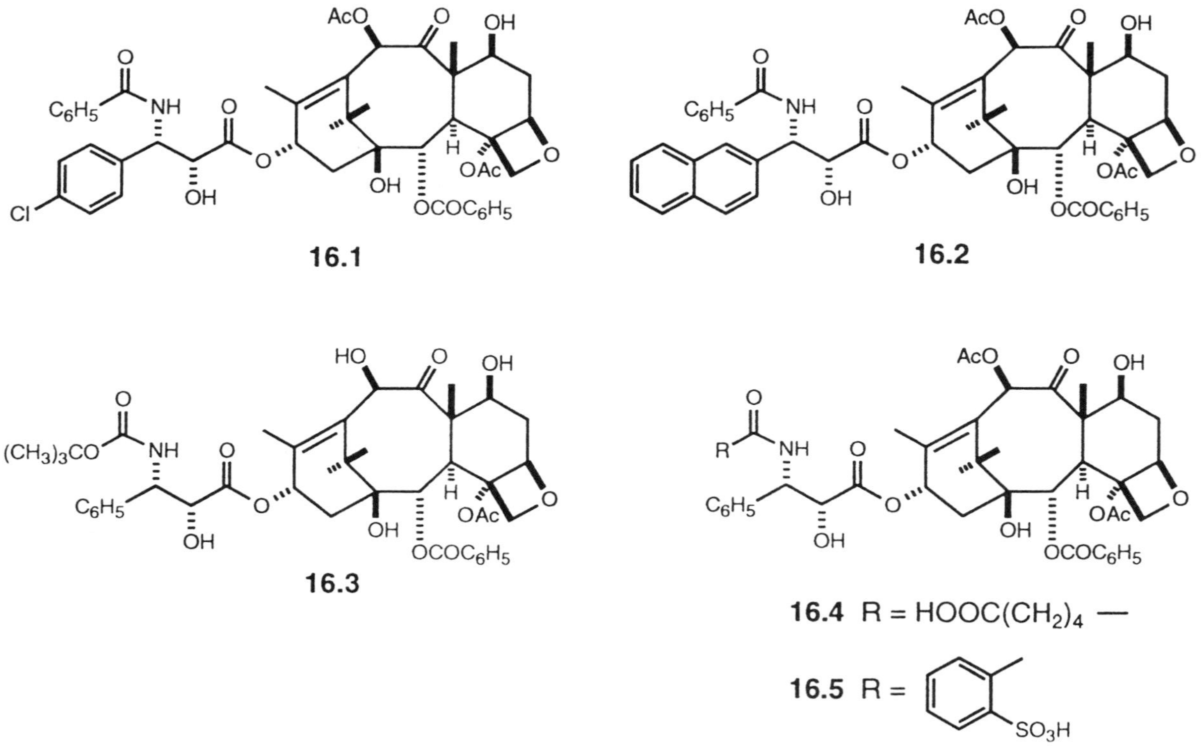

Figure 16 Paclitaxel analogs with variations in the side chain.

Various analogs with simplified side chains have been prepared, including 3-phenylpropionic acid (36) and phenyllactic acids (36,76) and *N*-benzoylisoserines (76). Those derivatives lacking the 3'-phenyl group were significantly less active than corresponding derivatives which retained this group, indicating the importance of the 3'-phenyl group for activity (76).

Various analogs that contained the 3'-phenyl group but which varied the position and stereochemistry of the hydroxyl and amino substituents were investigated by the French investigators (36). The major conclusion to emerge from this work was that the natural structure and stereochemistry of the paclitaxel side chain substituents is superior to any of the other possible variations in terms of bioactivity of the final product.

Various substituents of the 3'-phenyl group have been prepared, primarily by Georg et al. (63,77,78). Most of the derivatives prepared have similar to or lesser activity than paclitaxel in the tubulin assembly assay and in the National Cancer Institute's tumor panel. As one example, the 3'-(4-chlorophenyl) derivative **16.1** has up to 10,000-fold less activity than paclitaxel against various colon cancer cell lines (71), while the naphthyl derivative **15.2** is about sevenfold less active than paclitaxel as a tubulin-assembly promoter (71).

A number of modifications of the *N*-benzoyl group have also been made. One of these, docetaxel (**16.3**) (36), has been found to be more active than paclitaxel against J774.2 and P388 cells and also to be about five times as active against paclitaxel-resistant cells (79); it is currently in clinical trials both in France and the United States. Other modifications at the *N*-benzoyl position have been less successful, although some acidic substituents such as the glutaryl (**16.4**) and sulfobenzoyl (**16.5**) substituents were quite potent (36).

F. Summary

The results obtained to date on structure-activity relationships of paclitaxel can be summarized by the information given in Figure 17 (80).

V. CONCLUSION: RETROSPECT AND PROSPECT

The existence of a cytotoxic compound in *Taxus brevifolia* has been known now for thirty years, and the structure of paclitaxel itself has been known for over twenty years. In spite of this long history, it is only in recent years that interest in paclitaxel has blossomed, spurred in large measure by the first published report of its clinical activity against ovarian cancer (12). Evidence of this increased emphasis on paclitaxel research is the increasing number of paclitaxel-related publications appearing in the literature. My chemically oriented database, for example, which includes only a small number of the biologically related papers on paclitaxel,

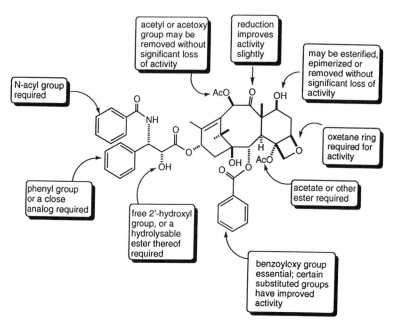

Figure 17   Summary of known structure-activity relationships of paclitaxel. Source: Ref. 80.

records an increase from a mere handful of papers a year in the 1970s to 25 in 1988, 29 in 1989, 31 in 1990, 46 in 1991, 76 in 1992, and 129 in 1993.

Viewed in retrospect, we can be very grateful for the pioneering studies of Drs. Wall and Wani and the workers at the National Cancer Institute and elsewhere who laid the foundation for the initial clinical studies on paclitaxel. They pioneered with work on the drug when it was not fashionable to do so, and their persistence has paid off handsomely. We can also be grateful for Dr. Horwitz's discovery of paclitaxel's unique mechanism of action, which has stimulated an enormous amount of biochemical and biological interest in paclitaxel and has given us an important tool for biological studies.

And what of the prospects for paclitaxel? Although it is not the "wonder drug" that some touted it as being (81), it is still a very important drug for ovarian cancer and breast cancer, and its full potential has yet to be seen as various treatment regimens and combination therapies are developed. The supply problem has essentially been solved, as semisynthetic material from 10-deacetylbaccatin III is combined with paclitaxel isolated directly from *T. brevifolia* bark and from needles of various varieties of *Taxus*. Looking ahead, it is very probable that either plant tissue culture or fungal culture will compete with the natural *Taxus* plant as a source of paclitaxel or of important precursors such as 10-deacetylbaccatin III.

In the future, however, paclitaxel will probably not be the drug of choice. The extensive work that has been carried out on structure-activity relationships of paclitaxel will surely lead in the not too distant future to one or more analogs with improved bioactivity in addition to the current analog docetaxel. These analogs will probably initially be made by the attachment of a modified side chain to baccatin III or a modified baccatin III derived from natural sources, but it is very possible that a simplified but active baccatin III analog could be synthesized more economically than it could be prepared from natural material.

In conclusion, the future prospects for therapeutically important new drugs based on the paclitaxel structure are excellent, and the next few years should continue to yield important advances in this exciting field.

REFERENCES

1. Kingston DGI, Molinero AA, Rimoldi JM. The taxane diterpenoids In: Herz W, Kirby GW, Moore RE, et al., eds. Progress in the Chemistry of Organic Natural Products. Vol. 61. Vienna: Springer-Verlag, 1993:1–206.
2. Nicolaou KC, Dai WM, Guy RK. Chemistry and biology of taxol. Angew Chem Int Ed 1994;33:15–44.
3. Wani MC, Taylor HL, Wall ME, et al. Plant antitumor agents: VI. The isolation and structure of taxol, a novel antileukemic and antitumor agent from *Taxus brevefolia*. J Am Chem Soc 1971;93:2325–2327.
4. Graf E. Taxin B, das Hauptalkaloid von *Taxus baccata* L. Archiv der Pharmazie (Weinheim, Germany) 1958; 291:443–449.
5. Graf E, Kirfel A, Wolff G-J, Breitmaier E. Die Aufklärung von taxin A aus *Taxus baccata* L. Liebigs Ann Chem 1982; 376–381.
6. Bauereis von R, Steiert W. Pharmakologische Eigenschaften von Taxin A und B. Arzneim Forsch 1959;9:77–79.
7. Rowinsky EK, McGuire WP, Guarnieri T, et al. Cardiac disturbances during administration of taxol. J Clin Oncol 1991;9:1704–1712.
8. Suffness M, Cordell GA. Antitumor alkaloids. In: Brossi A, ed. The Alkaloids. Vol. 25. New York: Academic Press, 1985:1–369.
9. Kingston DGI. Taxol, an exciting anticancer drug from Taxus brevifolia: An overview. In: Kinghorn AD, Balandrin MF, eds. Human Medicinal Agents from Plants. ACS Symposium Series 534. Washington, DC: American Chemical Society, 1993: 139–148.
10. Schiff PB, Fant J, Horwitz SB. Promotion of microtubule assembly *in vitro* by taxol. Nature 1979;277:665–667.
11. Kris MS, O'Connell JP, Gralla RJ, et al. Phase 1 trial of taxol given as 3-hour infusion every 21 days. Cancer Treat Rep 1986;70:605–607.
12. McGuire WP, Rowinsky EK, Rosenshein NB, et al. Taxol: A unique antineoplastic agent with significant activity in advanced ovarian epithelial neoplasms. Ann Intern Med 1989;111:273–279.
13. Cragg GM, Schepartz SA, Suffness M, Grever MR. The taxol supply crisis: New NCI

policies for handling the large-scale production of novel natural product anticancer and anti-HIV agents. J Nat Prod 1993;56:1657–1668.

14. Chmurny GN, Hilton BD, Brobst S, et al. ^{1}H and ^{13}C-NMR assignments for taxol, 7-*epi*taxol, and cephalomannine. J Nat Prod 1992;55:414–423.

15. Falzone JJ, Benesi AJ, Lecomte JTJ. Characterization of taxol in methylene chloride by NMR spectroscopy. Tetrahedr Lett 1992;33:1169–1172.

16. Dubois J, Guénard D, Guéritte-Voegelein F, et al. Conformation of taxotere and analogues determined by NMR spectroscopy and molecular modeling studies. Tetrahedron 1993;49:6533–6544.

17. Williams HJ, Scott AI, Dieden RA, et al. NMR and molecular modeling study of the conformations of taxol and of its side chain methyl ester in aqueous and non-aqueous solution. Tetrahedron 1993;49:6545–6560.

18. Vander Velde DG, Georg GI, Grunewald GL, et al. "Hydrophobic collapse" of taxol and taxotere solution conformations in mixtures of water and organic solvent. J Am Chem Soc 1993;115:11650–11651.

19. Mellado W, Magri NF, Kingston DGI, et al. Preparation and biological activity of taxol acetates. Biochem Biophys Res Commun 1984;124:329–335.

20. Miller RW, Powell RG, Smith CR Jr, et al. Antileukemic alkaloids from *Taxus wallichiana* Zucc. J Org Chem 1981;40:1469–1474.

21. Magri NF, Kingston DGI, Jitrangsri C, Piccariello T. Modified taxols: 3. Preparation and acylation of baccatin III. J Org Chem 1986;51:3239–3242.

22. Chen S-H, Huang S, Wei J, Farina V: The chemistry of taxanes: Reaction of taxol and baccatin derivatives with Lewis acids in aprotic and protic media. Tetrahedron 1993;49:2805–2828.

23. Samaranayake G, Magri NF, Jitrangsri C, Kington DGI. Modified taxols: 5. Reaction of taxol with electrophilic reagents, and preparation of a rearranged taxol derivative with tubulin assembly activity. J Org Chem 1991;56:5114–5119.

24. Chaudhary AG, Gharpure MM, Rimoldi JM, et al. Unexpectedly facile hydrolysis of the 2-benzoate group of taxol and synthesis of analogs with increased activities. J Am Chem Soc 1994;116:4097–4098.

25. Samaranayake G, Neidigh KA, Kingston DGI. Modified taxols: 8. Deacylation and reacylation of baccatin III. J Nat Prod 1993;56:884–898.

26. Farina V, Huang S. The chemistry of taxanes: Unexpected rearrangement of baccatin III during chemoselective debenzoylation with Bu$_3$SnOMe/LiCl. Tetrahedr Lett 1992; 33:3979–3982.

27. Wahl A, Guéritte-Voegelein G, Guénard D, et al. Rearrangement reactions of tax-anes: Structural modifications of 10-deacetylbaccatin III. Tetrahedron 1992;48:6965–6974.

28. Chaudhary AG, Rimoldi JM, Kingston DGI. Modified taxols: 10. Preparation of 7-deoxytaxol, a highly bioactive taxol derivative, and interconversion of taxol and 7-epitaxol. J Org Chem 1993;58:3798–3799.

29. Castellano EE, Hodder OJR. The crystal and molecular structure of the diterpenoid baccatin V, a naturally occurring oxetan with a taxane skeleton. Acta Cryst 1973; B29:2566–2570.

30. McLaughlin JL, Miller RW, Powell RG, Smith CR Jr. 19-Hydroxybaccatin III, 10-

deacetylcephalomannine, and 10-deacetyltaxol: New antitumor taxanes from *Taxus wallichiana*. J Nat Prod 1981;44:312–319.

31. Mathew AE, Mejillano MR, Nath JP, et al. Synthesis and evaluation of some water-soluble prodrugs and derivatives of taxol with antitumor activity. J Med Chem 1992; 35:145–151.

32. Magri NF, Kingston DGI. Modified taxols: 4. Synthesis and biological activity of taxols modified in the side chain. J Nat Prod 1988;51:298–306.

33. Deutsch HM, Glinski JA, Hernandez M, et al. Synthesis of congeners and prodrugs: 3. Water-soluble prodrugs of taxol with potent antitumor activity. J Med Chem 1989; 32:788–792.

34. Zhao Z, Kingston DGI, Crosswell AR. Modified taxols: 6. Preparation of water-soluble prodrugs of taxol. J Nat Prod 1991;54:1607–1611.

35. Nicolaou KC, Riemer C, Kerr MA, et al. Design, synthesis and biological activity of protaxols. Nature 1993;364:464–466.

36. Guéritte-Voegelein F, Guénard D, Lavelle F, et al. Relationships between the structure of taxol analogues and their antimitotic activity. J Med Chem 1991;34:992–998.

37. Magri NF, Kingston DGI. Modified taxols: 2. Oxidation products of taxol. J Org Chem 1986;51:797–802.

38. Chen S-H, Fairchild C, Mamber SW, Farina V. Taxol structure-activity relationship: Synthesis and biological activity of 10-deoxytaxol. J Org Chem 1993;58:2927–2928.

39. Chen SH, Huang S, Kant J, et al. Synthesis of 7-deoxy and 7,10-dideoxytaxol via radical intermediates. J Org Chem 1993;58:5028–5029.

40. Chaudhary AG, Kingston DGI. Synthesis of 10-deacetoxytaxol and 10-deoxytaxotere. Tetrahedr Lett 1993;34:4921–4924.

41. Holton RA, Somoza C, Chai KB. A simple synthesis of 10-deacetoxytaxol derivatives. Tetrahedr Lett 1994;35:1665–1668.

42. Chen SH, Wei JM, Vyas DM, et al. A facile synthesis of 7,10-dideoxytaxol and 7-epi-10-deoxytaxol. Tetrahedr Lett 1993;34:6845–6848.

43. Chen SH, Wei JM, Farina V. Taxol structure-activity relationships: Synthesis and biological evaluation of 2-deoxytaxol. Tetrahedr Lett 1993;34:3205–3206.

44. Chen SH, Huang S, Wei J, Farina V. Serendipitous synthesis of a cyclopropane-containing taxol analog via anchimeric participation of an unactivated angular methyl group. J Org Chem 1993;58:4520–4521.

45. Py S, Khuong-Huu F. A novel rearrangement of the taxane skeleton. Bull Soc Chim France 1993;130:189–191.

46. Klein LL, Maring CJ, Li L, et al. Synthesis of ring-B rearranged taxane analogs. J Org Chem 1994;59:2370–2373.

47. Chen SH, Combs CM, Hill SE, et al. The photochemistry of taxol: Synthesis of a novel pentacyclic taxol isomer. Tetrahedr Lett 1992;33:7679–7680.

48. Rao SS, Horwitz SB, Ringel I. Direct photoaffinity labeling of tubulin with taxol. J Natl Cancer Inst 1992;84:785–788.

49. Lowe J. Pacific Yew: Draft environmental Impact Statement. Portland, OR: USDA Forest Service, January 1993, p. 523.

50. Wheeler NC, Jech K, Masters S, et al. Effects of genetic, epigenetic, and environ-

mental factors on taxol content in *Taxus brevifolia* and related species. J Nat Prod 1992;55:432–440.

51. Stull DP, Jans NA. Current taxol production from yew bark and future production strategies. Second NCI Workshop on Taxol and *Taxus*. Alexandria, VA: National Cancer Institute, September 1992.

52. Witherup KM, Look SA, Stasko TG, et al. High performance liquid chromatographic separation of taxol and related compounds from *Taxus brevifolia*. J Liq Chromatogr 1989;12:2117–2132.

53. Castor TP. Improved isolation of taxol by supercritical fluid processing. Second NCI Workshop on Taxol and *Taxus*. Alexandria, VA: National Cancer Institute, September 1992.

54. Hansen RC, Holmes RG, Shugert RB Jr, et al. Harvesting, drying and storage of cultivated *Taxus* clippings: An exploratory study. Second NCI Workshop on Taxol and *Taxus*. Alexandria, VA: National Cancer Institute, September 1992.

55. Denis JN, Greene AE, Guénard D, et al. Highly efficient, practical approach to natural taxol. J Am Chem Soc 1988;110:5917–5919.

56. Christen AA, Bland J, Gibson DM. Cell culture as a means to produce taxol. Proc Am Assoc Cancer Res 1989;30:566.

57. Fett-Neto AG, DiCosmo F, Reynolds WF, Sakata K. Cell culture of *Taxus* as a source of the antineoplastic drug taxol. Biotechnology 1992;20:1572–1575.

58. Shuler ML, Hirasuna TJ, Willard DM. Kinetics of taxol production by tissue culture. Second NCI Workshop on Taxol and *Taxus*. Alexandria, VA: National Cancer Institute, September 1992.

59. Stierle A, Strobel G, Stierle D. Taxol and taxane production by *Taxomyces andreanae*, an endophytic fungus of Pacific yew. Science 1993;260:214–216.

60. Commercon A, Bezard D, Bernard F, Bourzat JD. Improved protection and esterification of a precursor of the taxotere and taxol side chains. Tetrahedr Lett 1992;33:5185–5188.

61. Didier E, Fouque E, Commerçon A. Expeditious semisynthesis of docetaxel using 2-trichloromethyl-1,3-oxazolidine as side-chain precursor. Tetrahedr Lett 1994;35:3063–3064.

62. Holton RA, Liu JH, Gentile LN, Beidiger RJ. Semi-synthesis of taxol. Second NCI Workshop on Taxol and *Taxus*. Alexandria, VA: National Cancer Institute, September 1992.

63. Georg GI, Cheruvallath ZS, Himes RH, Mejillano MR. Novel biologically active taxol analogues: baccatin III 13-(N-(p-chlorobenzoyl)-(2′R,3′S)-3′-phenyliso-serinate) and baccatin III 13-(N-benzoyl-(2′R,3′S)-3′-(p-chlorophenyl)isoserinate). Bioorg Med Chem Lett 1992;2:295–298.

64. Farina V, Hauck SI, Walker DG. A simple chiral synthesis of the taxol side chain. Synlett 1992;761–763.

65. Georg GI, Cheruvallath ZS, Harriman GCB, et al. An efficient semisynthesis of taxol from (3R,4S)-N-benzoyl-3[(t-butyldimethylsilyl)oxy]-4-phenyl-2-azetidinone and 7-(triethylsilyl)baccatin III. Bioorg Med Chem Lett 1993;3:2467–2470.

66. Holton RA. PCT Int Appl WO 93 06,079. Chem Abstr 1993;119:13954j.

67. Holton RA, Somoza C, Kim HB, et al. First total synthesis of taxol. 1. Functionalization of the B ring. J Am Chem Soc 1994;116:1597–1598.

68. Holton RA, Kim HB, Somoza C, et al. First total synthesis of taxol. 2. Completion of the C and D rings. J Am Chem Soc 1994;116:1599–1600.

69. Nicolaou KC, Yang Z, Lin JJ, et al. Total syntheses of taxol. Nature 1994;367: 630–634.

70. Kingston DGI. The chemistry of taxol. Pharm Ther 1991;52:1–34.

71. Georg GI, Boge TC, Cheruvallath ZS, et al. The medicinal chemistry of taxol. In: Suffness M, ed. Taxol: Science and Applications. Boca Raton, FL: CRC Press, 1994.

72. Lataste H, Sénilh V, Wright M, et al. Relationships between the structure of taxol and baccatine III derivatives and their *in vitro* action on the disassembly of mammalian brain and *Physarum* amoebal microtubules. Proc Natl Acad Sci USA 1984;81:4090–4094.

73. Klein LL. Synthesis of 9-dihydrotaxol: A novel bioactive taxane. Tetrahedr Lett 1993;34:2047–2050.

74. Neidigh KA, Gharpure MM, Rimoldi JM, Kingston DGI, Jiang YQ, Hamel E. Synthesis and biological evaluation of 4-deacetylpaclitaxel. Tetrahedr Lett 1994; 35:6839–6842.

75. Ojima I, Fenoglio I, Park YH, et al. Synthesis and structure-activity relationship (SAR) study of novel nor-seco taxol and taxotere analogs. In: Stony Brook Symposium on Taxol and Taxotere: New Hope for Breast Cancer Chemotherapy. State University of New York at Stony Brook, 1993, p.53.

76. Swindell CS, Krauss NE, Horwitz SB, Ringel I. Biologically active taxol analogues with deleted A-ring side chain substituents and variable C-2′ configurations. J Med Chem 1991;34:1176–1184.

77. Georg GI, Cheruvallath ZS, Himes RH, Mejillano MR. Semisynthesis and biological activity of taxol analogues: baccatin III 13-(N-benzoyl-(2′R,3′S)-3′-(p-tolyl)isoserinate), baccatin III 13-(N-p-toluoyl)-2′R,3′S)-3′-phenylisoserinate), baccatin III 13-(N-p-touoyl)-2′R,3′S)-3′-(p-trifluoromethylphenylisoserinate), and baccatin III 13-(N-(p-trifluoromethylbenzoyl)-2′R,3′S)-3′-phenylisoserinate). Bioorg Med Chem Lett 1992;2:1751–1754.

78. Georg GI, Cheruvallath ZS, Himes RH, et al. Synthesis of biologically active taxol analogues with modified phenylisoserine side chains. J Med Chem 1992;35:4230–4237.

79. Ringel I, Horwitz SB. Studies with RP56976 (taxotere): A semisynthetic analog of taxol. J Natl Cancer Inst 1991;83:288–291.

80. Kingston DGI. Taxol: The chemistry and structure-activity relationships of a novel anticancer drug. Trends Biotechnol 1994;12:222–227.

81. Kolata G. The aura of a miracle fades from a cancer drug. New York Times 1993; Nov 7:1, 28.

2

Molecular Mechanisms

ISRAEL RINGEL
The Hebrew University
Jerusalem, Israel

I. INTRODUCTION

Paclitaxel, a novel diterpenoid, was first isolated from the bark of *Taxus brevifolia*, and reported by Wani et al. (1) as an antileukemic agent. Paclitaxel is a potent inhibitor of cell replication, and it has been shown to inhibit specific functions in many nonmalignant tissues, most of which may be mediated through microtubule disruption (reviewed in 2–5). Recently, several cellular effects of paclitaxel are suspected to be unrelated to paclitaxel's direct action on microtubule function, and will be discussed later.

II. MECHANISM OF MICROTUBULE ASSEMBLY

Microtubules are a major component of the spindle fibers and the cytoskeleton of eukaryotic cells. They participate in a variety of cellular functions, such as mitosis, morphogenesis, motility, and intracellular organelle transport. They are cylindricallike structures several hundred angstroms in outside diameter and typically several micrometers long. Microtubules are assembled mainly from tubulin, a dimeric protein of ~110,000 MW, consisting of two polypeptide chains (α and β) of approximately identical molecular weight (reviewed by 6). Most species express multiple isoforms of these subunits by transcriptional activation of one or more members of the small multigene families that encode either subunit (reviewed by 7), and the level of tubulin expression is controlled through an autoregulatory pathway in which the concentration of tubulin subunits dictates the stability of tubulin mRNA (reviewed by 8). Microtubules purified by repeated cycles of polymerization and depolymerization contain tubulin and several co-purified proteins collectively referred to as microtubule-associated proteins (MAPs) (9,10). MAPs have been shown to be components of the mitotic spindle and other specialized cellular structures (11). These experimental data suggest that a number of the MAPs are important for microtubule stability and participate significantly in both the nucleation and elongation phases of the assembly reaction (12).

Tubulin has two binding sites for guanine nucleotides, one exchangeable and one nonexchangeable (13–15). Generally, GTP bound at the exchangeable site of the protein is required to initiate the assembly of microtubules and is hydrolyzed to GDP in the reaction process (16). Tubulin has several sites for drug binding (17, reviewed by 18) and probably most important biologically, has unique Ca^{2+} and Mg^{2+} binding sites (19). Microtubule assembly proceeds from a nucleation stage, through protofilament formation and lateral association of the protofilaments, into a sheet structure that curves into a cylindrical form (20). The elongation process occurs in an endwise manner where tubulin subunits are being added to both ends in vitro, although at different rates. The faster growing end is conventionally known as the plus end. At steady state, the microtubule polymers are at dynamic equilibrium with tubulin dimers in solution. The concentration of soluble dimers at steady state, defined as the critical concentration, represents the extent of polymer stability in diverse conditions. A low critical concentration indicates a more stable polymer.

In vivo mechanisms of microtubule assembly control are of considerable oncogenic interest. Antimicrotubule agents are among the most important anti-cancer drugs and have contributed to the therapy of most curable neoplasms. These drugs arrest cell division at metaphase by interfering with normal spindle formation.

III. PACLITAXEL ACTION ON MICROTUBULES

Antimicrotubule drugs, can be grouped into two classes based on their effects on microtubules. For most of them, their inhibitory action involves destabilization of the microtubule polymer and interference with the assembly competency of tubulin. Among these are the vinca alkaloids, colchicine, podophyllotoxin, and nocodazole, all of which bind to the tubulin dimer (reviewed by 18). Paclitaxel, on the other hand, was demonstrated to interfere with microtubule function by binding to the polymer and stabilizing it against depolymerization (21,22). Paclitaxel promotes the assembly of tubulin even under conditions that normally do not support microtubule polymerization. These include the absence of MAPs or exogenous GTP (23–25), low temperature (26), and mild alkaline pH (27). It promotes both the nucleation and elongation phases of the polymerization process, and can reduce the critical concentration of tubulin to almost zero (21,24,28). Paclitaxel slows the flux of tubulin from microtubule polymers in a concentration-dependent manner (29). The most profound effect of paclitaxel is on the dissociation rate constants at the two ends, while the association rate constant is hardly affected (29,30). The linkage-free energy provided by paclitaxel binding is approximately -3.0 kcal/mol of α,β-tubulin dimer, which results in a stable polymer even at conditions that normally do not support microtubule assembly (28). These properties of paclitaxel lead to the suppression of both treadmilling and dynamic instability (29,30).

Steady-state microtubules assembled in the presence of GTP bind paclitaxel with approximately the same stoichiometry as microtubules assembled in the presence of paclitaxel alone (22). Microtubule polymers bind paclitaxel with an apparent binding constant of $\sim 1 \times 10^{-6}$ (22), and binding saturation occurs at approximate stoichiometry with the tubulin dimer concentration (22,31). It was proposed that the binding of paclitaxel to microtubule ends changes the conformation of GDP-tubulin from inactive to active, allowing productive binding of tubulin dimers, polymer elongation, and a lower dissociation constant at the microtubule end (31). Paclitaxel binds to polymerized form of tubulin (22), and no evidence was found for paclitaxel interaction with an unpolymerized dimer (31). The same results were found for 7-acetyl paclitaxel (32). Paclitaxel stabilizes the formed polymers against depolymerization by Ca^{2+} (21), podophyllotoxin (27), and low temperature (26).

In the presence of paclitaxel, more and shorter microtubules are polymerized (21), with higher flexibility than GTP-assembled polymers (33,34). Purified tubulin-paclitaxel microtubules have a smaller mean diameter ($\sim$ 22 nm) than those induced by microtubule-associated proteins or glycerol ($\sim$ 24 nm), but nearly identical wall substructure. This is because the majority of paclitaxel-microtubules consist of only 12 protofilaments instead of the typical pattern of 13 protofilaments (35). Although the predominant conformation of paclitaxel-assembled tubulin is microtubules, a fraction of the polymers consist of non-microtubule forms like ribbons and hoops (21,22). These additional polymeric forms scatter light more than "normal" microtubule do at identical microtubule protein concentrations. The ribbons and hoops are less stable than regular microtubules, and they decompose more readily at mild alkaline pH (27).

Recent studies have demonstrated that both α- and β-tubulin exist as multiple isotypes (7), of which some are not as sensitive as others to paclitaxel action. β_{III} isotype of bovine brain tubulin has lower assembly competency (36) and removal of β_{III} enhances paclitaxel-induced microtubule assembly (37). Paclitaxel is less potent as an assembly promoter of plant tubulin compared to its effect on mammalian tubulin, probably due to major changes in amino acid sequences (38).

This suggests that paclitaxel, a product of plant metabolism, may interact poorly with plant microtubules (38). Plant tubulin (from maize and tobacco) may be subjected to numerous cycles of paclitaxel-induced polymerization and cold/ Ca^{2+}-induced depolymerization with little loss of polymerization competence (39). Microtubules assembled in the presence of GTP from pure yeast (*Saccharomyces cerevisiae*) tubulin were not stabilized by paclitaxel against Ca^{2+} action, and paclitaxel hardly assembled them by itself. Only hybrid microtubules containing substoichiometric amounts of bovine tubulin were stabilized by paclitaxel, allowing the isolation of a large number and variety of yeast proteins that associate with microtubules (40).

Although paclitaxel-stabilized microtubules are relatively stable, paclitaxel is being used as a tool for the purification of microtubules and MAPs (41,42). Disassembly of the polymers and removal of paclitaxel can be achieved by a combination of high concentrations of Ca^{2+} and low temperatures (43). In the absence of MAPs, paclitaxel-stabilized microtubules are slowly depolymerized at cold temperatures (25). A "pH shock" may also serve this purpose (27).

IV. PACLITAXEL BINDS PREFERENTIALLY TO β-TUBULIN

Photoaffinity labeling has been widely used to help with the determination of drug binding sites on proteins, typically by using a potent photoaffinity analog of the drug, for example, one bearing an azido or diazo moiety (44). Assuming that the photoaffinity analog binds in the same way as the natural substrate, then irradiation of the analog while bound to the protein will convert it to a reactive intermediate that will covalently label one or more amino acids in the region of the active site. Occasionally, a natural drug has a photoactive moiety that, upon irradiation, binds covalently to the macromolecule. Irradiation at 254 nm of a mixture of ^{3}H-GTP and tubulin (45,46) or of a ^{3}H-colchicine-tubulin complex (47) led directly to photoaffinity labeling by GTP or by colchicine, respectively, to the β subunit of tubulin. ^{3}H-paclitaxel was used directly to photolabel tubulin. A complex of microtubule protein and ^{3}H-paclitaxel was irradiated by ultraviolet light and analyzed by gel electrophoresis and autoradiography. The radiolabeled drug preferentially binds covalently to the β subunit of tubulin, and the binding can be competed with unlabeled paclitaxel (48). However, the low extent of photoincorporation of paclitaxel precluded the use of ^{3}H-paclitaxel as a probe for defining the paclitaxel binding site within β-tubulin. Several photoaffinity analogs of paclitaxel were synthesized, in which the photoreactive substituents are on the 7 position (49,50), 2-benzoate group (51), or in the A-ring side chain (52,53) of paclitaxel. ^{3}H-3'-(*p*-azidobenzamido)-paclitaxel, an analog with similar biological activities as paclitaxel (52), covalently binds to the N-terminal domain of β-tubulin after irradiation of the microtubule-drug complex (54). Paclitaxel competes with ^{3}H-3'-(*p*-azidobenzamido)-paclitaxel binding, suggesting that the photoaffinity analog and paclitaxel are binding at the same or overlapping sites. Formic acid cleavage of ^{3}H-3′-(p-azidobenzamido)-paclitaxel-photolabeled β-tubulin and subsequent protein sequence and mass analyses have identified the N-terminal 31 amino acids as the major site for ^{3}H-3′-(p-azidobenzamido)-paclitaxel photoincorporation (54). This region is essential for tubulin assembly process and Cys[12] has been implicated as an important component of the exchangeable GTP binding site (46). Paclitaxel stimulates phosphorylation of β-tubulin in both differentiated and undifferentiated N115 cells (55), which may correlate with its assembly properties.

V. EFFECT OF PACLITAXEL IN CELLS

Cells incubated with paclitaxel accumulate in the G_2 and M phases of the cell cycle and induce the expression of tubulin. At concentrations equivalent to ED_{50}, paclitaxel inhibited mitotic progression without arresting cells in mitosis (56). At its lowest effective concentrations, paclitaxel appears to block mitosis by kinetically stabilizing spindle microtubules and not by changing the mass of polymerized microtubules (57). Immunofluorescence studies utilizing tubulin antibodies reveal the presence of unusual bundles of polymers that are not usually associated with the microtubule organizing center (MTOC) (58,59). Asters are observed for cells in mitosis (59,60). It was suggested that bundle formation may correlate with the antitumor activity of paclitaxel (61). The mechanism of microtubule bundling by paclitaxel is not clear. Using extracts of xenopus eggs, Verde et al. showed that paclitaxel aster assembly requires phosphorylation, and that they do not grow from preformed centers, but rather by a reorganization of microtubules first crosslinked into bundles (60). Cytoplasmic dynein is also required for paclitaxel aster assembly (60), and it may crossbridge microtubules into bundles even in the absence of paclitaxel (62). Turner and Margolis reported that paclitaxel-induced microtubule bundling was mediated by a factor, a protein doublet of ~ 100 kDa, present in rat brain crude extracts (63). Studies performed on a variety of cell systems by several research groups revealed several proteins which have the capability of bundling microtubules even in the absence of paclitaxel. Among them is a 65-kDa MAP that forms crossbridge structures between adjacent microtubules in vitro (64), MAP2c, which at low levels of expression binds to microtubules radiating from the centrosomal MTOC, but at higher levels promotes the assembly of microtubules and the formation of bundles independently of the MTOC (65). Kinesin may have a second microtubule binding site, in addition to the site on the motor domain, which crossbridges microtubules (66). Tau (67), a 72-kDa MAP which is immunologically related to MAP2 (68), synapsin 1 (69), and several other proteins were found to be involved in the crossbridging of microtubules. Whether paclitaxel promotes bundle formation through a mediator factor or by a direct action on microtubules is yet to be resolved.

Paclitaxel exhibits profound cell cycle-independent effects on murine macrophages. It induces the release of tumor necrosis factor α (TNF-α) and activates the acute internalization of TNF-α (70,71), activities shared by bacterial lipopolysaccharide (LPS). Paclitaxel activates the expression of six LPS-inducible genes and induces tyrosine phosphorylation of several 41–45-kDa proteins, as LPS does (71,72). LPS antagonists block paclitaxel-induced signaling in murine macrophages, suggesting that paclitaxel stimulates macrophages through an LPS receptor-dependent mechanism (73). Ding et al. (74) found that LPS binds to β-tubulin, which may explain some of the similarities in action between paclitaxel and LPS.

REFERENCES

1. Wani MC, Taylor HL, Wall ME, et al. Plant antitumor agents. VI. The isolation and structure of taxol, a novel antileukemic and antitumor agent from *Taxus brevifolia*. J Am Chem Soc 1971;93:2325–2327.
2. Manfredi JJ, Horwitz SB. Taxol: an antimitotic agent with a new mechanism of action. Pharmacol Ther 1984;25:83–125.
3. Horwitz SB, Lothstein L, Manfredi JJ, et al. Taxol: mechanism of action and resistance. Ann NY Acad Sci 1986;466:733–744.
4. Horwitz SB. Mechanism of action of taxol. TIPS 1992;13:134–136.
5. Horwitz SB, Cohen D, Rao S, et al. Taxol: Mechanisms of action and resistance. J Natl Cancer Inst 1993;15:55–61.
6. Burns RG, Surridge CD. Tubulin: conservation and structure. In: Hyams JS, and Lloyd CW, eds. Microtubules. Wiley-Liss, Inc., 1994:3–31.
7. Raff EC. The role of multiple tubulin isoforms in cellular microtubule function. In: Hyams JS, Lloyd CW, eds. Microtubules. Wiley-Liss, Inc., 1994:85–109.
8. Cleveland DW, Theodorakis NG. Regulation of tubulin synthesis. In: Hyams JS, Lloyd CW, eds. Microtubules. Wiley-Liss, Inc., 1994:47–58.
9. Murphy DB, Johnson KA, Borisy GG. Role of tubulin-associated proteins in microtubule nucleation and elongation. J Mol Biol 1977;117:33–52.
10. Wiche G, Oberkanins C, Himmler A. Molecular structure and function of microtubule-associated proteins. Int Rev Cytol 1991;124:217–273.
11. Sherline P, Schiavone K. Immunofluorescence localization of proteins of high-molecular-weight along intracellular microtubules. Science 1977;198:1038–1040.
12. Johnson KA, Borisy GG. Kinetic analysis of microtubule self-assembly in vitro. J Mol Biol 1977;117:1–32.
13. Allende JE. GTP-mediated macromolecular interactions: the common features of different systems. FASEB J 1988;2:2356–2367.
14. Carlier M-F, Didry D, Pantaloni D. Microtubule elongation and GTP hydrolysis. Role of guanine nucleotides in microtubule dynamics. Biochemistry 1987;26:4428–4437.

15. O'Brien ET, Voter WA, Erickson HP. GTP hydrolysis during microtubule assembly. Biochemistry 1987;26:4148–4156.
16. Weisenberg RC, Deery WJ. Role of nucleotide hydrolysis in microtubule assembly. Nature 1976;263:792–793.
17. Dustin P. *Microtubules*. New York: Springer-Verlag, 1984.
18. Wilson L, Jordan MA. Pharmacological probes of microtubule function. In: Hyams JS, Lloyd CW, eds. Microtubules. Wiley-Liss, Inc., 1994:59–83.
19. Kirschner MW. Microtubule assembly and nucleation. Int Rev Cytol 1978;54:1–71.
20. Detrich HW III, Jordan MA, Wilson L, et al. Mechanism of microtubule assembly. Changes in polymer structure and organization during assembly of sea urchin egg tubulin. J Biol Chem 1985;260:9479–9490.
21. Schiff PB, Fant J, Horwitz SB. Promotion of microtubule assembly in vitro by taxol. Nature (Lond.) 1979;227:665–667.
22. Parness J, Horwitz SB. Taxol binds to polymerized tubulin in vitro. J Cell Biol 1981;91:479–487.
23. Schiff PB, Horwitz SB. Taxol assembles tubulin in the absence of exogenous GTP or microtubule associated proteins. Biochemistry 1981;20:3247–3252.
24. Kumar N. Taxol-induced polymerization of purified tubulin. J Biol Chem 1981;256:10435–10441.
25. Hamel E, del Campo AA, Lowe MC, et al. Interaction of taxol, microtubule associated proteins, and guanine nucleotides in tubulin polymerization. J Biol Chem 1981;256:11887–11894.
26. Thompson WC, Wilson L, Purich DL. Taxol induces microtubule assembly at low temperature. Cell Motility 1981;1:445–454.
27. Ringel I, Horwitz SB. Effect of alkaline pH on taxol-microtubule interactions. J Exp Pharm Ther 1991;259:855–860.
28. Howard WD, Timasheff SN. Linkages between the effects of taxol, colchicine, and GTP on tubulin polymerization. J Biol Chem 1988;263:1342–1346.
29. Wilson L, Miller HP, Farrell KW, et al. Taxol stabilization of microtubules in vitro: dynamics of tubulin addition and loss at opposite microtubule ends. Biochemistry 1985;24:5254–5262.
30. Caplow M, Zeeberg B. Dynamic properties of microtubules at steady state in the presence of taxol. Eur J Biochem 1982;127:319–324.
31. Diaz JF, Menendez M, Andreu JM. Thermodynamics of ligand-induced assembly of tubulin. Biochemistry 1993;28:10067–10077.
32. Takoudju M, Wright M, Chenu J, et al. Interaction of 7-acetyltaxol with different tubulin assemblies. FEBS Lett 1988;234:177–180.
33. Dye RB, Fink SP, Williams RC Jr. Taxol-induced flexibility of microtubules and its reversal by MAP-2 and Tau. J Biol Chem 1993;268:6847–6850.
34. Venier P, Maggs AC, Carlier MF, et al. Analysis of microtubule rigidity using hydrodynamic flow and thermal fluctuations. J Biol Chem 1994;269:13353–13360.
35. Andreu JM, Bordas J, Diaz JF, et al. Low resolution structure of microtubules in solution. Synchrotron X-ray scattering and electron microscopy of taxol-induced microtubules assembled from purified tubulin in comparison with glycerol and MAP-induced microtubules. J Mol Biol 1992;226:169–184.

36. Banerjee A, Roach MC, Trcka P, et al. Increased microtubule assembly in bovine brain tubulin lacking the type III isotope of β-tubulin. J Biol Chem 1990;265:1794–1799.

37. Lu Q, Luduena RF. Removal of beta III isotype enhances taxol induced microtubule assembly. Cell Struct Funct 1993;18:173–182.

38. Morejohn LC, Fosket DE. Taxol-induced rose microtubule polymerization in vitro and its inhibition by colchicine. J Cell Biol 1984;99:141–147.

39. Bokros CL, Hugdahl JD, Hanesworth VR, et al. Characterization of the reversible taxol-induced polymerization of plant tubulin into microtubules. Biochemistry 1993; 32:3437–3447.

40. Barnes G, Louie KA, Botstein D. Yeast proteins associated with microtubules in vitro and in vivo. Mol Biol Cell 1992;3:29–47.

41. Vallee RB. Purification of brain microtubules and microtubule-associated protein 1 using taxol. Methods Enzymol 1986;134:104–115.

42. Vallee RB, Collins CA. Purification of microtubules and microtubule-associated proteins from sea urchin eggs and cultured mammalian cells using taxol, and use of exogenous taxol-stabilized brain microtubules for purifying microtubule-associated proteins. Methods Enzymol 1986;134:116–127.

43. Collins CA, Vallee RB. Temperature-dependent reversible assembly of taxol-treated microtubules. J Cell Biol 1987;105:2847–2854.

44. Bayley H, Knowles JR. Photoaffinity labeling. Methods Enzymol 1977;46:69–114.

45. Nath JP, Eagle GR, Himes RH. Direct photoaffinity labeling of tubulin with GTP. Biochemistry 1985;24:1555–1560.

46. Shivanna BD, Mejillano MR, Williams TD, et al. Exchangable GTP binding site of β-tubulin. J Biol Chem 1993;268:127–132.

47. Wolff J, Knipling L, Cahnmann HJ, et al. Direct photoaffinity labeling of tubulin with colchicine. Proc Natl Acad Sci USA 1991;88:2820–2824.

48. Rao S, Horwitz SB, Ringel I. Direct photoaffinity labeling of tubulin with taxol. J Natl Cancer Inst 1992;84:785–788.

49. Carboni JM, Farina V, Rao S, et al. Synthesis of a photoaffinity analog of taxol as an approach to identify the taxol binding site on microtubules. J Med Chem 1993;36: 513–515.

50. Rimoldi JM, Kingston DG, Chaudhary AG, et al. Modified taxols 9: Synthesis and biological evaluation of 7-substituted photoaffinity analogues of taxol. J Natl Prod 1993;56:1313–1330.

51. Chaudhary AG, Gharpure MM, Rimoldi JM, et al. Unexpectedly facile hydrolysis of the 2-benzoate group of taxol and syntheses of analogs with increased activities. J Am Chem Soc 1994;116:4097–4098.

52. Swindell CS, Heerding JM, Krauss NE, et al. Characterization of two taxol photoaffinity analogs bearing azide and benzophenone-related photoreactive substituents in the A-ring side chain. J Med Chem 1994;37:1446–1449.

53. Combeau C, Commercon A, Mioskowski C, et al. Predominant labeling of β- over α-tubulin from porcine brain by a photoactivable taxoid derivative. Biochemistry 1994;33:6676–6683.

54. Rao S, Krauss NE, Heerding JM, et al. 3'-(p-Azidobenzamido)taxol photolabels the N-terminal 31 amino acids of β-tubulin. J Biol Chem 1994;269:3132–3134.
55. Gard DL, Kirschner MW. A polymer-dependent increase in phosphorylation of beta-tubulin accompanies differentiation of a mouse neuroblastoma cell line. J Cell Biol 1985;100:764–774.
56. Long BH, Fairchild CR. Paclitaxel inhibits progression of mitotic cells to G_1, phase by interference with spindle formation without affecting other microtubule functions during anaphase and telephase. Cancer Res 1994;54:4355–4361.
57. Jordan MA, Toso RJ, Thrower D, et al. Mechanism of mitotic block and inhibition of cell proliferation by taxol at low concentrations. Proc Natl Acad Sci USA 1993;90: 9552–9556.
58. Schiff PB, Horwitz SB. Taxol stabilizes microtubules in mouse fibroblast cells. Proc Natl Acad Sci USA 1980;77:1561–1565.
59. DeBrabander M, Gevens G, Nuydens R, et al. Taxol induces the assembly of free microtubules in living cells and blocks the organizing capacity of the centrosomes and kinetochores. Proc Natl Acad Sci USA 1981;78:5608–5612.
60. Verde F, Berrez JM, Antony C, et al. Taxol-induced microtubule asters in mitotic extracts of Xenopus eggs: requirement for phosphorylated factors and cytoplasmic dynein. J Cell Biol 1991;112:1177–1187.
61. Rowinsky EK, Cazenave LA, Donehower RC. Taxol: a novel investigational anti-microtubule agent. J Natl Cancer Inst 1990;82:1247–1259.
62. Amos LA. Brain dynein crossbridges microtubules into bundles. J Cell Sci 1989; 93:19–28.
63. Turner PF, Margolis RL. Taxol-induced bundling of brain-derived microtubules. J Cell Biol 1984;99:940–946.
64. Chang Jie J, Sonobe S. Identification and preliminary characterization of a 65 kDa higher-plant microtubule-associated protein. J Cell Sci 1993;105:891–901.
65. Weisshaar B, Doll T, Matus A. Reorganisation of the microtubular cytoskeleton by embryonic microtubule-associated protein 2 (MAP2c). Development 1992;116:1151–1161.
66. Andrews SB, Gallant PE, Leapman RD, et al. Single kinesin molecules crossbridge microtubules in vitro. Proc Natl Acad Sci USA 1993;90:6503–6507.
67. Scott CW, Klika AB, Lo MM, et al. Tau protein induces bundling of microtubules in vitro: comparison of different tau isoforms and a tau protein fragment. J Neurosci Res 1992;33:19–29.
68. Takeuchi M, Hisanaga S, Umeyama T, et al. The 72-kDa microtubule-associated protein from porcine brain. J Neurochem 1992;58:1510–1516.
69. Bennett AF, Baines AJ. Bundling of microtubules by synapsin 1. Eur J Biochem 1992; 206:783–792.
70. Ding H, Porteu F, Sanchez E, et al. Shared actions of endotoxin and taxol on TNF receptors and TNF release. Science 1990;248:370–372.
71. Manthey CL, Brandes ME, Perera PY, et al. Taxol increases steady-state levels of lipopolysaccharide-inducible genes and protein-tyrosine phosphorylation in murine macrophages. J Immunol 1992;149:2459–2465.

72. Carboni JM, Singh C, Tepper MA. Taxol and LPS induce similar tyrosine phospho-
    proteins in macrophages. J Cell Biol 1991;115:18a.
73. Manthey CL, Qureshi N, Stutz PL, et al. Lipopolysaccharide antagonists block taxol-
    induced signaling in murine macrophages. J Exp Med 1993;178:695–702.
74. Ding A, Sanchez E, Tancinco M, et al. Interactions of bacterial lipopolysaccharide
    with microtubule proteins. J Immunol 1992;148:2853–2858.

3

Mechanisms of Resistance

SUSAN BAND HORWITZ, SRINIVASA RAO,
CHIA-PING HUANG YANG, and GEORGE A. ORR
Albert Einstein College of Medicine
Bronx, New York

I. INTRODUCTION

The emergence of drug resistance is a significant problem that develops during the treatment of human malignancies with cancer chemotherapeutic agents. The problem is not that useful antitumor drugs are unavailable, but rather that tumor cells can, by a variety of methods, develop resistance and replicate in the presence of cytotoxic agents. Malignant cells are clever and are determined to survive, by one method or another. There are innumerable mechanisms by which cells may become resistant to a single drug.

Many laboratories, including our own, have become intrigued by drug resistance. As part of our research programs, we have isolated and studied cell lines selected for resistance to cytotoxic agents. In some cases this has involved mutagenesis followed by selection, and in other situations selection has taken place in the absence of mutagenesis. Such cell lines are useful for examining the biochemical and genetic changes that occur in cells growing in tissue culture under stressful conditions. Some of these cell lines will replicate in concentrations of drug that are thousands of fold greater than are required to inhibit the growth of a parental drug-sensitive cell line. Although these concentrations of drug are much higher than a cancer cell would be exposed to in vivo, such cells often exaggerate their differences thereby making it easier for scientists to direct and answer their questions concerning drug resistance. Although resistant cells growing in tissue

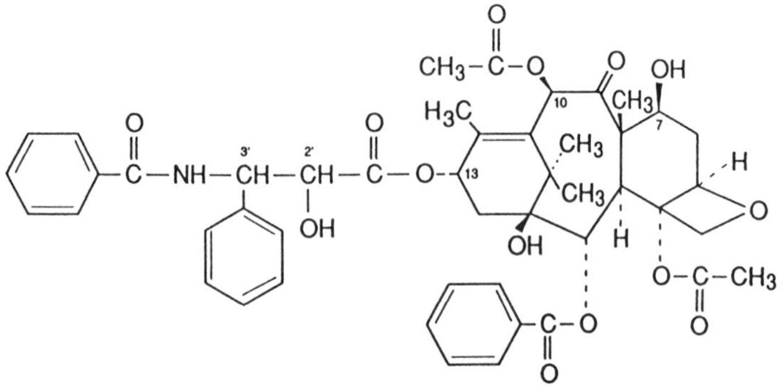

Figure 1 Structural formula of paclitaxel.

culture may provide clues, mechanisms of resistance must eventually be dissected in vivo. Many variables, some completely unknown, may influence the acquisition of drug resistance in human tumors. It is difficult to study drug resistance in the patient, but a necessary task if scientists and physicians are to overcome drug resistance when it occurs or, more important, reduce the emergence of drug resistance.

Paclitaxel is a drug of considerable current interest because of its activity in a number of human malignancies and its unusual chemical structure and mechanism of action (1). The drug has been approved by the Food and Drug Administration for the treatment of ovarian and breast carcinomas and is demonstrating promising activity in carcinomas of the lung, head and neck, bladder, esophagus and testes (2). Paclitaxel, originally isolated from the bark of the slow-growing Western yew, *Taxus brevifolia* (3), is a complex diterpene having a taxane ring structure with a four-membered oxetane ring and an ester side chain at position C-13 (Fig. 1). Unfortunately, as is the case with other anticancer drugs, tumors become resistant to paclitaxel, and the ease with which this happens is very disappointing. Although there is essentially no information on the mechanisms of paclitaxel resistance that are important in human tumors, paclitaxel-resistant cell lines are being studied in laboratories and such research is providing information that can be pursued in vivo. Two such mechanisms of resistance will be reviewed in this chapter.

II. PACLITAXEL AND THE MULTIDRUG RESISTANCE (MDR) PHENOTYPE

Because of its natural product origin and hydrophobic nature, paclitaxel is an excellent compound to use for the selection of cells that have the MDR phenotype.

The latter includes the overproduction of P-glycoprotein, an integral membrane protein that acts as a drug-efflux pump to maintain the intracellular concentration of drug below cytotoxic levels (4–6). Such cells have an amplification of the DNA that encodes P-glycoprotein and/or an overexpression of the mRNA for P-glycoprotein. As its name implies, the MDR phenotype refers to cells that demonstrate cross-resistance to a large variety of hydrophobic compounds to which the cell has never been exposed. Although the phenomenon of cross-resistance can be the result of different biochemical changes occurring in the cell, resistance to paclitaxel and the development of cross-resistance in our cells is related to the overproduction of P-glycoprotein (7).

A highly paclitaxel-resistant cell line, J7.T1, has been isolated in our laboratory from drug-sensitive J774.2 cells, a macrophage-like murine cell line. This cell line, which was selected in a stepwise fashion with paclitaxel in the absence of mutagenesis, is over 900-fold resistant to the drug and displays the MDR phenotype (7,8). Analysis of the accumulation of radiolabeled paclitaxel in the sensitive and resistant cells clearly indicated that there was a dramatically reduced accumulation of the drug in the J7.T1 cell line (Fig. 2). In the mouse, there are two functional genes, *mdr*1a and *mdr*1b, each of which codes for a related but distinct P-glycoprotein isoform. The paclitaxel-resistant J7.T1 cell line was unusual in that both genes were amplified and their gene products were overproduced in nearly equal quantities (Fig. 3).

P-glycoprotein is the hallmark of the MDR phenotype and a member of the ATP-binding cassette (ABC) superfamily of membrane transporters. The glycoprotein is composed of approximately 1280 amino acid residues that contain a 140-kDa protein core and approximately 15–30 kDa of N-linked carbohydrate that are clustered in the first extracellular loop (8–12). Hydropathy plot analysis has suggested that P-glycoprotein is composed of two homologous halves, each of which contains six putative transmembrane spanning domains and a nucleotide binding fold (Fig. 4). The latter contains the consensus Walker motifs that represent the areas with the greatest amino acid sequence homology between the two halves of the molecule and between other ABC transporters. However, there is substantial conservation between the two halves of the molecule that are connected by a 60–70-amino-acid segment referred to as the linker region. It is known that P-glycoprotein is phosphorylated in vivo and also in vitro by both protein kinase A and protein kinase C, and there is some experimental evidence that the function of P-glycoprotein may be regulated by its state of phosphorylation. Recent studies have found that the major phosphorylation sites in P-glycoprotein are present in the linker regions of both murine and human P-glycoproteins (13,14). Studies are being done to determine the significance of the phosphorylation that occurs at specific serines in the linker region as it relates to the transport activities of P-glycoprotein.

In J7.T1 cells, P-glycoprotein is responsible for a major portion of the

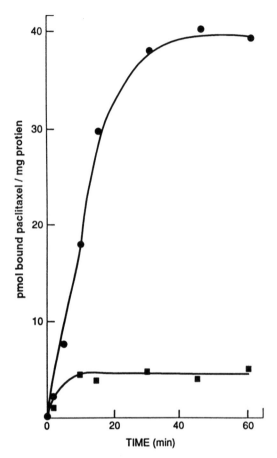

Figure 2 Accumulation of [³H]paclitaxel in J774.2 and J7.T1 cells. Confluent 35-mm plates of cells were incubated with 2 mL of medium containing 0.3 μM [³H]paclitaxel at 37°C for the indicated times. Cells were washed three times with ice-cold phosphate-buffered saline and lysed with 1 mL 1 N NaOH for 16 hr. An aliquot of cell lysate was neutralized with an equal volume of glacial acetic acid, and radioactivity was determined. Control (●), J7.T1 (■). Each point represents the average of four determinations. (From Ref. 7, p. 3856; with permission.)

paclitaxel-resistance that is observed in cells growing in tissue culture. P-glyco-protein has been identified in many human tumors and its concentration has been observed to increase after treatment with some antitumor drugs (15). Although at present no data implicate P-glycoprotein as a determinant of paclitaxel resistance in human tumors, the glycoprotein is clearly one viable candidate.

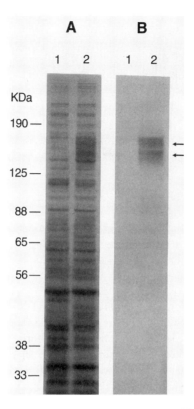

Figure 3 Two isoforms of P-glycoprotein are overproduced in the murine paclitaxel-resistant J7.T1 cell line. Proteins from a plasma-membrane-enriched subcellar fraction were resolved by SDS-PAGE and silver-stained (A) or transferred to nitrocellulose (B). Twenty-five micrograms of protein was loaded in each lane. In B, the blot was probed with a P-glycoprotein-specific peptide polyclonal antibody (Oncogene Science, Uniondale, New York). (Lanes 1) Parental drug-sensitive cells (murine J774.2 macrophage-like cells); (Lanes 2) paclitaxel-resistant J7.T1 cells. (From Ref. 24, p. 55; with permission.)

III. PACLITAXEL AND THE MICROTUBULE

All the available evidence indicates that the major intracellular target for paclitaxel is the microtubule, an organelle composed of α- and β-tubulin heterodimers. When cells are incubated with paclitaxel, discrete bundles of stable microtubules are formed in the cell. These bundles result from a reorganization of the micro-tubule cytoskeleton (16). Microtubules are not static but rather exist in a state of dynamic equilibrium with their subunits. It is believed that paclitaxel acts by altering the normal equilibrium and shifting it in favor of the formation of the

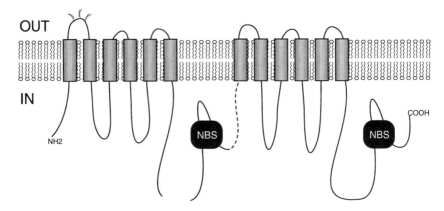

Figure 4   Structure of P-glycoprotein. Each half of P-glycoprotein is referred to as a cassette and contains six transmembrane spanning domains followed by a nucleotide binding site (NBS). The two cassettes are connected by a linker region (dashed line).

microtubule polymer from its subunits, the α- and β-tubulins (17,18). Microtubules are required for normal cell replication and function. They are a major component of the mitotic spindle and absolutely essential for normal cell division. In addition, they are needed for maintaining cell shape and motility and for transport between organelles within the cell. Therefore, a drug such as paclitaxel that alters the normal dynamic behavior of microtubules will dramatically influence normal cell behavior and replication.

A mutation or a posttranslational alteration in tubulin that has the potential to result in a modification or elimination of the paclitaxel binding site could be responsible for the emergence of a paclitaxel-resistant cell population. A series of mutant Chinese hamster ovary cells that are resistant to paclitaxel have been characterized (19–21). Altered α- and/or β-tubulin has been identified by abnormal migration patterns on two-dimensional gel electrophoresis. It is not known whether these changes are the result of mutations or posttranslational modifications such as phosphorylation or acetylation. Other Chinese hamster cells developed a dependence on paclitaxel and actually require the drug for normal growth.

Figure 5   High-performance electrophoresis chromatographic analysis of [^{3}H]3'-(p-azidobenzamido)paclitaxel-photolabeled β-tubulin (A) and its formic acid digestion products (B). Intact β-tubulin was resolved on a 7% polyacrylamide gel (A) and digested β-tubulin on a 12% polyacrylamide gel containing 6 M urea (B). In each case, 75,000 dpm in a total volume of 25 μL was loaded. Electrophoresis was conducted either at 0.3 mA for 30 min followed by 1.5 mA for 5 hr (A) or at 0.4 mA for 30 min followed by 1.3 mA for 5 hr

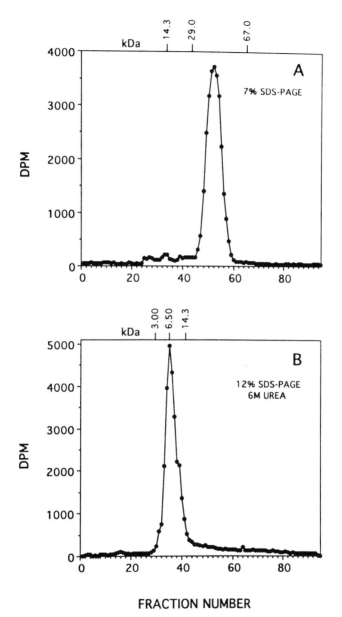

(B). Fractions were counted by liquid scintillation spectrometry. Insulin (3 kDa, A/B chains), aprotinin (6.5 kDa), lysozyme (14.3 kDa), carbonic anhdrase (29 kDa), and bovine serum albumin (67 kDa) were used as markers. (From Ref. 23, p. 3134; with permission.)

Although it has been known that the cellular target for paclitaxel is the microtubule, only recently has information on the binding site for the drug become available. Experiments done by direct photoaffinity labeling of microtubule protein with [^{3}H]paclitaxel resulted in the preferential labeling of the β-subunit of tubulin (22). Since the extent of photoincorporation was low, it was impractical to define the binding site for [^{3}H]paclitaxel in β-tubulin. However, the availability of 3'-(p-azidobenzamido)paclitaxel, a photoaffinity analog with similar biological properties as paclitaxel, has allowed further delineation of the paclitaxel-binding site.

To locate the binding site for [^{3}H]3'-(p-azidobenzamido)paclitaxel, photo-labeled β-tubulin was digested with formic acid, thereby taking advantage of the fact that formic acid cleaves Asp-Pro bonds. There are two such bonds in β-tubulin, at amino acids 31–32 and 304–305. The results of such experiments can be summarized in an electrophoretic profile in which it is clear that the intact β-tubulin gave rise to a single radiolabeled formic acid digestion product (Fig. 5). To determine the identity of this radiolabeled peptide, it was sequenced and proven to be the conserved N-terminus of β-tubulin. Electrospray mass spectroscopy was done to confirm that formic acid had cleaved at the Asp^{31}-Pro^{32} bond. The combination of these two methods established that one domain of the paclitaxel-binding site in β-tubulin is the N-terminal 31 amino acids (23). This knowledge provides for the first time a defined segment of β-tubulin in which to search for mutations in the binding site for paclitaxel. PCR-based methodology will be used to sequence the N-terminal domain of β-tubulin in paclitaxel-resistant cell lines and human tumor samples from patients who have acquired resistance to paclitaxel. Such studies may provide evidence of mutations that are responsible for paclitaxel resistance.

IV. SUMMARY

From experiments done in the laboratory with paclitaxel-resistant cell lines, there are at least two mechanisms that could be responsible for the development of paclitaxel resistance. The presence of the MDR phenotype could eliminate intracellular paclitaxel, resulting in a paclitaxel-resistant cell line. Alternatively, a mutation in the microtubule binding site for paclitaxel could result in elimination of the intracellular target for paclitaxel. Undoubtedly there are more than these two mechanisms that could be responsible for paclitaxel resistance. In addition, the role of these mechanisms in conferring resistance to paclitaxel in the clinic is not known at this juncture. It is important to analyze resistant human tumors because it is only in this way that paclitaxel resistance will be understood. Strategies for overcoming or inhibiting the emergence of paclitaxel resistance will be possible only with a thorough understanding of the factors involved in the development of such resistance in human tumors.

ACKNOWLEDGMENTS

Research that originated in the authors' laboratory was supported, in part, by U.S. Public Health Service Grant CA 39821.

REFERENCES

1. Horwitz SB. Mechanism of action of Taxol. Trends Pharmacol Sci 1992;13:134–136.
2. Donehower RC, Rowinsky EK. Paclitaxel. In: DeVita VT Jr, Hellman S, Rosenberg SA, eds. Principles and practices of oncology updates. Vol. 8, Philadelphia: Lippincott, October 1994.
3. Wani MC, Taylor HL, Wall ME, et al. Plant antitumor agents. VI. The isolation and structure of Taxol, a novel antileukemic and antitumor agent from *Taxus brevifolia*. J Am Chem Soc 1971;93:2325–2327.
4. Endicott JA, Ling V. The biochemistry of P-glycoprotein-mediated multidrug resistance. Annu Rev Biochem 1989;58:137–171.
5. Gottesman MM, Pastan I. Biochemistry of multidrug resistance mediated by the multidrug transporter. Annu Rev Biochem 1993;62:385–427.
6. Kirschner LS, Greenberger LM, Hsu SI-H, et al. Biochemical and genetic characterization of the multidrug resistance phenotype in murine macrophagelike J774.2 cells. Biochem Pharmacol 1992;43:77–87.
7. Roy SN, Horwitz SB. A phosphoglycoprotein associated with Taxol-resistance in J774.2 cells. Cancer Res 1985;45:3856–3863.
8. Greenberger LM, Lothstein L, Williams SS, Horwitz SB. Distinct P-glycoprotein precursors are overproduced in independently isolated drug-resistant cell lines. Proc Natl Acad Sci USA 1988;85:3762–3766.
9. Chen CJ, Chin JE, Ueda K, et al. Internal duplication and homology with bacterial transport proteins in the *mdr*1 (P-glycoprotein) gene from multidrug-resistant human cells. Cell 1986;47:381–389.
10. Gross P, Heriah YB, Croop JM, Housman DE. Isolation and expression of a complementary DNA that confers multidrug resistance. Nature 1986;232:728–731.
11. Greenberger L, Williams SS, Horwitz SB. Biosynthesis of heterogeneous forms of multidrug resistance-associated proteins. J Biol Chem 1987;262:13685–13689.
12. Richert ND, Aldwin L, Nitecki D, et al. Stability and covalent modification of P-glycoprotein in multidrug-resistant KB cells. Biochemistry 1988;27:7607–7613.
13. Orr GA, Han EK-H, Browne PC, et al. Identification of the major phosphorylation domain of murine *mdr*1b P-glycoprotein: analysis of the protein kinase A and protein kinase C phosphorylation sites. J Biol Chem 1993;268:25054–25062.
14. Chambers TC, Pohl J, Raynor RL, Kuo JF. Identification of specific sites in human P-glycoprotein phosphorylated by protein kinase C. J Biol Chem 1993;268:4592–4595.
15. Goldstein LJ, Galski H, Fojo A, et al. Expression of a multidrug resistance gene in human cancers. J Natl Cancer Inst 1989;81:116–124.
16. Schiff PB, Horwitz SB. Taxol stabilizes microtubules in mouse fibroblast cells. Proc Natl Acad Sci USA 1980;77:1561–1565.

17. Schiff PB, Fant J, Horwitz SB. Promotion of microtubule assembly in vitro by Taxol. Nature 1979;277:665–667.
18. Schiff PB, Horwitz SB. Taxol assembles tubulin in the absence of exogenous GTP or microtubule associated proteins. Biochemistry 1981;20:3247–3252.
19. Cabral F, Abraham I, Gottesman MM. Isolation of a Taxol-resistant Chinese hamster ovary cell mutant that has an alteration in α-tubulin. Proc Natl Acad Sci USA 1981;78:4388–4391.
20. Schibler MJ, Cabral F. Taxol-dependent mutants of Chinese hamster ovary cells with alterations in α- and β-tubulin. J Cell Biol 1986;102:1552–1531.
21. Cabral F, Barlow SB. Mechanisms by which mammalian cells acquire resistance to drugs that affect microtubule assembly. FASEB J 1989;3:1593–1599.
22. Rao S, Horwitz SB, Ringel I. Direct photoaffinity labeling of tubulin with Taxol. J Natl Cancer Inst 1992;84:785–788.
23. Rao S, Krauss NE, Heerding JM, et al. 3'-(p-azidobenzamido)taxol photolabels the N-terminal 31 amino acids of β-tubulin. J Biol Chem 1994;269:3132–3134.
24. Proceedings of the Second National Cancer Institute Workshop on Taxol and Taxus. In: Ihde DC, ed. Journal of the National Cancer Institute Monographs, Vol. 15 Washington, DC US Government Printing Office, 1993.

4

Combination with Other Agents: Preclinical Data

WILLIAM C. ROSE and CRAIG R. FAIRCHILD
Pharmaceutical Research Institute
Bristol-Myers Squibb Company
Princeton, New Jersey

I. IN VITRO CYTOTOXICITY DATA

A. Introduction

Paclitaxel, a natural plant product isolated from the bark of the western yew (*Taxus brevifolia*), has recently been approved in its clinical formulation for the treatment of refractory ovarian cancer, and is showing promising activity in malignant melanoma, breast cancer, and lung cancer (1). Although paclitaxel has been demonstrated to be a clinically useful anticancer agent, not all patients' tumors respond to the drug, and those that do usually relapse. Therefore, combinations of paclitaxel with other antitumor agents are a logical approach to improve clinical antitumor responses. Indeed, for more than two decades it has been recognized that the heterogeneous nature of cancer and its ability to develop drug resistance provides a strong rationale for combination chemotherapy (2). In this section the available data on paclitaxel in combination with other anticancer agents in vitro is reviewed as a backdrop for paclitaxel-drug combination studies that have been done in vivo, which are discussed later in this chapter.

Before discussing the data from the various laboratories that have conducted research on paclitaxel-drug combinations, the end points used to determine in vitro cytotoxicity will be described. In this review, *cytotoxicity* is used in the broad sense of the term to include both growth inhibition as well as cell death. Among the assays used to determine cytotoxicity are various cell staining techniques (e.g., tetrazolium, neutral red, and sulphorodamine B dyes), cell counting, tritiated thymidine uptake, and colony formation. All but the latter assay measure primarily inhibition of cell growth, and only the colony formation assay measures both inhibition of cell growth and cell death because it indicates that cells have undergone multiple rounds of mitotic division. In the studies discussed in this section, some of the investigators examining paclitaxel-based drug combinations actually measured cytotoxicity by colony forming assay while the others evaluated effects on cell growth.

Analysis of drug combination data is complicated by a lack of universally accepted terminology and methodology (3). An often applied definition of the term *synergy* as it relates to cytotoxicity data is an effect of two or more drugs used in combination (sequentially or simultaneously) that is greater in magnitude than the sum of the effects produced by the same concentrations of those drugs used individually; the sum of the individual effects is referred to as the *additivity threshold*. Antagonism occurs when the effect of the combination is less than additive. (Some authors also use the terms *supraadditive* and *subadditive*, which we have translated herein as *synergy* and *antagonism*, respectively.) However, if either (or any) drug in the combination is used at a concentration where its dose-response curve is nonlinear (or not evaluated), a simple algebraic summation of effects may yield a spurious conclusion. To avoid such pitfalls, many investigators have relied on either of two approaches to characterize the cytotoxic effects of combination chemotherapy (synergy, additivity, antagonism): the isobologram (4) and the median-effect plot/combination index (5). A description of those methods is beyond the scope of this chapter, but if the studies to be described do not mention having included dose-response titrations or having had their data analyzed by one of those methods or comparable versions of them (6), then the validity of the conclusions drawn should be particularly well scrutinized. The effects of all the paclitaxel-based drug interactions to be discussed are summarized in Table 1.

B. Paclitaxel plus Cisplatin

The effects of paclitaxel in combination with cisplatin (cDDP) were reported initially by Citardi et al. (7). When mouse leukemia L1210 cells resistant to paclitaxel were incubated with 1 μM paclitaxel for 24 hr before a 30-min exposure to cDDP, the concentration of cDDP required to produce a 90% cytotoxic effect was decreased from 47 μM (in the absence of paclitaxel) to 13 μM. However, if the agents were given simultaneously for 24 hr, or cDDP was given first for 30 min followed by paclitaxel for 24 hr, there were inconsequential changes in the concentrations of cDDP required to yield 90% cytotoxic effects. No description was provided of the cytotoxic effects of paclitaxel alone or the particular cytotoxicity assay used. Although the authors did not describe their data in terms of synergy or antagonism, they demonstrated the superiority of the paclitaxel $\rightarrow$ cDDP sequence when compared to the other regimens. The paclitaxel $\rightarrow$ cDDP

Table 1 Summary of in Vitro Cytotoxicity Data for Paclitaxel in Combination with Other Chemotherapeutic Agents

Paclitaxel plus[a]	Sequence	Cell line(s)	Outcome	Reference
ADR	Paclitaxel first	MCF-7, A549	Antagonism[b]	13
	Paclitaxel first	MCF-7	Antagonism	14
	Paclitaxel first	MAM 16/C	Additive	14
	Concomitant	MCF-7	Antagonism	14
	Concomitant	MAM 16/C	Additive	14
	Concomitant	OVCAR-3. Caov-4	Additive	15
	Paclitaxel last	MCF-7	Antagonism[c]	14
	Paclitaxel last	MAM 16/C	Synergy	14
m-AMSA	Paclitaxel first	MCF-7, A549	Antagonism[b]	13
L-BSO	Paclitaxel last	MCF-7, A549	Antagonism[d]	16
	Concomitant	MCF-7, A549A	No effect[c]	16
cDDP	Paclitaxel first	L1210	Synergy?[b,e]	7
	Paclitaxel first	L1210	Synergy	8
	Paclitaxel first	A2780/CP70	Synergy[b]	11
	Paclitaxel first	Fresh ovarian tumors	Antagonism[b]	12
	Concomitant	L1210	No synergy[b,e]	7
	Concomitant	Fresh ovarian tumors	Antagonism	12
	Paclitaxel last	L1210	No synergy[b,e]	7
	Paclitaxel last	L1210	Antagonism	8
	Paclitaxel last	Fresh ovarian tumors	Antagonism[b]	12
EDX	Paclitaxel first	SKBR-3	Antagonism	24
	Concomitant	SKBR-3	Additive	24
	Paclitaxel last	SKBR-3	Synergy	24
EM	Concomitant	DU145	Synergy[b]	20
INFβ	Paclitaxel last	MCF-7, ACHN, UO-31, OVCAR-4, OVCAR-5	Synergy	26
Tiazofuran	Concomitant	PANC-1, OVCAR-5, H125, 3924A	Synergy	19
TOP	Paclitaxel first	MCF-7	Antagonism	14
	Paclitaxel first	MAM 16/C	Synergy	14
	Paclitaxel last	MCF-7	Additive	14
	Paclitaxel last	MAM 16/C	Synergy	14
VBL	Concomitant	DU145	Additive[b]	20
DHVD$_3$	Concomitant	MCF-7	Synergy	25
VP-16	Paclitaxel first	MCF-7, A549	Antagonism[b]	13

[a]ADR, doxorubicin; m-AMSA, amsacrine; L-BSO, L-buthionine sulfoximine; cDDP, cisplatin; EDX, edatrexate; EM, estramustine; INFβ, interferon β, TOP, topotecan; VBL, vinblastine; DHVD3, 1,25-dihydroxyvitamin D$_3$; VP-16, etoposide.
[b]No formal drug combination analysis was described in the reference.
[c]In the reference, an error was made describing this interaction as "supraadditive"; in fact, it was subadditive (S. M. Schmid, Southern Research Institute, Birmingham, AL; personal communication).
[d]L-BSO is a chemosensitizer and was used at a nontoxic concentration. Therefore, the outcome given is relative to the effect of paclitaxel alone.
[e]The cytotoxic potency of cDDP was greatly enhanced when the drug was applied following paclitaxel; however, in the absence of data pertaining to paclitaxel alone, only suppositions regarding synergy or antagonism can be made.

combination did not enhance the interstrand DNA cross-linking produced by cDDP alone as assessed using an alkaline elution technique.

Recently, Jekunen et al. (8) demonstrated a synergy when human ovarian 2008 cells were exposed to paclitaxel for 19 hr before a 1-hr concurrent treatment with paclitaxel and cDDP. Conversely, if cDDP was given first for 1 hr followed immediately by 20 hr of paclitaxel, antagonism was observed. These investigators examined the effect of paclitaxel on cellular cDDP uptake, membrane integrity, and glutathione and metallothionein levels to explain the mechanism of action for the synergistic paclitaxel-cDDP regimen. None of these parameters was affected by paclitaxel applied at a concentration which caused a 50% reduction in colony formation. Interestingly, in a cDDP-resistant 2008 subline (2008/C13*5.25), the sequence paclitaxel → cDDP was synergistic while cDDP → paclitaxel was antagonistic, just as had been observed in the parental cell line. In these studies, synergistic or antagonistic cytotoxicity was assessed by combination analysis.

Although the combination sequence paclitaxel → cDDP appeared to be the most cytotoxic regimen in two studies (7,8), the reason for this effect was unknown. Because resistance to cDDP can result from increased repair of DNA lesions due to DNA alkylation, studies were performed to assess the repair process in cells treated with paclitaxel and cDDP. Dabholkar et al. (9) examined the expression of two excision repair genes (ERCC1 and XPAC) in a cDDP-resistant human ovarian carcinoma cell line (A2780/CP70). When paclitaxel was given for 24 hr before a 1-hr exposure to cDDP, they saw no effect on the transcription of either repair gene when examined between 0 and 7 days after drug exposure. Likewise, no effect was seen with either simultaneous drug exposure or cDDP → paclitaxel. However, the paclitaxel-cDDP drug combinations did result in modest inhibitions of DNA adduct repair of cDDP-induced lesions in A2780/CP70 cells (10). When cells were treated for 24 hr with a concentration of paclitaxel capable of inhibiting cell growth by 10% (i.e., an IC_{10}) (10 nM), followed immediately by 1 hr of 200 μM cDDP, 14% of the adducts were removed, compared to 29% after treatment with cDDP alone and 20% when cDDP was followed by paclitaxel. When a 24-hr incubation in drug-free medium was included between the paclitaxel → cDDP regimen, adduct repair was even further reduced, to 3%. This effect appeared to be reversible as the repair levels returned to baseline (31%), when the length of the drug-free interval was increased to 72 hr. These investigators subsequently reported that maximum inhibition of DNA repair (which occurred with 24-hr incubation in drug-free medium) was paralleled by a maximum (and synergistic) increase in cytotoxicity for these combination schedules (11), and that the enhanced cytotoxicity, as measured by metabolism of a tetrazolium dye, returned to baseline when the drug-free period was extended to 72 hr. No formal drug interaction analysis was described.

Although the authors of the previous reports have demonstrated that paclitaxel → cDDP can be synergistic, data from another study lead to the conclusion that the opposite is true. When paclitaxel was added prior to, at the same time, or within 6 hr following cDDP versus 44 fresh human ovarian tumors, Kern and Morgan (12) observed antagonistic inhibition. Additive cytotoxicity was observed when cDDP was added 24 to 48 hr prior to paclitaxel. Cytotoxicity was assessed by cellular tritiated thymidine incorporation, but the durations of the various drug exposures were not mentioned. The reason for the different findings by these investigators is unclear; however, their results were obtained with primary human tumors, while in other studies human cell lines were used, and the method of data analysis was not described.

C. Paclitaxel plus Etoposide

Hahn et al. (13) examined the effect of paclitaxel in combination with etoposide (VP-16) in human MCF-7 breast and A549 lung carcinoma cells. These cells were pretreated with 10 nM paclitaxel for 24 hr, then incubated with various concentrations of VP-16 for 1 hr; cytotoxicity was assessed by clonogenic assay. Upon correcting the data for paclitaxel-induced cell killing, the authors concluded that the resulting cytotoxicity was less than additive (i.e., antagonistic), although no formal method of data analysis was mentioned.

D. Paclitaxel plus Doxorubicin

The combination of paclitaxel plus doxorubicin (ADR) was studied in human (MCF-7) and mouse (MAM 16/C) breast carcinoma cell lines by Waud et al. (14). Cell growth inhibition was assessed by neutral red dye uptake. These investigators observed supraadditive (synergistic) cytotoxicity when ADR was given before paclitaxel (24-hr exposure for each drug) against MAM 16/C cells, but they found additive or subadditive (antagonistic) cytotoxicity with all other regimens evaluated against either cell line. The data were analyzed using the Prichard-Shipman (6) approach of evaluating drug interactions. Additive cytotoxicity was also observed by Saunders et al. (15) with paclitaxel and ADR combinations versus human OVCAR-3 and Caov-4 ovarian carcinoma cell lines. The two drugs were given concurrently, but the times of exposure were not reported, and the growth inhibition data were subjected to analysis using an isobologram. Hahn et al. (13) evaluated paclitaxel plus ADR in human MCF-7 breast and A549 lung carcinoma cell lines by colony formation assay. Pretreatment of these cell lines with 10 nM paclitaxel for 24 hr followed by various concentrations of ADR for 1 hr resulted in subadditive (antagonistic) cytotoxicity, but the method of drug interaction analysis used to arrive at this conclusion was not described.

E. Paclitaxel plus Amsacrine [4'-(9-acridinylamino)methane-sulfon-m-anisidide]

The combination of paclitaxel and amsacrine (m-AMSA) was examined in human MCF-7 breast and A549 lung carcinoma cell lines (13). This drug combination yielded antagonistic cytotoxicity when the cells were pretreated with 10 nM paclitaxel for 24 hr, followed by incubation with various concentrations of m-AMSA for 1 hr. No mention was made of the method used to analyze the drug interaction cytotoxicity data.

F. Paclitaxel plus Topotecan

Paclitaxel combined with the camptothecin analog topotecan (TOP) was studied in human (MCF-7) or mouse (MAM 16/C) breast cancer cell lines by Waud et al. (14) using neutral red dye uptake to determine cell growth inhibition. When 24 hr of exposure to TOP preceded 24 hr of exposure to paclitaxel, additive cytotoxicity was observed versus MCF-7 cells; subadditive (antagonistic) cytotoxicity was observed when paclitaxel preceded TOP. However, versus MAM 16/C cells, either sequence of drug exposures resulted in supraadditive (synergistic) cytotoxicity. Drug interaction data were subjected to analysis using the Prichard-Shipman method (6).

G. Paclitaxel plus L-Buthionine Sulfoximine

The glutathione-lowering drug L-buthionine sulfoximine (L-BSO) is of interest as a chemosensitizer, particularly in the chemotherapy of ovarian cancer. Accordingly, Liebmann et al. (16) investigated the effect of L-BSO on paclitaxel's cytotoxicity. They found that pretreatment with L-BSO at 5 mM (a noncytotoxic concentration) for 24 hr prior to paclitaxel lowered intracellular glutathione to undetectable levels and produced a threefold increase in survival of MCF-7 cells and a tenfold increase in survival of A549 cells, compared to the cells treated with paclitaxel alone (10 to 50 nM for 24 hr). The intracellular accumulation of paclitaxel was not affected. When cells were treated with paclitaxel alone, the majority of them became arrested in the G$_2$/M phase of the cell cycle; however, concurrent treatment with L-BSO produced a threefold increase in the percentage of cells in S-phase. These results lead one to suggest that the mechanism responsible for the antagonistic influence of L-BSO on the cytotoxicity caused by paclitaxel could be due to its effect on the cell cycle via decreased glutathione levels. Interestingly, glutathione depletion by L-BSO with 1-chloro-2,4-dinitrobenzene altered microtubule structure and led to a loss of microtubules in human 3T3 cells (17). Furthermore, preincubation of 3T3 cells with paclitaxel before glutathione depletion prevented the dissagregation of microtubules. However, glutathione depletion by L-BSO did not affect the morphology of microtubules or the binding of ^{3}H-paclitaxel in either MCF-7 or A549 cells. Further studies will be required to determine the role of glutathione in the antagonism of paclitaxel cytotoxicity by L-BSO.

H. Paclitaxel plus Tiazofurin

The guanine nucleotide GTP is required for microtubule assembly. Tiazofurin is an inhibitor of inosine monophosphate dehydrogenase and disrupts GTP metabolism (18), although it is not clear if it also can disrupt the polymerization of microtubules in the cell. Paclitaxel blocks tubulin assembly by stabilizing the formation of microtubules. Therefore, if combined, these two compounds could provide a block of mitotic spindle formation in two different steps in the assembly process, although presumably these are opposing actions. Taniki et al. (19) evaluated the combination of these two drugs in human pancreatic (PANC-1), ovarian (OVCAR-5) and lung (H125) carcinoma cells and a rat hepatoma cell line (3924A). Using a combination index analysis to determine if a synergy between paclitaxel and tiazofurin existed, these investigators found synergistic cytotoxicity in all the cell lines when both drugs were applied concurrently.

I. Paclitaxel plus Vinblastine

Vinblastine (VBL) is a clinically established anticancer drug that is known to inhibit tubulin assembly. It was tested in combination with paclitaxel by Speicher et al. (20) and cytotoxicity was assessed by colony forming assay following a 14-day continuous drug exposure. When 0.5 nM paclitaxel, a concentration that caused 20% inhibition of cell survival, was combined simultaneously with various concentrations of VBL (0.1 to 0.5 nM), the combinations failed to increase the levels of cytotoxicity in a human prostatic carcinoma cell line (DU145) beyond that associated with the collective effects of the individual drugs. No formal analysis of the data was described, but we interpreted the results as indicative of an additive drug interaction.

J. Paclitaxel plus Estramustine

Estramustine (EM) is used clinically to treat advanced hormone-refractory prostate carcinoma. This unique molecule, which is a combination of estradiol and nornitrogen mustard, acts by binding noncovalently to microtubule-associated proteins and induces microtubule disassembly and cell death. (This is in contrast to VBL, which binds directly to tubulin.) The effect of combining 0.5 nM paclitaxel, a concentration capable of 20% inhibition of cell survival, with various concentrations of EM (1 to 5 μM) was examined on the clonogenic survival of DU145 human prostatic carcinoma cells (20). The authors concluded that a greater than additive (synergistic) effect occurred, although no formal drug combination analysis was described.

This combination might have been expected to produce a block in G2/M due to the drugs' combined effect on microtubules; however, it appeared that the combination of EM and paclitaxel resulted in an increased number of cells in S phase and no mitotic blockade (20). Several investigators have proposed that microtubules can influence DNA synthesis by regulation of mitogenic signals (21,22). Similarly, Speicher et al. (20) suggest that paclitaxel plus EM produces a disruption of cytoskeleton and nuclear matrix communication, with subsequent effects on the control of DNA synthesis. Such activities could account for the alteration of the number of cells in S phase and a reduction in the number of cells blocked in mitosis. In addition, micronucleation and aberrant mitotic figures increased with the paclitaxel-EM combination, possibly due to disruption of the mitotic spindle, which can lead to reversion to an interphase state without completion of mitosis or cytokinesis (23).

K. Paclitaxel plus Edatrexate

A new dihydrofolate reductase inhibitor edatrexate (EDX), which is currently in clinical trials, was combined with paclitaxel and tested against the human breast adenocarcinoma cell line SKBR-3 (24). Drug interactions were determined using a combination index-isobologram analysis of data from a 7-day cell growth inhibition assay. Synergism was demonstrated when treatment with EDX (for as long as 3 hr) was followed immediately by 24 to 27 hr of exposure to paclitaxel. When the reverse schedule was used, mild antagonism was demonstrated. Concurrent exposure of cells to paclitaxel and EX for as long as 3 hr was additive. The mechanism for the observed synergism is currently unknown.

L. Paclitaxel plus 1,25-Dihydroxyvitamin D$_3$

Saunders et al. (25) have investigated the combination of paclitaxel with 1,25-dihydroxyvitamin D$_3$ (DHVD$_3$) the most active natural metabolite of vitamin D$_3$. This cytostatic vitamin D$_3$ metabolite has been shown to have preclinical activity against breast cancer both in vitro and in vivo. Synergistic activity was observed after a 3-day simultaneous exposure of MCF-7 breast cells to these two drugs. The growth inhibition data were analyzed by isobologram.

M. Paclitaxel plus Interferon β

The biological response modifier interferon β (INFβ) was used in combination with paclitaxel against five human carcinoma cell lines: MCF-7 breast, ACHN and UO-31 renal, and OVCAR-4 and OVCAR-5 ovarian (26). Cytotoxicity was assessed by a dye staining assay and the results were analyzed by Prichard-Shipman (6) or isobole methodology. Supraadditive (synergistic) cytotoxicity was demonstrated in all cell lines, with optimal activity occurring when INFβ preceded paclitaxel (the times of exposure were not reported). The relationship between paclitaxel and INFβ with regards to cell growth and cytotoxicity remains to be explored.

II. IN VIVO ANTITUMOR DATA

A. Introduction

Paclitaxel-based combination chemotherapy studies from several laboratories involving different tumor models have been described in recent years. In assessing the antitumor data from those many diverse experiments, we have evaluated them for therapeutic synergy as defined by Venditti and Goldin (27) and expounded upon further by many others (28–31). Briefly, to qualify as therapeutically synergistic, a drug combination must be therapeutically superior to each optimally applied single agent in the combination. If the treatment periods used for the combination and single-drug therapies differ appreciably, then adjustments should be made in evaluating their respective data. Any therapeutic superiority claimed should reflect a biologically meaningful difference and toxicity limitations should be applied uniformly to all treatments.

Operationally, a typical end point for "biologically meaningful" has been ≥ 1 log cell kill (LCK), usually determined by improvements in tumor (re)growth delays, although life span increases (e.g., as reflected by %T/C values) have also been used. Biologically meaningful results should be evaluated for their statistical significance but one does not always find such verification among data presentations. Whenever provided or whenever they could be determined, LCK values were used to compare the effectiveness of treatment regimens. The formula for determining LCK is as follows: LCK = T − C(in days)/(3.32) (TVDT), where T − C represents the relative time for treated (T) and control (C) mice to grow tumors of a predetermined target size, and TVDT is the tumor volume doubling time of tumors in the control group measured (typically) just prior to achieving their tumor target size.

A large part of the combination chemotherapy data available for review was derived from a few laboratories, and the specific methodologies used are worth reviewing. For example, at Bristol-Myers Squibb (BMS), Rose (32,33) used the murine Madison 109 lung carcinoma (M109) in both staged and unstaged settings to assess several paclitaxel-based drug combinations. Throughout those studies, all paclitaxel doses, regardless of their level, were administered IV in a vehicle containing 10% polyoxyethylated castor oil/10% ethanol/80% saline (in one experiment, the proportions were 12.5% each of polyoxyethylated castor oil and ethanol), in 0.01 mL/g of body weight; a maximum of one such paclitaxel injection was administered per day. Paclitaxel was always given on a consecutive daily injection schedule based on schedule dependency data indicating this to be a most advantageous treatment regimen against the tumor model (33). No result of therapy was used if it was accompanied by more than one drug-associated death in a treatment group and any mouse dying before achieving a 1-g tumor target size was presumed to have died due to drug toxicity. Antitumor activity was judged on the basis of increases in lifespan (%T/C values) and gross LCK based on all mice in a treatment group except those dying of drug toxicity. All the data from the SC M109 combination chemotherapy studies are summarized in Table 2.

LoRusso et al. (34,35) used the murine MAM 16/C adenocarcinoma to evaluate several paclitaxel-based combination chemotherapies. In each of those studies, paclitaxel was prepared as a fixed stock solution of 8 mg/mL in 50% polyoxyethylated castor oil/50% ethanol. Following dilution of this stock solution with varying

Table 2   Effect of Paclitaxel-Based Combination Chemotherapy Versus SC Madison 109 Lung Carcinoma

Experiment no.	Optimal treatments[a] [dose (mg/kg/d), route, schedule] Paclitaxel	Other drug	Maximum effects[b] Med. ST, % T/C	LCK	Outcome of experiment
A	48, IV, qd 1 → 5	—	147	1.4	
	—	cDDP: 8, IP, d 1 & 5	123	0.6	NS
	—	VP-16: 120, IP, d 1 & 5	126	1.2	NS
	36, IV, qd 1 → 5	cDDP: 6, IP, d 1 & 5	155	1.8c	NS
	24, IV, qd 1 → 5	VP-16: 60, IP, d 1 & 5	158	1.5	NS
B	24/36, IV, qd 1 → 5	—	173	1.2	
	—	ADR: 7.5/10, IV, d 1 & 5	170	1.2	
	—	CYT: 160, IP, d 1 & 5	139	0.7	
	36, IV, qd 1 → 5	ADR: 5, IV, d 1 & 5	168	1.5	NS
	16, IV, qd 1 → 5	ADR: 7.5, IV, d 1 & 5	175	1.4	NS
	24, IV, qd 1 → 5	CYT: 80, IP, d 1 & 5	161	1.3	NS
C	24, IV, qd 1 → 5	—	140	0.8	
	—	MTX: 45, IP, d 1 & 5	109	0	
	—	PMM: 180, IP, d 1 & 5	85	0	
	18, IV, qd 1 → 5	MTX: 30, IP, d 1 & 5	137	0.8	NS
	24, IV, qd 1 → 5	PMM: 80, IP, d 1 & 5	138	0.8	NS
D	24, IV, qd 5 → 9	—	145	1.6	
	—	BLEO: 30U, IP, qd 5 → 9	110	0.6	
	—	CIM: 100, IP, qd 5 → 9	103	0	
	24, IV, qd 5 → 9	BLEO: 20U, IP, qd 5 → 9	128	2.1	NS
	18, IV, qd 5 → 9	CIM: 100, IP, qd 5 → 9	151	1.4	NS
E	48, IV, qd 4 → 8	—	154	1.5	
	—	6-TG: 12, IP, d 4, 6 & 8	144	0.8	
	24, IV, qd 4 → 8	6-TG: 5, IP, d 4, 6 & 8	165	1.6	NS

[a]Regimens showing the best therapeutic effects, or, if inactive, the maximum tolerated dose or highest dose tested. When two dose levels (e.g., X/Y) are indicated, one was responsible for the best % T/C value and the other the best LCK value. No result of therapy is shown if it was associated with more than one drug-related death. Paclitaxel was administered once daily on the days indicated. When given on the same day as another drug, paclitaxel was given either 1 hr prior to the other drug (Expts A, B & C), 30 to 60 min after the other drug (Expt. D), or simultaneously (Expt. E). ADR, doxorubicin; cDDP, cisplatin; CYT, cyclophosphamide; BLEO, bleomycin, administered in units (U)/kg/day; CIM, cimetidine; MTX, methotrexate; PMM, pentamethylmelamine; VP-16, etoposide; 6-TG, 6-thioguanine.

[b]Med. ST, median survival time; LCK, gross $\log_{10}$ cell kill.

[c]$P < 0.05$ versus optimum effect of concomitantly evaluated paclitaxel.

[d]NS, no synergy

Source: Adapted from Refs. 32 and 33 and courtesy of Rose WC, unpublished data.

proportions of warm saline, paclitaxel was administered IV, 0.2 mL/mouse. The maximum concentration of polyoxyethylated castor oil and ethanol contained in the injected volumes was 15% of each. In order to administer doses of paclitaxel in excess of approximately 23 to 25 mg/kg/day, it was necessary to administer "split doses," that is, two injections of paclitaxel per day. To eliminate a treatment variable, all paclitaxel injections regardless of dose level were consequently administered as split doses. It is important to appreciate this methodology because of the potential influence of just the polyoxyethylated castor oil and ethanol administered each day upon host toxicity. The amounts of polyoxyethylated castor oil and ethanol delivered with the higher doses of paclitaxel evaluated approached one-half a lethal quantity. Thus, the potential for a compromised host was substantial when one considers that two such injections per day were administered whenever paclitaxel was given.

Two other points of methodology involving the data of LoRusso et al. (34,35) need to be related. Consistent with National Cancer Institute (NCI) guidelines, treated groups of mice experiencing greater than a 20% loss in body weight were considered to have had an excessively toxic treatment and were not included by LoRusso et al. in determining and comparing therapeutic results. Dr. LoRusso was most generous in sharing the detailed data she and her colleagues presented, and we have taken the liberty of including one result of therapy in which a 22% weight loss occurred (but no drug-associated deaths). We have also chosen to include for illustration another group of mice that had been excluded by LoRusso et al. due to an observed transient neurotoxicity (but again, no drug-associated deaths). Lastly, LoRusso et al. calculated their gross LCK values by the same formula described above, but they included dying mice only; tumor-free mice (cures) alive at the end of an experiment were described separately and no other life-span data were considered. We have used their values when presenting their data. The antitumor effects reflecting delay in tumor growth data are presented in Table 3.

Waud et al. (14) also used the SC MAM 16/C model to explore paclitaxel-based combination chemotherapies. Paclitaxel was dissolved in polyoxyethylated castor oil/ethanol and further diluted with saline to an unspecified final concentration(s) of each component prior to IV administration. Antitumor activity was assessed on the basis of *net* LCK, which served as an adjustment made to the tumor growth delay data to take into account (i.e., attempt to normalize) treatments of varying duration. Highlights of the antitumor data from these investigations are also provided in Table 3.

B. Paclitaxel plus Etoposide

This combination was evaluated by Rose (32,33) using the unstaged SC M109 lung carcinoma model (experiment A, Table 2). Following optimal treatment with 48 mg/kg/inj of paclitaxel on a consecutive daily injection schedule, a T/C of 147%

Table 3 Effect of Paclitaxel-Based Combination Chemotherapy Versus SC Staged Mammary 16/C Adenocarcinoma

Experiment no.	Optimal Treatments[a] [dose (mg/kg/d), route, schedule]		Max. LCK (C/T)[b]	Outcome of experiment
	Paclitaxel	Other drug(s)		
A	31, IV, d 6, 8, 11, & 13	—	3.3	
	34, IV, d 6 & 11	VP-16: 21, IV, d 6, 8, 11, & 13	3.3	
	—	VP-16: 25, IV, d 8 & 13	3.5	No synergy
B	31, IV, d 3, 7, 11, 15, 19, 23, & 27	—	5.5 (1/6)	Synergy
	56, IV, d 3, 11, 19, & 27	VP-16: 33, IV, d 3, 7, 11, 15, 19, 23, & 27	6.2 (1/7)	Synergy
	34, IV, d 3, 11, 19, & 27	VP-16: 25, IV, d 7, 15, & 23	- (5/8)	Synergy
	21, IV, d 3, 11, 19, & 27	VP-16: 25, IV, d 7, 15, & 23	- (6/8)	
	—	VP-16: 25, IV, d 7, 15, & 23	- (4/6)	
C	47, IV, d 4, 8, 12, 16, & 20	—	4.9 (0/6)	
	30, IV, d 4, 8, 12, 16, & 20	5-FU: 40, IV, d 4, 8, 12, & 16	4.3 (1/6)	
	—	5-FU: 19, IV, d 8 & 16	0	
D	19, IV, d 4, 12, & 20	—	4.6 (1/7)	No synergy
	50,[c] IV, d 5, 9, 13, 17, & 21	ADR: 7.5,[d] IV, d 5, 9, 13, 17, & 21	4.9 (0/6)	
	31, IV, d 5, 9, 13, 17, & 21	ADR: 4.6, IV, d 5, 9, 13, 17, & 21	4.6 (0/7)	
E	48, IV, d 5, 13, & 21	—	6.7 (0/6)	
	—	ADR: 8, IV, d 9 & 17	3.6 (0/6)	
	30, IV, d 5, 13, & 21	ADR: 8, IV, d 9 & 17	5.9 (0/6)	Synergy?
	30, IV, d 5, 13, & 21	ADR: 5, IV, d 9 & 17	6.2 (0/8)	Synergy?
	30, IV, d 2, 6, 10, 14, 18, & 22	CYT: 68, IP, d 2, 6, 10, 14, 18, & 22; ADR: 4.4, IV, d 2, 6, 10, 14, 18, & 22	3.7 (4/8)	Synergy?
	15, IV, d 2, 6, 10, 14, 18, & 22	CYT: 54, IP, d 6, 14, & 22; ADR: 6, IV, d 6, 14, & 22	5.3 (2/6)	
			- (6/6)	
	15, IV, d 2, 10, & 18		1.7 (0/5)	No synergy
	15, IV, d 2, 10, & 18		3.1 (0/5)	No synergy
			1.7 (2/7)	No synergy
			2.2 (3/8)	No synergy

	Paclitaxel regimen (mg/kg)	Second-agent regimen (mg/kg)	Max net LCK[b]	Conclusion
F₁	7.6, IV, d 2, 10, & 18	ADR: 6, IV, d 6, 14, & 22	1.4 (4/7)	No synergy
	30, IV, d 2, 10, & 18	CYT: 34, IP, d 6, 14, & 22 + ADR: 5.6, IV, d 6, 14, & 22	6.3 (2/8)	No synergy
	15, IV, d 2, 10, & 18	CYT: 34, IP, d 6, 14, & 22 + ADR: 5.6, IV, d 6, 14, & 22	4.9 (4/8)	No synergy
F₂	38.7, IV, qd 3 → 7	—	1.5	
			3.5	
	10, IV, qd 3 → 7	ADR: 18, IV, d 2	3.5	No synergy
	22.5, IV, qd 3 → 7	ADR: 12, IV, d 2	1.5	
	—	ADR: 27, IV, d 3	6.7	
F₃	15, IV, qd 3 → 7	ADR: 18, IV, d 3	5.0	No synergy
	38.7, IV, qd 2 → 6	—	3.1	
			7.7	
	22.5, IV, qd 2 → 6	ADR: 18, IV, d 7	7.7	
	48, IV, d 3, 7, &11	ADR: 18, IV, d 7	1.4	
	—	TOP: 13.2, IP, d 3, 7, & 11	0.1	
G₁	32, IV, d 3, 7, & 11 (0 & 4 hr)	TOP: 5.8, IP, d 3, 7, & 11 (8 & 12 hr)	1.7	No synergy
	48, IV, d 3, 7, & 11		1.1	
G₂	9.4, IV, d 3, 7, & 11 (8 & 12 hr)	TOP: 13.2, IP, d 3, 7, & 11	0.4	No synergy
	14.2, IV, d 3, 7, & 11 (8 & 12 hr)	TOP: 1.8, IP, d 3, 7, & 11 (0 & 4 hr)	1.8	Synergy?
	72, IV, d 3, 7, & 11	TOP: 5.8, IP, d 3, 7, & 11 (0 & 4 hr)	1.8	Synergy?
G₃	—	TOP: 19.8, IP, d 3, 7, & 11	2.1	
	48, IV, d 3, 7, & 11 (0 & 4 hr)	TOP: 3.8, IP, d 3, 7, & 11 (0 & 4 hr)	1.2	No synergy
			1.8	No synergy

[a]Regimens yielding the best therapeutic effects or, if not active, the maximum tolerated dose or highest dose tested. No regimen is presented if it caused more than one death in the treated group. All paclitaxel doses were administered in split amounts on the days indicated except in experiment F: VP-16, etoposide; ADR, doxorubicin; CYT, cyclophosphamide; 5-FU, 5-fluorouracil; TOP, topotecan.

[b]Maximum gross log cell kill (LCK) of dying mice only, with cures shown separately, for experiments A through E. Maximum net LCK for experiments F and G.

[c]Associated with an 18% body weight loss and transient neurotoxicity (but no deaths).

[d]Associated with a 22% body weight loss (but no deaths).

Source: Adapted from Refs. 34 and 35 in experiments A through E and from Ref. 14 in experiments F and G.

accompanied by a 1.4 LCK was obtained. Etoposide (VP-16) was also active; a dose of 120 mg/kg/inj given IP on days 1 and 5 post–tumor implant caused a maximum T/C of 126% and 1.2 LCK. In combination chemotherapy trials, both drugs were administered on the same treatment schedules as had been applied when they were used singly. On days when both drugs were given, paclitaxel was injected 1 hr prior to VP-16. The most effective combination regimen tested involved 24 mg/kg/inj of paclitaxel given with 60 mg/kg/inj of VP-16, but the T/C of 158% and 1.5 LCK obtained were not significantly superior to the optimum effects of paclitaxel alone.

Two experiments involving the compounds mentioned above were conducted by LoRusso et al. (34,35) using the staged SC MAM 16/C model (experiments A and B, Table 3). In the initial study (experiment A), paclitaxel was given every second or third day beginning on day 6 post–tumor implant for a total of 4 days of treatment, and a maximum of 3.3 LCK was achieved. The same maximum effect was obtained following treatment with VP-16 on the same schedule. Optimum intermittent treatment on an alternating drug schedule using paclitaxel plus VP-16 produced a maximum 3.5 LCK. Thus, while the individual drugs were quite effective against advanced-stage MAM 16/C tumors, intermittent, alternating combination chemotherapy provided no therapeutic advantage.

In the second experiment (experiment B, Table 3), in which treatment initiation was not as delayed as in experiment A, intermittent and prolonged therapy with paclitaxel, q4d × 7 beginning on day 3 post–tumor implant, resulted in 5.5 LCK and one of six cures at an optimal dose of 31 mg/kg/day (an higher dose was too lethal). The cumulative exposure of 217 mg/kg of paclitaxel was 75% greater than the total dose tolerated in the previous experiment (124 mg/kg), although the amount of drug administered (and the amounts of polyoxyethylated castor oil and ethanol delivered) on each treatment day was identical. It would appear the use of a q4d regimen permitted the extra paclitaxel to be given, and one might suppose the recovery period between drug (and vehicle) exposures contributed to the acceptability of the treatments. Optimal therapy with VP-16 was even more efficacious than paclitaxel. A dose of 33 mg/kg/day, delivered on the same q4d × 7 schedule, caused 6.2 LCK plus one of seven cures. This was the highest dose level of VP-16 evaluated and it caused no deaths and no weight loss. Several combination regimens provided cure rates in the 63% to 75% range, an improvement over the solo cures seen when applying either drug alone. Each of the combination therapies involved intermittent, alternating drug treatments with 4 days between injections. These data possibly support a claim for therapeutic synergy between paclitaxel and VP-16.

Pending confirmation of the experiment just described and assuming that the highest dose of VP-16 evaluated was, in fact, a maximum tolerated dose (MTD), one other question that can reasonably be asked is whether either drug alone might have proven more effective if some other schedule of treatment (but of the same overall duration) had been used. The doubling time of the MAM 16/C tumor is about one day, and the schedule dependency study done in the SC M109 tumor model (33), which has a similar rapid doubling time, indicated consecutive daily treatments were most advantageous. Possibly, then, some form of intermittent, multiple courses of such treatments might be tried. But the amount of polyoxyethylated castor oil and ethanol which accompanied each day's paclitaxel treatments in the MAM 16/C experiments may well have precluded any attempt at a more frequent drug administration regimen.

C. Paclitaxel plus 5-Fluorouracil

The combination of paclitaxel plus 5-fluorouracil (5-FU) was evaluated by LoRusso et al. (34,35) in the staged SC MAM 16/C adenocarcinoma model (experiment C, Table 3). Using a q4d × 5 treatment schedule, optimal paclitaxel therapy consisting of approximately 47 mg/kg/day caused 4.9 LCK. Two-thirds of this amount of paclitaxel still provided for 4.3 LCK plus one of six cures. In contrast, 5-FU was inactive in this model. The best intermittent, alternating combination chemotherapy regimens tried using these two drugs provided for only 4.6 LCK and one of seven cures; this result was no better than those associated with the better solo paclitaxel therapies and hence no therapeutic synergy was found.

D. Paclitaxel plus Doxorubicin

Rose (32,33) evaluated the combination of paclitaxel and doxorubicin (ADR) against unstaged SC M109 lung carcinoma (experiment B, Table 2). Consecutive daily injections of paclitaxel resulted in optimal effects which included a T/C of 173% and 1.2 LCK. Doxorubicin, administered IV on days 1 and 5 post–tumor implant, yielded a maximum T/C of 170% and 1.2 LCK. Thus, the two drugs were similarly effective in this tumor model. Combination chemotherapies involving paclitaxel plus ADR made use of the same treatment schedules as had been applied with each drug singly on days when both drugs were given, paclitaxel injections preceded ADR by 1 hr. Optimal combination drug therapies resulted in a maximum T/C of 175% and LCK of 1.5. These results were not meaningfully superior to the best effects of the individual drugs.

LoRusso et al. (34,35) described two experiments in which the combination of paclitaxel plus ADR was evaluated in the staged SC MAM 16/C adenocarcinoma model. Highlights of both of these studies are shown in Table 3 (experiments D and E), although the latter experiment, it should be noted, included yet another drug, cyclophosphamide. In experiment D, 50 mg/kg/day of paclitaxel delivered q4d × 5 resulted in 4.9 LCK. LoRusso et al. chose to consider this dose level as frankly toxic, based on a profound albeit transient neurotoxicity accompanied by 18% body weight loss. We have included the data associated with the dose level of 50 mg/kg/day because no deaths attributed to drug toxicity were observed. At the next lower dose of paclitaxel evaluated, 31 mg/kg/day, a 4.6 LCK was obtained. Similarly, the highest dose of ADR evaluated, 7.5 mg/kg/day q4d × 5 IV, yielded an LCK value of 6.7, causing a 22% loss in body weight (but no deaths). LoRusso et al. felt this dose of ADR was too toxic, in accordance with NCI guidelines, and instead presented the data obtained using the next lower dose of ADR (approximately 4.6 mg/kg/day), a 3.7 LCK, as the drug's maximum therapeutic effect. Since no deaths attributed to drug administration occurred at the higher dose level of ADR, we have chosen to consider the data from both the aforementioned ADR regimens.

In the combination setting, paclitaxel was administered q8d × 3 beginning on day 5 postimplant; ADR was also administered intermittently q8d × 2, alternating with paclitaxel, such that one of the drugs was given every fourth day. When 8 mg/kg/day of ADR was given in combination with either 30 or 48 mg/kg/day of paclitaxel, the resulting LCK values were 5.9 to 6.2. These results qualified, according to LoRusso et al. (34,35), as therapeutically synergistic based on their ≥ 1 LCK superiority to the 4.6 LCK associated with the best effect obtained with "acceptable" levels of solo drug, in this case 31 mg/kg/day of paclitaxel. However, they would not be deemed synergistic combinations if one were to compare them to the 6.7 LCK associated with 7.5 mg/kg/day of ADR. Another combination treatment group is also worthy of mention, one receiving 30 mg/kg/day of paclitaxel plus 5 mg/kg/day of ADR. This regimen resulted in a 50% cure rate and a 3.7 LCK among dying mice only. (When evaluating preclinical antitumor data, one should not overemphasize the importance of cures when they occur in the midst of therapies generating generally high LCK values. The mean difference between a > 6 LCK effect without any cures and one that produces even 50% cures may be ≤ 0.5 LCK.) But what is noteworthy about the combination drug regimen producing this 50% cure rate is the fact that higher dose levels of one or both drugs were neither curative nor obviously excessively toxic. (Is "more not better" when paclitaxel is involved?) In summary, LCK values of 5.9 to 6.2, or even a 50% cure rate, achieved with combination chemotherapy would not be considered therapeutically synergistic if compared to the 6.7 LCK achieved with ADR alone but *would* be considered synergistic if compared to the 4.6 LCK achieved with paclitaxel alone. Aside from the different outcomes which stem from different definitions of acceptable toxicity levels, the experiment must be repeated to confirm whatever claims are to be made.

In the second MAM 16/C experiment conducted by LoRusso et al. (34,35) involving the combination of paclitaxel plus ADR (experiment E, Table 3), treatments were initiated on day 2 postimplant ("early-stage" tumors). The MTD of paclitaxel was 30 mg/kg/day administered q4d × 6 and it produced a 5.3 LCK plus two of six cures. At one-half this dose level, 15 mg/kg/day, on the same schedule, 100% of the mice were cured. Thus, the most efficacious result involving paclitaxel was found with a dose level less than the drug's MTD. Doxorubicin produced 3.1 LCK at its optimal dose, 4.4 mg/kg/day, applied IV on the same treatment schedule. It is obviously difficult to establish therapeutic synergies when one drug is completely curative; nevertheless, combination chemotherapies should be expected at least to be able to match the efficacy of the best drug given alone, and any failure to do so should provoke skepticism as to the merit of the combination used. Applying the same intermittent alternating treatment schedules described in experiment D, none of the combinations evaluated involving paclitaxel plus ADR yielded more than three of eight or four of seven cures. One must question the claim for therapeutic synergy between paclitaxel and ADR in this model (experiment D) if the same approach fails in another experiment (experiment E) against a similar tumor burden.

The same MAM 16/C tumor model was used by Waud et al. (14) to evaluate paclitaxel plus ADR (Table 3). In one experimental series, ADR was given initially on day 2 postimplant followed by paclitaxel given qd 3 → 7. The most effective combination regimen applied in this manner involved 12 mg/kg of ADR plus 10 mg/kg/day of paclitaxel; this treatment caused 3.5 LCK. In comparison, ADR alone yielded 3.5 LCK and paclitaxel alone produced 1.5 LCK. Thus, no therapeutic synergy was realized using this treatment protocol despite the indication from in vitro studies (discussed above) that this particular sequence (and not the reverse) was supraadditive against MAM 16/C cells. Attempts to obtain a synergistic interaction with these drugs were also made using the reverse sequence of administration as well as one form of simultaneous drug administration. When paclitaxel, 22.5 mg/kg/day, was administered consecutively on days 2 → 6 and ADR, 18 mg/kg, was given on day 7 only, a maximum 7.7 LCK was obtained, but this was no better than the 7.7 LCK found using 26 mg of ADR/kg alone. Similarly, treatment with 18 mg of ADR/kg on day 3 plus 15 mg of paclitaxel/kg/day, qd 3 → 7, resulted in 5.0 LCK, but this was inferior to the 6.7 LCK obtained using 26 mg/kg of ADR alone. Waud et al. (14) concluded, and we concur, that in the manner they were evaluated, paclitaxel and ADR were not synergistic versus MAM 16/C adenocarcinoma.

E. Paclitaxel plus Cyclophosphamide

Paclitaxel and cyclophosphamide (CYT) were evaluated singly and in combination by Rose (32,33) against the unstaged SC M109 lung carcinoma (experiment B, Table 2). Cyclophosphamide was modestly effective in this tumor model, causing a maximum T/C of 139% accompanied by 0.7 LCK following IP treatments on days 1 and 5 post–tumor implant of 160 mg/kg/inj. Consecutive daily administration of paclitaxel however, resulted in a maximum T/C of 173% and 1.2 LCK. When the two drugs were evaluated in combination, the same treatment schedules were used as had been applied when each drug was given singly. On days when both drugs were administered, paclitaxel preceded CYT by 1 hr. The optimal combination treatment regimen tested, consisting of 24 mg/kg/inj of paclitaxel plus 80 mg/kg/inj of CYT, yielded a maximum T/C of 161% accompanied by 1.3 LCK. These results were not meaningfully superior to the best effects of paclitaxel alone.

The combination of paclitaxel plus CYT was also evaluated by LoRusso et al. (34,35) in the SC early-stage MAM 16/C adenocarcinoma model (experiment E, Table 3). Paclitaxel alone, at a dose of 15 mg/kg/day administered q4d × 6, beginning on day 2 postimplant, was 100% curative; at twice this dose level, the apparent MTD of paclitaxel in this experiment, 5.3 LCK accompanied by two of six mice cured were obtained. Cyclophosphamide alone, 68 mg/kg/day IP, on the same schedule, caused a modestly active 1.7 LCK. The most effective drug combination regimen, consisting of alternating, intermittent exposure to each drug, such that mice were treated with one of the two drugs every fourth day, produced 1.7 LCK plus two of seven cures. In the manner evaluated, paclitaxel plus CYT were not synergistic in this tumor model.

F. Paclitaxel plus Doxorubicin plus Cyclophosphamide

LoRusso et al. (34,35) conducted an ambitious experiment in which paclitaxel plus the above-mentioned drugs were evaluated singly and in concert versus SC early-stage MAM 16/C adenocarcinoma (experiment E, Table 3). The effects of each drug alone, and ADR and CYT in combination with paclitaxel are described above in the appropriate sections involving those drug combinations. Suffice it to say here that the administration of paclitaxel on an intermittent treatment schedule alternating with both ADR plus CYT (such that either paclitaxel or the other two drugs were administered to mice every fourth day, beginning on day 2 post-implant) was not therapeutically synergistic in this model. The best effects demonstrated using this three-drug combination were 6.3 LCK with two of eight cured mice, or 4.9 LCK with a 50% cure rate. Paclitaxel alone, at one-half its MTD, produced a 100% cure rate.

G. Paclitaxel plus Topotecan

The combination of IV paclitaxel with the camptothecin derivative topotecan (TOP), given IP, was evaluated by Waud et al. (14) in a series of related experiments involving the SC MAM 16/C adenocarcinoma (Expt. G, Table 3). Each drug was administered twice daily, 4 hr between injections, on Days 3, 7 and 11 post-tumor implant. When given in combination, the same treatment protocol was applied, but the drugs were given either simultaneously or sequentially with 4 hr separating the administration of the two drugs. In the protocol calling for paclitaxel to be given first followed by TOP (Expt. G_1), paclitaxel was administered on Days 3, 7 and 11, followed four hours later on each of those days by sequential injections of TOP. When this experiment was performed, 48 mg/kg/day of paclitaxel alone produced 1.4 LCK and 13.2 mg/kg/day of TOP yielded only 0.1 LCK; in comparison, the optimum combination regimen, 32 mg/kg/day of paclitaxel plus 5.8 mg/kg/day of TOP, produced 1.7 LCK. Thus, in contrast to the in vitro data (discussed above) of Waud et al. (14) in which this particular sequence of drug exposure was shown to be supraadditive, no synergy was observed in vivo.

Simultaneous drug treatments (experiment G_3) likewise failed to achieve a synergistic effect. Some enhancement of therapeutic activity was found, however, when the paclitaxel injections were initiated 4 hr following TOP (experiment G_2). Whereas TOP alone, 13.2 mg/kg/day, produced a minimal effect of 0.4 LCK, and paclitaxel alone, 48 mg/kg/day, caused 1.1 LCK, two different combination regimens yielded 1.8 LCK values. The hint of success obtained with this TOP → paclitaxel intermittent treatment regimen must be confirmed and then extended to other tumor models.

Waud and colleagues (Southern Research Institute, Birmingham, AL, personal communication) have recently completed some additional experiments using paclitaxel with TOP in the MAM 16/C tumor model in an attempt to confirm and extend the suggestion of synergy reported previously (14) and excerpted in Table 3. Upon repeating the same experimental protocol that they had found to be successful originally (TOP → paclitaxel, on a split-dose schedule), only a modest (about 0.6 LCK) improvement over the best effect of either compound given individually was obtained, thus confirming the suggestion of synergy. Additional experiments involving non–split dose TOP → paclitaxel regimens, and using both simultaneous as well as paclitaxel → TOP sequences, failed to uncover a therapeutically synergistic combination treatment.

H. Paclitaxel plus Cisplatin

The combination of paclitaxel plus cisplatin (cDDP) was evaluated by Rose (32, 33) versus unstaged SC M109 lung carcinoma (experiment A, Table 2). Consecutive daily treatments with 48 mg/kg/inj of paclitaxel resulted in a maximum T/C of 147% and 1.4 LCK. In comparison, cDDP produced only borderline activity, achieving a maximum T/C of 123% and 0.6 LCK following IP injections of 8 mg/kg/inj on days 1 and 5 post–tumor implant. When the two drugs were evaluated together, the same treatment schedules were utilized as had been applied when both drugs were given singly. On days when both paclitaxel and cDDP were injected, the former was given 1 hr before cDDP. The best effects obtained using paclitaxel plus cDDP were a T/C of 155% accompanied by 1.8 LCK. This LCK value (reflecting primary tumor growth delay), but not the increase in life span, was significantly ($p < 0.05$) greater than the LCK caused by paclitaxel alone. In practical terms, however, the improvement, even if experimentally reproducible, was less than 0.5 LCK and thus of limited likely utility. Furthermore, the enhanced activity was observed at only that one particular combination drug regimen, and it was a maximum tolerated level.

I. Paclitaxel plus Methotrexate

This combination was evaluated by Rose (33) using the unstaged SC M109 lung carcinoma (experiment C, Table 2). Maximally tolerated doses of methotrexate (MTX) administered IP on days 1 and 5 post–tumor implant failed to achieve an active result against this tumor model. Optimal consecutive daily therapy with paclitaxel produced a T/C of only 140% and 0.8 LCK, slightly more modest levels of activity than typically seen with this drug. Using the same treatment schedules as when they were applied singly, various combinations of MTX and paclitaxel were evaluated. On days when both were given, paclitaxel preceded MTX by 1 hr. The most effective combination of the two drugs, 24 mg/kg/inj of paclitaxel plus 30 mg/kg/inj of MTX, produced only a T/C of 137% accompanied by 0.8 LCK. No synergy was observed with these two drugs against the SC M109 tumor when they were applied in the manner evaluated.

J. Paclitaxel plus Pentamethylmelamine

Rose (33) evaluated these two drugs individually and in combination using the unstaged SC M109 lung carcinoma (Expt. C, Table 2). Paclitaxel alone, adminis-tered on a consecutive daily injection schedule, produced a maximum T/C of 140% and a 0.8 LCK. Pentamethylmelamine (PMM) was given IP on Days 1 and 5 post-tumor implant and was inactive at all the doses evaluated. Combination regimens were applied using the same treatment schedules that had been used with each drug when it was given singly. On days when both drugs were administered, paclitaxel was given 1 hr before PMM. No combination involving these two drugs yielded therapeutic results superior to that caused by optimal paclitaxel therapy alone.

K. Paclitaxel plus Bleomycin

The combination of paclitaxel plus bleomycin (BLEO) was evaluated by Rose (33) versus the staged SC M109 tumor model (Expt. D, Table 2). Paclitaxel, 24 mg/kg/ inj, was administered on a consecutive daily injection schedule, beginning on Day 5 post-tumor implant, and achieved a maximum T/C of 145% accompanied by a 1.6 LCK. BLEO, administered IP on the same schedule, failed to produce an active extension in lifespan and succeeded in causing a delay in primary tumor growth which reflected only a 0.6 LCK (a borderline result with respect to activity). Combination regimens involving these two drugs were evaluated using the same qd 5 → 9 treatment schedules that were used with each drug tested individually; paclitaxel was always given 30 to 60 min following each BLEO injection. The most effective combination chemotherapy regimen consisted of 24 mg/kg/inj of paclitaxel plus 20U/kg/inj of BLEO. It produced a maximum T/C of 128% accompanied by a 2.1 LCK, but this increase in LCK value was not significant statistically ($p > 0.05$) and probably of limited significance biologically.

L. Paclitaxel plus Cimetidine

When paclitaxel is administered clinically, it is typically given in conjunction with several other agents whose purpose is to mitigate or circumvent the often accompanying hypersensitivity reactions. One of these agents is H_2-histamine antagonist cimetidine (CIM). Rose (33) evaluated the potential influence of this compound on paclitaxel's antitumor activity using the staged SC M109 lung carcinoma model (experiment D, Table 2). Paclitaxel alone caused a maximum T/C of 145% and 1.6 LCK following consecutive daily treatment with 24 mg/kg/inj. Cimetidine alone, using the same schedule of treatment, was not active. When both drugs were given in combination on the same consecutive daily treatment schedule with CIM preceding each paclitaxel injection by 30 to 60 min, the maximum therapeutic effects of 155% T/C and 1.4 LCK were not significantly different than those obtained using paclitaxel alone.

The lack of influence of CIM on paclitaxel's antitumor activity (33) was actually encouraging, given the widespread use of this histamine antagonist to mitigate the often seen hypersensitivity reactions associated with the clinical administration of paclitaxel. The preclinical data also are consistent with the recently reported observation that CIM did not influence the mean steady-state plasma levels of paclitaxel measured in patients with recurrent ovarian adenocarcinoma (36).

M. Paclitaxel plus 6-Thioguanine

The combination of paclitaxel plus the purine antagonist 6-thioguanine (6-TG) was evaluated versus the staged SC M109 lung carcinoma (Rose W.C., unpublished data). Optimal treatment with 48 mg/kg/inj of paclitaxel, using a consecutive daily injection schedule beginning on day 4 post–tumor implant, resulted in a maximum T/C of 154% accompanied by 1.5 LCK. An intermittent injection schedule was used to administer 6-TG and optimal therapy with 12 mg/kg/inj produced a maximum T/C of 144% and 0.8 LCK. Paclitaxel was given in combination with 6-TG using the same treatment schedules as were used with each drug when it was given individually. On days when both drugs were given, they were administered within 5 min of each other. The maximum therapeutic effects following combination chemotherapy were a 165% T/C and 1.6 LCK (experiment E, Table 2). These results were not significantly different from the best effects obtained using paclitaxel alone.

III. FUTURE DIRECTIONS

Conversations and correspondence with numerous investigators indicate that it is their intention to evaluate paclitaxel in combination settings in vitro with most of the known marketed anticancer drugs and several others being developed. These future studies will often include sequence analyses and a range of concentrations of each drug; hopefully, a formal analysis for the presence of synergy will always be performed. Should these investigations result in the discovery of synergistic interactions, it would be useful to extend any initial observation to additional cell lines to determine the ubiquity of the finding.

Future in vivo paclitaxel-based combination chemotherapy studies at BMS will include selected other drugs (e.g., VP-16, cDDP, ADR, and BLEO) in solid tumor models other than SC M109. We will also explore treatment schedules other than the variety applied thus far, including the use of intermittent, sequential drug combination therapies with which LoRusso et al. (34,35) had preliminary success. Unconfirmed data involving paclitaxel plus ADR in a murine pulmonary squamous cell carcinoma model, ASB XIV, suggest that intermittent and alternating drug therapies may be therapeutically synergistic (Rose, W.C., unpublished data). Considering the synergy seen in vitro between EM and paclitaxel (20), this combination is also deserving of evaluation in vivo, and perhaps other alkylating agents such as mitomycin C and a nitrosourea should also be evaluated with paclitaxel.

Following through on leads developed in vitro (24), Sirotnak and associates (Memorial Sloan-Kettering Institute, New York, NY, personal communication) intend to evaluate paclitaxel in combination with EDX, probably in the SKBR-3 human mammary tumor model, the same tumor used in their initial cytotoxicity studies.

IV. DISCUSSION

Based on the in vitro data pertaining to paclitaxel-based drug interactions, cytotoxic effects were enhanced either when tumor cells were exposed initially to paclitaxel, followed sometime thereafter by introduction of the other drug in the combination being studied, or when the reverse sequence of exposure was applied, or when concomitant treatments were used. Each of these sequences was either a success or failure, depending on the drugs and tumor cells involved. Many of the published accounts have appeared only as abstracts; consequently it has often been difficult to discern how the claims for synergy or enhanced cytotoxicity were made and if the methodologies used were sufficiently rigorous to support the conclusions reached.

In designing combination chemotherapies of likely merit, one strives to include drugs which are active when used individually, have different mechanisms of action, and have different toxicity patterns (37,38). The unique mechanism of action by which paclitaxel exerts its antitumor activity makes it an obvious candidate for inclusion in such combination regimens. Additionally, the demonstrable activity observed in many tumor models when paclitaxel is used alone (32), and the lack of appreciable degeneration of activity with modestly decreasing dose (i.e., good activity at other than just the MTD), should also contribute to successful interactions. Paclitaxel was certainly active in the two tumor models (M109 and MAM 16/C) used for most of the combination chemotherapy evaluations presented; in the majority of situations, the other drug combined with pacli-taxel was also active when used alone. Therefore, it has been most unexpected to realize but a paucity of therapeutic synergies when evaluating the effects of the many paclitaxel-based combination chemotherapies attempted.

Of the few possible synergies described, even they have not always had the benefit of confirmation from the discovering laboratory, let alone multicenter acclamation. When these few successful drug combinations are reevaluated, one must also attempt to optimize each solo drug's administration. It should be noted that a particular treatment schedule used effectively with a drug in a combination chemotherapy setting need not represent an optimum treatment schedule when that same drug is used individually. Furthermore, with respect to toxicity limita-tions, although their definitions may vary among laboratories, it is important that they be applied uniformly throughout an experiment, whether they involve weight-loss nadirs, lethality, or transient neurotoxicity. Knowing the likely MTD levels of particular drug combinations also allows one to focus the scope of confirmatory experiments upon potentially optimal treatment groups, with smaller increments between dose levels and increased group size. Additionally, given the toxicity associated with the polyoxyethylated castor oil/ethanol-containing vehicles, future confirmatory studies might benefit from an approach which limits the exposure of the mice to no more than once-daily injections of reduced quantities of these noxious ingredients.

ACKNOWLEDGMENTS

We would like to express our appreciation toward the following individuals who provided us with details regarding either or both their published or presented data and unpublished or in-progress experimental results: Dr. William R. Waud, Dr. Patricia LoRusso, and Dr. Frank M. Sirotnak. We also thank Dr. Anna Maria Casazza for her review of the manuscript and helpful suggestions.

REFERENCES

1. Rowinsky EK, Cazenave CA, Donehower RC. Taxol: A novel investigational anti-microtubule agent. J Natl Cancer Inst 1990;82:1247–1259.
2. Frei E III. Combination cancer chemotherapy: Presidential address. Cancer Res 1972; 32:2593–2607.
3. Berenbaum MC. Criteria for analyzing interactions between biologically active agents. Adv Cancer Res 1981;35:269–335.
4. Sabath LD. Synergy of antibacterial substances by apparently known mechanisms. Antimicrob Agents Chemother 1968;1967:210.
5. Chou TC, Talay P. Quantitative analysis of dose-effect relationships: The combined effects of multiple drugs or enzyme inhibitors. Adv Enzyme Regul 1984;22:27–55.

6. Prichard MN, Shipman C. A three-dimensional model to analyze drug-drug inter-actions. Antiviral Res 1990;14:181–206.

7. Citardi MJ, Rowinsky EK, Schaefer KL, Donehower RC. Sequence-dependent cyto-toxicity between cisplatin and the antimicrotubule agents taxol and vincristine. Proc Am Assoc Cancer Res 1990;34:2431.

8. Jekunen A, Christen R, Shalinsky D, Howell SB. Synergistic interaction between cisplatin and taxol in human ovarian carcinoma cells in vitro. Proc Am Assoc Cancer Res 1993;34:1773.

9. Dabholkar M, Yu JJ, Parker RJ, et al. Effect of taxol and cisplatin on the expression of excision repair genes in human ovarian cancer cells. Proc Am Assoc Cancer Res 1993; 34:2127.

10. Parker R, Lee KB, Dabholkar M, et al. Influence of taxol:cisplatin sequencing on cisplatin-DNA adduct repair in human ovarian cancer cells. Proc Am Assoc Cancer Res 1993;34:2122.

11. Lee KB, Parker R, Dabholkar M, et al. Taxol effect on cisplatin sensitivity and cisplatin cellular accumulation in human ovarian cancer cells. Proc Am Assoc Cancer Res 1993;34:2114.

12. Kern DH, Morgan CR. Apparent in vitro antagonism between cisplatin and taxol. Proc Am Assoc Cancer Res 1993;34:1788.

13. Hahn SM, Liebmann JE, Goldspiel BR, et al. Taxol in combination with doxorubicin, etoposide, and m-AMSA: Possible antagonism in vitro. Proc Am Assoc Cancer Res 1992;33:2634.

14. Waud WR, Schmid SM, Plowman J. *In vitro* and *in vivo* combination chemotherapy evaluations of taxol with doxorubicin or topotecan. Presented at the Second NCI Work-shop on Taxol and *Taxus*. Alexandria, VA: National Cancer Institute, September 1992.

15. Saunders DE, Christensen C, LoRusso PM, et al. Inhibition of ovarian carcinoma cells by taxol combined with vitamin D and adriamycin. Proc Am Assoc Cancer Res 1992;33:2641.

16. Liebmann JE, Hahn SM, Cook JA, et al. Glutathione depletion by L-buthionine sulfoximine antagonizes taxol cytotoxicity. Cancer Res 1993;53:2066–2070.

17. Leung MF, Chou IN. Relationship between 1-chloro-2,4,-dinitrobenzene-induced cytoskeletal perturbations and cellular glutathione. Cell Biol Toxicol 1989;5:51–66.

18. Streeter DG, Miller JP. The *in vitro* inhibition of purine nucleotide biosynthesis by 2-β-D-ribofuranosylthiazole-4-carboxamide. Biochem Biophys Res Comm 1981; 103:1409–1412.

19. Taniki T, Prajda N, Hata Y, et al. Synergistic action of taxol and tiazofurin in human ovarian, pancreatic and lung carcinoma cells. Proc Am Assoc Cancer Res 1993; 34:1769.

20. Speicher LA, Barone L, Tew KD. Combined antimicrotubule activity of estramustine and taxol in human prostatic carcinoma cell lines. Cancer Res 1992;52:4433–4440.

21. Ball RL, Carney DH, Albrecht T. Taxol inhibits stimulation of cell DNA synthesis by human cytomegalovirus. Exp Cell Res 1990;191:37–44.

22. Otto AM, Ulrich MO, Zumbe A, et al. Microtubule-disrupting agents affect two differents regulating the initiation of DNA synthesis in Swiss 3T3 cells. Proc Natl Acad Sci 1981;78:3063–3067.

23. Jordan MA, Thrower D, Wilson L. Mechanism of inhibition of cell proliferation by vinca alkaloids. Cancer Res 1991;51:2212–2222.
24. Chou TC, Otter GM, Sirotnak FM. Combined effects of edatrexate with taxol or taxotere. Proc Am Assoc Cancer Res 1993;34:1783.
25. Saunders DE, Christensen C, Williams JR, et al. Additive and synergistic growth inhibition of MCF-7 breast cancer cells by 1,25 dihydroxyvitamin D_2 in binary combination with taxol, retinoic acid and dexamethasone. Proc Am Assoc Cancer Res 1993;34:1787.
26. Schmid SM, Garrett BD, Coffield RT, Harrison SD. Combination interferon beta (IFN beta)/taxol in vitro with cell lines of various histogenesis: supraadditive effects. Proc Am Assoc Cancer Res 1992;33:2646.
27. Venditti JM, Goldin A. Drug synergism in antineoplastic chemotherapy. In: Goldin A, Hawking F, eds. Advances in Chemotherapy. Vol. 1. New York: Academic Press, 1964:397–498.
28. Schabel FM Jr, Trader MW, Laster WR Jr, et al. Patterns of resistance and therapeutic synergism among alkylating agents. In: Schonfeld H, ed. Fundamentals in Cancer Chemotherapy/Antibiotics and Chemotherapy. Vol. 23. Basel: Karger, 1978:200–215.
29. Schabel FM Jr. Synergism and antagonism among antitumor agents. In: Pharmacological Basis of Cancer Chemotherapy. Baltimore: Williams & Wilkins, 1975:595–623.
30. Corbett TH, Griswold DP Jr, Wolpert MK, et al. Design and evaluation of combination chemotherapy trials in experimental animal tumor systems. Cancer Treat Rep 1979;63:799–801.
31. Carter SK. Planning combined therapy: The interaction of experimental and clinical studies. Cancer Chemother Rep 1974;4:(part 2) 3–11.
32. Rose WC. Taxol: A review of its preclinical in vivo antitumor activity. Anti-Cancer Drugs 1992;31:311–321.
33. Rose WC. Taxol-based combination chemotherapy and other in vivo preclinical antitumor studies. Presented at the Second NCI Workshop on Taxol and Taxus. Alexandria, VA: National Cancer Institute, September 1992.
34. LoRusso P, Demchik LL, Plowman J, et al. Preclinical activity and toxicity of taxol combinations. Presented at the Second NCI Workshop on Taxol and Taxus. Alexandria, VA: National Cancer Institute, September 1992.
35. LoRusso PM, Demchik LL, Plowman J, et al. Preclinical activity and toxicity of taxol combinations. Proc Am Assoc Cancer Res 1993;34:301.
36. Reed E, Sarosy G, Jamis-Dow C, et al. Cimetidine does not influence taxol steady-state plasma levels. Proc Am Assoc Cancer Res 1993;34:395.
37. Carter SK. Principles of combination chemotherapy. In: Hellman K, Carter SK, eds. Fundamentals of Cancer Chemotherapy. New York: McGraw-Hill, 1987:48–57.
38. Schabel FM Jr. New experimental drug combinations with potential clinical utility. Biochem Pharmacol 1974;23(suppl 2):163–176.

5

Interaction with Ionizing Radiation

PETER B. SCHIFF, RUTH GUBITS,
SHARAFADEEN KASHIMAWO, and CHARLES R. GEARD
College of Physicians & Surgeons of Columbia University
New York, New York

I. INTRODUCTION

For several decades, oncologists have been combining radiotherapy and chemotherapy for the management of patients with malignant disease. The rationale for this combined-modality approach has been an attempt to increase local control through the lethal cytotoxic interaction of the two modalities and to reduce distant failure and thus improve disease-free and overall survival. A major challenge has been to identify systemic agents with significant clinical activity that also have the capacity for potentiating the cytotoxic effects of radiation therapy. The identification of correct combinations and sequences of various treatments without significantly increasing toxicity is a major challenge. The interaction between radiation and chemotherapy can be divided into three general categories (1). The first is spatial cooperation (2), that is, delineating separate targets or sites within the body for radiation and chemotherapy, so that the effects of the two agents lead to an additive response. The second category is enhancement, or any observable improvement that is greater than that seen with either chemotherapy or radiotherapy alone. Finally, there may be a diminution or decrease in effectiveness which is less than that observed with either modality alone.

Radiosensitizers are chemical or pharmacological agents that enhance the lethal effects of radiation in a greater than additive fashion. The aim of all radiosensitizers is to move the tumor control curve to lower doses of radiation by

Schiff et al.

sensitizing tumor cells while not significantly affecting the normal tissue complication curve (see Fig. 1). Radiosensitizers are divided into two broad groups or
categories: nonhypoxic and hypoxic cell sensitizers. Examples of hypoxic cell
sensitizers are metronidazole, misonidazole, and etanidazole. Although these
nitro imidazoles were developed primarily as radiosensitizers, they have also been
shown to be effective chemosensitizers. Examples of nonhypoxic cell sensitizers
include the halogenated pyrimidines.

   Paclitaxel is the prototype of a new class of antitumor compounds that target
microtubules. It is purified from the bark of the Pacific yew tree, *Taxus brevifolia*.
Alternative methods of producing paclitaxel are in various stages of development.
Its chemical structure and antitumor activity in rodents were reported in 1971 (3).
The semisynthetic compound taxotere is the second in this important new class of
drugs. Paclitaxel's principal mode of action is its potent microtubule stabilizing
activity and ability to promote microtubule assembly, resulting in cells accumulating with a G2/M phase DNA content (4,5). Using tissue culture and xenograft
systems, the drug has proved cytotoxic against a variety of human malignant cell

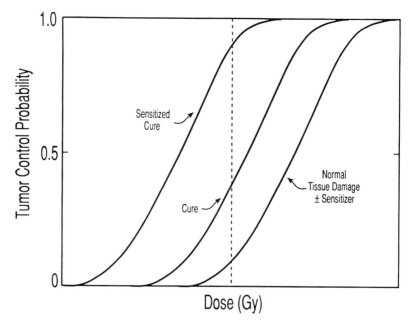

Figure 1   Strategy of radiosensitizers. The addition of a radiosensitizer is expected to shift
the tumor control curve to the left while not significantly moving the normal tissue
complication curve.

types. Recent laboratory data from our department have shown paclitaxel to be a potent radiosensitizer (4–6). Several clinical trials have shown it to have activity against refractory ovarian cancer, breast cancer, melanoma, head and neck cancer, and lung cancer (7). It is particularly attractive to combine radiation therapy with a chemotherapeutic agent like paclitaxel, thus permitting the possibility of increased local control for some tumors while at the same time addressing occult metastatic disease.

Pharmacokinetic studies have shown mean peak plasma concentrations of paclitaxel to range between 3.1 to 4.1 μM with 6-hr infusion (210 to 250 mg/m^2), 0.72 to 0.94 μM with 24-hr infusion (200 to 250 mg/m^2), and 0.05 to 0.08 μM with 96-hr infusion (120 to 160 mg/m^2) schedules (8). Mean alpha and beta half-lives have ranged between 0.27 and 0.5 hr and from 1.3 to 8.6 hr, respectively. The peak and steady-state plasma values reported are all significantly higher than the drug levels required to achieve the known in vitro effects on microtubules (4), cytotoxicity (4–6), and radiation sensitizing activity (6,9). Hepatic metabolism and biliary excretion appear to dominate clearance of the drug.

II. RADIOBIOLOGICAL STUDIES

It is generally accepted that the G2 and M phases of the cell cycle are the most radiosensitive when compared to other phases of the cell cycle. The molecular basis of these differences is not well understood. One important mediator may be the p53 tumor suppressor protein, which is involved in mediating apoptotic cell death induced by both radiation (10) and chemotherapeutic agents (11). Based on paclitaxel's mechanism of action, we postulated that the drug could function as a radiosensitizer. Tissue culture studies performed in our department on several human tumor cell lines have shown a potential benefit from this combined treatment (6,9). Radiation sensitizing activity has been noted in a human astrocytoma cell line, human breast carcinoma cell line, and human melanoma cell line, but not a human cervical carcinoma cell line (Fig. 2). Radiation sensitizing activity has also been reported in other cell lines, as can be seen in Table 1. In 9 of 13 cell lines where the combined effects of paclitaxel and radiation have been evaluated on cellular proliferation capacity, resultant levels of cell kill indicate supraadditivity. However, in all cell lines, results are at least additive, indicating that paclitaxel does not antagonize the effect of ionizing radiation.

In Figure 2, the sensitizer enhancement ratio (SER) at the 10% cell survival level varies from 1.8 for astrocytoma to 1.5 for the breast cancer cells, to 1.2 for the melanoma cells and no effect (i.e. 1.0) for the cervical carcinoma cells. Of these cell lines, the melanoma cells are the most radioresistant, while the cervical carcinoma cells are the most radiosensitive; hence, the ability of paclitaxel to sensitize is not related to its levels, since the values of 1.8, 1.5, and 1.0 were found with 10 nM paclitaxel for 24 hr and 1.2 with 40 nM for 24 hr.

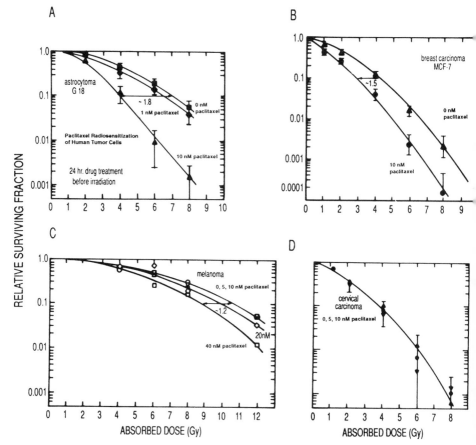

Figure 2 Effects of radiation alone (Cs-137 gamma rays at a dose rate of 1.1 Gy/min) or of radiation and paclitaxel (pretreatment for 24 hr) on cell survival of astrocytoma (G18) (A), breast carcinoma (MCF-7) (B), melanoma (HTB-72) (C), and cervical carcinoma (HTB-31) (D) cells. Results are normalized to control levels (radiation alone) or of the paclitaxel pretreatment (paclitaxel plus radiation). Deviation of the survival curves from superimposability indicates a sensitizing effect which can be expressed as a sensitizer enhancement ratio (SER) and which ranges from 1.8 (astrocytoma) to 1.5 (breast carcinoma) to 1.2 (melanoma) to 1.0 or no effect (cervical carcinoma).

It should be noted also that there are considerable differences in cellular sensitivity to paclitaxel alone (Table 2). Here it can be seen that there is an order-of-magnitude difference in cellular sensitivity for the human tumor cells, while the rodent cells are relatively unaffected by a treatment of 10 n*M* paclitaxel for 24 hr. The interaction between paclitaxel and ionizing radiation appears, therefore, to be

Table 1 Taxol Radiosensitizer Activity in Human Tumor and Rodent Tissue Culture

Tumor type	Cell lines	Interaction	References
Brain (astrocytoma)	G18	Supraadditive[a]	6,9
Breast	MCF-7	Supraadditive[a]	17, 18
	T47D	Supraadditive[a]	18
Cervix	HTB-31, HTB-35	Additive[a]	19,20
Melanoma	SK-Mel-28, HTB-72	Supraadditive[a]	19
Ovary	BG-1, SKOV-3, OVCAR-3	Supraadditive[b]	21
Lung	A549	Additive[a]	17
Pancreas	Shaw	Supraadditive[a]	17
Bone marrow	HL-60	Supraadditive[a]	22
Fibroblast—mouse	C3H 10T1/2	Additive[a]	23

[a]Clonogenic.
[b]Nonclonogenic.

both concentration- and time-dependent. The time-dependence does, however, appear to be related to the accumulation of paclitaxel-treated cells in the radiosensitive G2 and M phases of the cell cycle (Fig. 3). Here it can be seen that the effects of paclitaxel alone are dependent on the time of treatment (Fig. 3A), where significant effects of a 10-nM treatment on plating efficiency are seen at the same time (16 hrs) that the majority of cells have progressed through the cell cycle and accumulated with a G2/M DNA content (Fig. 3B). Further, it is at 24 hrs that the greatest effect of radiation (6 Gy) and paclitaxel (10 nM) is seen (Fig. 3C), corresponding to a population in which nearly all cells had a G2/M DNA content

Table 2 Taxol Cytotoxicity in Different Cell Lines (10 nM, 24 hr)

Cell line	Surviving fraction	References
Brain: G18	0.04	6,9
Breast: MCF-7	0.15	18
T47D	0.37	18
Cervix: HTB-31	0.08	19,20
HTB-35	0.15	19,20
Melanoma: HTB-72	0.48	19
Lung: A549	0.04	17
Ovary A2780	0.14	24
hamster CHO	>0.90	24
Mouse fibroblast: C3H 10T1/2	>0.90	23

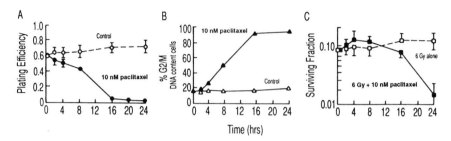

Figure 3   Effects of different times of treatment of 10 nM paclitaxel on the plating efficiency of astrocytoma cells (Fig. 3A). Control plating efficiencies are relatively constant at about 60%, while there is a continual decline with paclitaxel time of treatment. B. Flow cytometric estimates of the fraction of cells with a G2/M DNA content are shown for various times with 10 nM paclitaxel. Control levels of G2/M cells stay relatively constant at about 20% over the 24-hr period, while paclitaxel-treated cells approach 100% with a G2/M DNA content. C. The effects of radiation alone (6 Gy) on cell surviving fraction and of radiation delivered to cells at various times of treatment with 10 nM paclitaxel. At 24 hr, there is a considerable difference in surviving fraction between radiation alone, which stays relatively constant at about 10% cell survival, and radiation plus paclitaxel (about 2% cell survival).

(Fig. 3B). Certainly in this instance the majority of cells are killed by paclitaxel alone, but those cells surviving it show an enhanced sensitivity to the effects of ionizing radiation compatible with their being accumulated in the radiosensitive G2/M phase of the cell cycle.

In order to examine molecular changes associated with radiosensitization by paclitaxel, we asked whether there were differences in radiation-induced gene expression in tumor cells that were either untreated or pretreated with paclitaxel prior to gamma radiation. The group of genes known as cellular immediate early genes is rapidly and transiently inducible by ultraviolet and ionizing radiation (12,13) as well as numerous other extracellular stimuli (14,15). In the G18 astrocytoma cells, we found that six genes in this class were inducible by treatment with serum or the protein kinase C activator TPA, while none were inducible by paclitaxel (16). Treatment with 20 Gy of gamma radiation resulted in a significant induction of the TIS8 immediate early gene, also known as *egr*-1 or *zif*268 (Fig. 4, closed squares), but not the c-*fos*, c-*jun*, or TIS1 genes. Pretreatment of identical cultures with a dose of paclitaxel that was previously shown to radiosensitize these cells resulted in a significant suppression of radiation-induced TIS8 gene expression (Fig. 4, open squares). The TIS8 gene encodes a transcriptional activator protein, which is thought to participate in signal transduction pathways by altering the expression of specific target genes that, in turn, allow cells to respond to toxic treatments such as ionizing radiation. If TIS8 were to mediate an early step in the pathway leading to recovery from radiation damage, then suppression of its

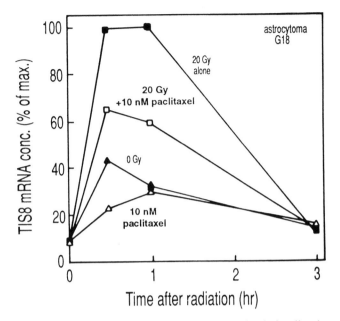

Figure 4 Effect of paclitaxel pretreatment on gene expression in irradiated astrocytoma cells. Tissue cultures of G18 human astrocytoma cells were irradiated with 20 Gy of gamma rays at a dose rate of 1.18 Gy/min either with or without pretreatment for 24 hr with 10 n*M* paclitaxel. Parallel cultures were mock irradiated by removal from the incubator and placement in the chamber of the inactive irradiator either with or without paclitaxel pretreatment. Separate cultures were collected at different times after irradiation or mock irradiation. Total RNA was isolated from the cells and assayed for TIS8 and β-actin mRNA content by Northern blot analysis and scanning densitometry. Relative levels of TIS8 mRNA were normalized to those of β-actin mRNA in the same sample to correct for differences in gel loading. The values are expressed as a percentage of the maximum level observed in the experiment. Note that a radiosensitizing dose of paclitaxel partially suppresses the rapid, transient induction to TIS8 mRNA that occurs after radiation.

induction, such as that observed after paclitaxel treatment, could lead to enhanced radiation sensitivity.

III. POTENTIAL CLINICAL APPLICATIONS

Our laboratory observations led us to design a phase I clinical trial combining paclitaxel and radiation for treatment of women with locally advanced breast cancer (NCI T92-0059), which has been initiated at the Columbia-Presbyterian Medical Center. Patients were classified according to the TNM system of the

American Joint Committee on Cancer (AJCC). Those with lesions labeled $T_3N_{1-2}M_0$, $T_4N_{(any)}M_0$, or $T_{(any)}N_3M_0$ without prior treatment are eligible. Patients on study receive 6 weekly 3-hr infusions of paclitaxel during their radiation therapy (5040 cGy/28 fx) followed by a modified radical mastectomy (when possible) or additional radiation therapy to 7500 cGy. The final phase of the study includes 6 cycles of CAF chemotherapy. This protocol is actively accruing patients. A second study is currently under way at our institution and the Johns Hopkins Oncology Center. This phase II protocol (NCI T93-0065) is a clinical and pharmacological study of preirradiation paclitaxel administered as a 96-hr infusion in adults with newly diagnosed glioblastoma multiforme. One of this study's goals is to determine possible paclitaxel activity in newly diagnosed patients with glioblastoma multiforme without prior treatment. It will most likely be a prelude to a combined radiation/paclitaxel study in a similar group of patients. Other centers are studying the combination of paclitaxel and radiation for lung cancer, cancer of the esophagus, and head and neck cancer. Although all of these studies use conventional external beam radiotherapy, other possible radiation modalities might include brachytherapy, stereotactic radiosurgery, colloid particles of chromic P-32, or radiolabeled antibodies.

IV. CONCLUSIONS

Paclitaxel is the prototype of a new class of antitumor compounds that targets microtubules. Several clinical trials have shown it to have palliative activity against refractory ovarian cancer, breast cancer, melanoma, head and neck cancer, and lung cancer. However, optimal doses and schedules have not yet been defined. Trials currently in progress will start to address these issues. A considerable number of laboratory studies suggest that paclitaxel may be effective in combined treatment regimens for a number of tumor types. Well-designed trials combining paclitaxel with other chemotherapeutic agents or radiation (where there are laboratory indications that paclitaxel can function as a radiosensitizer) will further define optimal use of this novel antitumor compound and the new generation of derivative paclitaxel-based compounds.

REFERENCES

1. John MJ, Flam MS, Legha SS, Phillips TL. Chemoradiation: An Integrated Approach to Cancer Treatment. Philadelphia:1993.
2. Steel GG, Peckam MJ. Exploitable mechanisms in combined radiotherapy-chemotherapy: The concept of additivity. Int J Radiat Oncol Biol Phys 1979;5:85.
3. Wani MC, Taylor HL, Wall ME, et al. Plant antitumor agents: VI. The isolation and structure of taxol, a novel antileukemic and antitumor agent from *Taxus brevifolia*. J Am Chem Soc 1971;93:2325–2327.

4. Schiff PB, Fant J, Horwitz SB. Promotion of microtubule assembly *in vitro* by taxol. Nature 1979;277:665–667.
5. Schiff PB, Horwitz SB. Taxol stabilizes microtubules in mouse fibroblast cells. Proc Natl Acad Sci 1980;77:1561–1565.
6. Tishler RB, Schiff PB, Geard CR, Hall EJ. Taxol: A novel radiation sensitizer. Int J Radiat Oncol Biol Phys 1992;22:613–617.
7. Rowinsky EK, Onetto N, Canetta RM, Arbuck SG. Taxol: The first of the taxanes, an important new class of antitumor agents. Semin Oncol 1992;19:646–662.
8. Rowinsky EK, Donehower RC. The clinical pharmacology of paclitaxel (Taxol). Semin Oncol 1993;20:16–25.
9. Tishler RB, Geard CR, Hall EJ, Schiff PB. Taxol sensitizes human astrocytoma cells to radiation. Cancer Res 1992;52:3495–3497.
10. Lowe SW, Schmitt EM, Smith SW, et al. p53 is required for radiation-induced apoptosis in mouse thymocytes. Nature 1993;362:847–849.
11. Lowe SW, Ruley HE, Jacks T, Housman DE. p53-dependent apoptosis modulates the cytotoxicity of anticancer agents. Cell 1993;74:957–967.
12. Fornace AJ. Mammalian genes induced by radiation: Activation of genes associated with growth control. Annu Rev Genet 1992;26:507–526.
13. Weichselbaum RR, Hallahan DE, Sukhatme V, et al. Biological consequences of gene regulation after ionizing radiation exposure. J Natl Cancer Inst 1991;83:480–484.
14. Curran T. The fos Oncogene. New York: Elsevier, 1988.
15. Gubits RM, Burke RE, Yu H, et al. IEG induction after neonatal hypoxia-ischemia. Mol Brain Res 1993;18:228–238.
16. Gubits RM, Geard CR, Schiff PB. Expression of immediate early genes after treatment of human astrocytoma cells with radiation and taxol. Int J Radiat Oncol Biol Phys 1993;27:637–642.
17. Liebmann J, Cook J, Teague D, et al. Taxol mediated radiosensitization in human tumor cell lines. Presented at the Second NCI Workshop on Taxol and Taxus. Alexandria, VA: National Cancer Institute, 1992.
18. Schiff PB. Personal Communication, 1992.
19. Geard CR, Jones JM, Schiff PB. Taxol and radiation. J NCI Monographs 1993;15:89–94.
20. Geard CR, Jones JM. Radiation and taxol effects on synchronized human cervical carcinoma cells. Int J Radiat Oncol Biol Phys 1994;29:565–569.
21. Steren A Sevin B., Perras J. et al. Taxol sensitizes human ovarian cancer cells to radiation. Gynecol Oncol 1993;48:252–258.
22. Choy H, Rodriguez FF, Koester S, et al. Investigation of taxol as a potential radiation sensitizer. Cancer 1993;71:3774–3778.
23. Hei TK, Hall EJ. Taxol, radiation, and oncogenic transformation. Cancer Res 1993;53:1368–1372.
24. Lopes NM, Adams EG, Pitts TW, Bhuyan BK. Cell kill kinetics and cell cycle effects of taxol on human and hamster ovarian cell lines. Cancer Chemother Pharmacol 1993;32:235–242.

6

Pharmacology and Metabolism

ERIC K. ROWINSKY
Johns Hopkins Oncology Center
and Johns Hopkins Hospital
Johns Hopkins University School of Medicine
Baltimore, Maryland

I. INTRODUCTION

Although paclitaxel may be one of the most important anticancer agents to be developed over the last two decades, with prominent clinical activity demonstrated to date in ovarian, breast, lung (both non-small cell and small cell), head and neck, germ cell, esophogeal, and bladder carcinomas, there has been a relative lack of pharmacological data available compared with other agents in similar phases of development. This was particularly true when paclitaxel entered clinical development in 1983, at which time preclinical pharmacological data were limited to studies involving a few rabbits. This scarcity of information was due in part to the difficulties in developing sensitive analytical assays to detect and measure the full range of drug and metabolite concentrations achieved in both small animals and humans, especially since early clinical development was restricted to prolonged infusion schedules, which are associated with lower drug concentrations. The recent development of more sensitive analytical assay methods, the use of shorter infusion schedules, and the availability of radiolabeled pharmaceuticals have led to new insights regarding tissue distribution, metabolism, pharmacokinetic and pharmacodynamic behavior, as well interactions with other antineoplastic and nononcological agents. This chapter reviews the pharmacology of paclitaxel as ascertained from limited preclinical animal studies, early clinical trials of prolonged infusion schedules, and more recent clinical studies evaluating shorter infusion schedules.

II. ANALYTICAL METHODS

Detailed pharmacological studies of paclitaxel were not performed as an integral part of preclinical drug development in animals; therefore only limited pharmacological information was available to investigators when paclitaxel entered early clinical development. Preclinical pharmacological data are often useful in guiding further clinical development, particularly with respect to selecting optimal schedules of administration. The lack of preclinical pharmacological studies with paclitaxel was largely due to the agent's unique structural characteristics, which precluded using highly sensitive analytical detection modalities. Although several analytical methods were published before clinical trials began, these assays were generally tedious and insensitive; therefore they were not applicable for use in large clinical investigations. The only pharmacological information that was available before clinical trials began was obtained by Hamel et al. (1). Hamel and colleagues developed a unique biochemical assay that exploited the ability of paclitaxel to induce tubulin to form cold-resistant polymers that hydrolyze GTP at 0°C. However, the lower limits of sensitivity of the biochemical assay was only 0.1 μmol/L, which is suboptimal for ascertaining accurate pharmacokinetic information from clinical trials employing prolonged infusions schedules. In preclinical studies in rabbits, paclitaxel was demonstrated to be almost entirely bound to plasma proteins (92%). However, protein binding was readily reversible and the agent was rapidly cleared from serum in a biexponential fashion. In a single rabbit receiving a rapid intravenous bolus of paclitaxel, distribution and elimination half-lives were reported to be 2.7 and 45 min, respectively (1).

Several reverse-phase high-performance liquid chromatographic (HPLC) methods were subsequently developed during early phase I investigations, permitting the characterization of the pharmacokinetic behavior of paclitaxel on both brief and prolonged schedules of administration (2–9). These HPLC methods utilized similar extraction and analytical procedures; however, the variable extraction efficiencies, relatively insensitive ultraviolet (UV) detection modalities, and other assay performance characteristics limited the sensitivity of most early HPLC methods, rendering them unreliable, especially for the pharmacological monitoring of patients receiving lower doses of paclitaxel infused over prolonged infusion ($\geq$ 24 hr) durations. More recently, Wall et al. described a modified HPLC assay procedure which utilizes a substantially longer analytical column and appears to have increased sensitivity compared with earlier procedures (10). In addition, investigators at the Netherlands Cancer Institute and Bristol-Myers Squibb described a highly sensitive HPLC assay with a lower limit of detection of 6 ng/mL (6 nmol/L) in plasma and 8 ng/mL (9 nmol/L) in urine (11,12). This method differed from previous methods in that it employed a selective solid-phase extraction technique using a solid-phase extraction, a long analytical column, and UV detection at 227 nm (12). It also permit the simultaneous detection of metabolites. The feasibility of increasing the sensitivity of traditional analytical methods using HPLC-electrospray mass spectrometry has also been reported (13).

In an attempt to increase the sensitivity and improve the clinical applicability of analytical procedures, various immunological assays have been developed using rapid and sensitive competitive inhibition enzyme immunoassay (CIEIA) techniques, primarily for quantitating concentrations of taxanes in plant extracts (14–17). Immunological assays, which had been reported to be more sensitive (0.1–0.3 nmol/L) than available HPLC methods (14–17), may be useful in the pharmacological monitoring of patients during large multicenter trials, particularly those utilizing prolonged (24–96 hr) infusion schedules which result in plasma concentrations that approach or are below the lower limits of sensitivity for HPLC. The applicability of the CIEIA methods for clinical monitoring has been substantiated to date in a phase II study of 96-hr paclitaxel infusions in patients with brain tumors (18). Initially, immunoassays utilized polyclonal antisera; however, these immunological assays employing monoclonal antibodies to the taxane ring have also become available (14,16; Grothaus P., personal communication; September 1993). The degree of cross-reactivity of these antibodies between paclitaxel, metabolites, and other taxane analogs has not been reported.

III. PHARMACOKINETIC BEHAVIOR IN HUMANS (ADULTS)

A. Pharmacokinetic Studies of Prolonged Paclitaxel Infusions

Early phase I trials and accompanying pharmacological trials of paclitaxel primarily focused on the assessment and development of prolonged infusion schedules due to a high incidence of major acute hypersensitivity reactions (HSRs) noted with shorter infusion schedules during early drug development (2–9,19–21). Most early pharmacological data were derived from studies that utilized prolonged 6- and 24-hr infusion schedules and employed similar extraction and HPLC procedures to quantitate paclitaxel concentrations in biological samples. As previously noted, the variable extraction efficiencies, limits of sensitivity (lower limits, 0.05 μmol/L), as well as other technical characteristics of these assays generally rendered them unreliable, especially for detailed and large-scale pharmacological monitoring (see Section II, Analytical Methods, above).

Pertinent pharmacokinetic parameters derived from early studies as well as more recent ones using prolonged infusions in adults with advanced cancers are summarized in Table 1 (3–9,12,19,21–23). Substantial interpatient variability was generally noted, but neither nonlinear nor dose-dependent behavior was observed over the broad dose ranges evaluated in early clinical studies. Instead, both peak

Table 1 Pharmacokinetic Parameters from Prolonged Infusion Trials in Adults[a]

Schedule (site) [Ref]	Model	$T_{1/2}$ (hr) $\alpha/\beta/\gamma$	Cl (mL/min/m²)	C_{max} (μmol/L) (Dose)	Vd_{ss} (L/m²)	MRT (hr)	Urine (% dose)
6-hr infusion (San Antonio) [8]	Biphasic	0.49/4.3/–	232	2.0–6.7 (175–275 mg/m²)	48.5	11.8	8.2
6-hr infusion (Einstein) [5]	Biphasic	0.32/8.6/–	100	3.2–8.1 (175–275 mg/m²)	55	8.6	5.2
24-hr infusion (Einstein) [6]	Biphasic	0.27/3.9/–	359	0.6–0.94 (200–275 mg/m²)	182	19.9	1.4
1–6-hr infusion qd × 5d (Wisconsin) [4]	Biphasic	–/1.3/–	833	0.06–0.37 (15–40 mg/m²)	81	–	6.6
1–6-hr infusion (Hopkins) [3]	Biphasic	0.27/6.4/–	253	1.3–13.0 (60–265 mg/m²)	67	5.6	5.9
24-hr infusion (Hopkins) [7]	–	–	–	1.6–3.5 (250–390 mg/m²)	–	–	–
24-hr infusion + cisplatin (Hopkins) [9]	–	–	363	0.21–0.83 (110–200 mg/m²)	–	–	–

24-hr infusion + cisplatin + G-CSF (Hopkins) [19]	—		228	0.52–3.4[b] (135–350 mg/m²)	—	—	—
24-hr infusion (Netherlands Cancer Inst) [12]	Triphasic	0.12/2.1/20.4	383	0.23–0.43 (135 & 175 mg/m²)	657	30.1	—
96-hr infusion (NCI) [21]	—		470	0.053–0.077 (120–160 mg/m²)	—	—	—
24-hr infusion (NCI Japan)[a] [22]	Biphasic	–/11.5/–	344	0.14–0.69 (49.5–180 mg/m²)	202	24.3	<15
24-hr infusion (Aichi) [23]	Biphasic	–/17.5/–	262	0.1–0.75 (50–200 mg/m²)	286	24.9	8.7
Mean[a]		0.29/6.95[b]/–	344		182	15.2	5.5
(SD)		(0.13)/(5.4)/–	(219)		(238)	(9.9)	(2.5)

Abbreviations: C_{max}, peak plasma concentration; Cl, systemic clearance; $T_{1/2\alpha}$, alpha half-life; $T_{1/2\beta}$, beta half-life; $T_{1/2\gamma}$, gamma half-life; Vd_{ss}, volume of distribution at steady-state; MRT, mean residence time.

[a] Means do not include data from reports that are not in final manuscript form. Studies in italics signify that data have been reported in abstract form only.

[b] Means of half-lives specified as either beta half-lives or terminal half-lives in studies with biphasic pharmacokinetics.

plasma paclitaxel concentrations (C_{max}) and areas under concentration-time curves (AUC) correlated well with paclitaxel doses. In most early studies of paclitaxel administered on prolonged infusion schedules, plasma disappearance of paclitaxel was generally characterized by a biphasic elimination model. In those studies in which biphasic disposition has been characterized and final results have been reported, mean alpha and beta half-lives have ranged from 0.27 to 0.49 hr (cumulative mean, 0.34 hr) and 1.3 to 8.6 hr (cumulative mean, 4.9 hr), respectively (3–6,8). Mean residence times (MRT) ranging from 5.6 to 30.1 hr (cumulative mean, 15.2 hr) have also been reported (3–6,8,12).

B. Pharmacokinetic Studies of Short Paclitaxel Infusions (Adults)

The results of a pivotal phase III multicenter study performed by the National Cancer Institute of Canada Clinical Trial Group (NCI CTG) in previously treated patients with ovarian cancer (24) has prompted a reevaluation of paclitaxel on shorter administration schedules, especially 3-hr infusion schedules, which were largely abandoned during paclitaxel's early development. This randomized prospective study demonstrated that the incidence of major HSRs is low and, more importantly, equivalent in patients receiving paclitaxel over 3 and 24 hr following premedication with corticosteroids and H_1- and H_2-histamine antagonists. Antitumor activity was also found to be equivalent on both schedules.

From a pharmacological perspective, the results of the NCI CTG study and more recent trials in adults (12,25,26; Noe D.A. and Rowinsky E.K., unpublished results) and children (27,28) indicate that paclitaxel's pharmacokinetics may be nonlinear, with C_{max} and AUC values increasing disproportionately with increasing doses. Nonlinear pharmacokinetic behavior is particularly evident with the agent administered over shorter periods. These results are not necessarily discrepant from earlier results of prolonged infusion studies, which indicated that the pharmacokinetics are linear. Instead, when drugs that truly behave in a nonlinear, saturable, Michaelis-Menton fashion are administered over long durations, plasma concentrations are generally low. If plasma levels are significantly lower than K_m, the Michaelis-Menton constant, elimination and/or tissue distribution processes are not saturated and pharmacokinetics appear linear (first-order). However, nonlinear (zero-order) pharmacokinetics become more apparent when the identical agent is administered over progressively shorter durations, resulting in higher plasma concentrations that approach or exceed K_m. At these higher plasma concentrations, elimination and/or tissue distribution processes become saturated. Nonlinear pharmacokinetic behavior may be due to either saturable elimination processes, saturable tissue distribution, or a combination of both. Thus far, disproportionate increases in C_{max} and AUC values with increasing doses of paclitaxel have indicated that elimination is in part saturable; however, a significant component of paclitaxel's nonlinear behavior also appears to be due to saturable tissue distribution processes that may occur as a result of drug transfer between compartments and/or saturable tissue binding of drug (28–30; Noe D.A. and Rowinsky E.K., unpublished results). The K_m for distribution appears lower than that for elimination, indicating that tissue saturation occurs at lower doses (<175 mg/m^2 over 3 hr) than saturation of elimination mechanisms (≥175 mg/m^2 over 3 hr) (28,30; Noe D.A. and Rowinsky E.K., unpublished results).

Paclitaxel's nonlinear pharmacokinetic profile may have several important clinical implications. First, it is possible that dose escalations, especially on shorter (e.g., 3-hr) administration schedules, will result in disproportionate increases in both AUC and C_{max} values as well as disproportionate increases in toxicity. Similarly, dose reductions may result in disproportionate decreases in AUC and/or C_{max} values, thereby possibly decreasing antitumor activity. Thus, it will be important to define these nonlinear pharmacokinetic and pharmacodynamic relationships clearly in the future.

Pharmacokinetic parameters from adult cancer patients participating in several trials that employed shorter infusion schedules are depicted in Table 2 (12,25,26). Plasma disposition data of some patients participating in more recent studies using more sensitive HPLC assays have been well described by both biphasic and triphasic models (11,12,30; Noe D.A. and Rowinsky E.K., unpublished results).

C. Pharmacokinetic Studies in Children

Preliminary plasma disposition data from phase I evaluations performed in children with solid tumors and leukemias have revealed pharmacological behavior which is essentially similar to that reported in adults (27–29). In a Pediatric Oncology Group (POG) study of paclitaxel 200 to 420 mg/m^2 administered over 24 hr, the pharmacological behavior of the agent was well described by a two-compartment model that incorporated both saturable tissue distribution and binding (27,28). Similar to adult studies, the K_m for tissue distribution was lower than that for elimination, indicating that tissue saturation occurs at lower plasma concentrations and paclitaxel doses compared to the saturation of elimination mechanisms. Although end-of-infusion paclitaxel concentrations generally increased with increasing doses (Pearson's correlation coefficient $[R^2] = 0.27$, $p = 0.005$), there was considerable overlap in this parameter at all dose levels (27). In this trial, median parameter estimates were as follows: (Vd$_c$, 8.3 L/m^2 (2.9–20 L/m^2), Vd$_{ss}$, 50.9 L/m^2 (18.9–260 L/m^2), Vm$_{10}$, 31.9 μmol-hr^{-1} (2.9–47.4 μmol-hr^{-1}), Km$_{10}$, 2.16 μmol/L (0.64–4.81 μmol/L), Vm$_{12}$, 26.9 μmol-hr^{-1} (6.0–142.7 μmol-hr^{-1}), K$_{21}$, 0.254 hr^{-1} (0.052–1.04 hr^{-1}), clearance 135 mL/min/m^2 (72–518 mL/min/m^2, and time >0.1 μmol/L, 40 hr (26–71 hr) (28). Paclitaxel concentrations in all patients exceeded estimated Km_{pc} values early in the infusion. In another trial in children with refractory leukemias in which paclitaxel 250 to 500 mg/m^2 was administered over 24 hr, pharmacokinetics were optimally modeled by both biphasic and triphasic open models (29). Terminal elimination half-life values were reported to range from 4.6 to 17 hr, whereas mean total

Table 2 Pharmacokinetic Parameters from Short Infusion Trials in Adults[a]

Schedule (Investigator) [Ref]	Model	Cl (mL/min/m²)	Mean C_{max} (μmol/L) (Dose)	VD Vd_{ss} (L/m2)	VD Vd_c (L/m2)	Other mean parameters
3-hr infusion (Huizing et al.) [12]	Three compartment	294 and 211	2.5 and 4.3 (135 and 175 mg/m²)	98.6	—	MRT = 8.1 hr
3-hr infusion (Gianni et al.) [25,30]	*Three compartment saturable drug transfer to one of the peripheral compartments and first-order transfer to the other*	190–246	3.3–7.6 (135–225 mg/m²)	—	3.8 (V_1)	$V_{m12} = 0.30$ μmol-min⁻¹ $K_{m12} = 0.23$ μM
3-hr infusion (Schiller et al.) [26]		132	7.0–12.5 (210–300 mg/m²)	—	5.0	$T_{1/2} = 9.7$ hr
3-hr infusion (Noe DA and Rowinsky) [unpublished results]	*Two compartment saturable drug binding in the peripheral compartment*	*239*	*4.75 (175 mg/m²)*	—	*4.3*	*Ka = 0.29 hr⁻¹-μmol⁻¹ Kd = 0.48 hr⁻¹ sites = 100 μmol $T_{1/2} = 14.6$ hr*

Abbreviations: C_{max}, peak plasma concentration; Cl, systemic clearance; $T_{1/2}$, terminal half-life of elimination; Vd_c, volume of distribution for the central compartment; Vd_{ss}, volume of distribution at steady state; MRT, mean residence time; V_m and K_m, Michaelis-Menton constants; Ka, K_{m12}, and Kd, intercompartmental rate constants.
[a]Studies in italics signify that data has not been published in manuscript form.

clearance and steady-state volume of distribution (Vd_{ss}) values were 334 mL/min/m^2 and 85 L/m^2, respectively.

IV. TISSUE DISTRIBUTION

Mean Vd_c and Vd_{ss} values have generally been reported to be large. In 6- to 24-hr infusion studies in which final results have been reported, mean Vd_c values have ranged from 8.6 to 19.2 L/m^2 (cumulative mean, 13.8 L/m^2) and mean Vd_{ss} values have ranged from 48.2 to 657 L/m^2 (cumulative mean, 182 L/m^2) (Table 1) (3–6,8). Similarly, large values for both Vd_c (4.5–5 L/m^2) and Vd_{ss} (98.6 L/m^2) have been reported in recent studies involving patients who received paclitaxel over 3 hr (Table 2) (12,25,26). These values are much larger than the volume of total body water, indicating that paclitaxel is extensively bound to plasma proteins and/or other tissue elements, possibly tubulin as well as other tissue proteins. Plasma protein binding, as determined by both equilibrium dialysis and ultrafiltration, has also been demonstrated to be extensive, ranging from 95% to greater than 97% over a wide range of drug concentrations (14,16,17). In one study in which the binding of paclitaxel to human plasma and to individual plasma proteins was studied by equilibrium dialysis, approximately 95% of the drug was demonstrated to be protein-bound (31). At clinically relevant concentrations (0.1–0.6 μmol/L), protein binding was found to be concentration-independent, indicating nonspecific hydrophobic binding. Human serum albumin and alpha 1–acid glycoprotein contributed equally to the binding, with a minor contribution from lipoproteins. None of the drugs that are commonly administered with paclitaxel—including dexamethasone, diphenhydramine, ranitidine, doxorubicin, 5-fluorouracil, and cisplatin—altered protein binding (31). In addition, protein binding was found to decrease red blood cell uptake of the agent dramatically. Despite extensive binding to plasma proteins, paclitaxel is readily eliminated from the plasma compartment, suggesting lower-affinity, reversible binding.

The tissue distribution of paclitaxel has not been extensively studied in either humans or animals to date. Limited data from phase I trials in which limited sampling was performed from various compartments following intravenous administration indicate that paclitaxel distributes to third-space fluid collections such as ascites. In one report, biologically relevant concentrations of paclitaxel (> 0.1 μmol/L) were measured in ascites 7 hr after the beginning of a 6-hr infusion (5). Drug concentrations in the ascitic fluid increased for several hours thereafter and reached a maximum concentration of approximately 40% above concurrent plasma levels 12 hr after the beginning of the infusion. This ratio was sustained for at least 12 hr. The penetration of paclitaxel into the central nervous system has also been demonstrated to be negligible, which may explain paclitaxel's virtual lack of central nervous system toxicity (7). In a phase I study in which high doses of paclitaxel (up to 390 mg/m^2) were administered to adults with refractory leukemias, the majority of whom did not have leukemic involvement of the central nervous system, paclitaxel was not detected in cerebrospinal fluid sampled at the end of 24-hr infusions, which is the time that peak plasma concentrations are achieved (7). Interestingly, paclitaxel was able to be measured in brain tumors in patients receiving 3-hr infusions of paclitaxel before tumor resection, whereas the drug was not detected in adjacent normal brain tissues (32).

The preliminary results of tissue distribution studies in animals have been reported (33–36). These studies assessed the tissue distribution of paclitaxel using radiolabeled compound. Lesser et al. sampled tissues 2 hr after the administration of ^{3}H-paclitaxel to rats (33). Following whole tissue extraction and autoradiography, tissue/plasma paclitaxel ratios were high in almost all tissues sampled (including liver, 90; heart, 80; lung, 77; muscle, 23; and spleen, 89). Ratios were particularly high in tissues that are involved in organ barrier filtration (including the portal triad, 323; renal medulla, 263; choroid plexus, 105; and glomeruli, 259). Interestingly, these studies demonstrated either no penetration or very limited penetration of the radioisotope into testes and brain, which are generally considered "tumor sanctuary" sites (33–36). Both Eiseman et al. and Klecker et al. also demonstrated widespread tissue distribution of ^{3}H-paclitaxel in mice and rats (34,36). In both species, the highest tissue concentrations were observed in liver, kidney, and lung, with lower concentrations found in heart and skeletal muscle. In both species, drug penetration into classic tumor sanctuary sites was low. Although peripheral neurotoxicity is a principal dose-limiting nonhematological effect of paclitaxel, radioactivity has not been detected in the peripheral nervous system of rats after treatment with ^{3}H-paclitaxel (33). Radioactivity has also not been detected in brain tumor xenografts in rabbits following the administration of ^{3}H-paclitaxel (Lesser G, unpublished results; January 1994).

V. PHARMACODYNAMICS: DRUG ACTIVITY

In adult studies in which final results have been reported, peak plasma paclitaxel concentrations (C_{max}) achieved with paclitaxel administered at clinically relevant doses have ranged from 2.5 to 12.9 μmol/L with 3-hr infusions (135–300 mg/m^2) (12,25,26,30); 2.2 to 13.0 μmol/L with 6-hr infusions (170–275 mg/m^2) (3,5,8); 0.23 to 0.94 μmol/L with 24-hr infusions (135–275 mg/m^2) (6,9,12,19); and 0.053 to 0.077 μmol/L with the 96-hr infusion schedule (120–160 mg/m^2) (20,21). Plasma concentrations achieved at the end of 24-hr infusions (C_{max}) have been calculated to be nearly equivalent to the steady-state values (C_{ss}) ($C_{24 h} = 0.97 C_{ss}$) using the mean kinetic parameter values for drug disposition and elimination derived from early pharmacological studies at the Johns Hopkins Oncology Center (JHOC) (9). C_{max} and C_{ss} values achieved following the administration of paclitaxel on 3- to 24-hr infusion schedules were several orders of magnitude higher than paclitaxel concentrations (0.01–0.1 μmol/L) capable of inducing relevant cytotoxic and microtubule effects in vitro, such as microtubule bundle formation as well as radiation enhancement (34–38). Several cooperative group randomized prospective trials that are incorporating pharmacological assessment of relationships between pertinent pharmacological parameters, toxicity, and clinical activity are currently being performed in patients with ovarian, breast, and lung cancers and hematological malignancies.

Paclitaxel concentrations (0.1–10 μmol/L) that are clinically achievable have been demonstrated to induce two distinct morphological effects on microtubules in human leukemia cells in vitro (37–41). First, paclitaxel-treated cells form abundant arrays of disorganized microtubules that are often aligned in parallel bundles. Microtubule bundles are formed during all phases of the cell cycle. Second, paclitaxel induces the formation of abnormal spindle asters during the mitotic phases (G_2 and M). Whereas mitotic cells normally have two spindle asters that are organized by microtubule organizing centers or centrioles, paclitaxel-treated mitotic cells form large numbers of abnormal asters that do not require centrioles for enucleation. Although the precise mechanisms that account for inherent resistance to paclitaxel have not been clearly defined, the sensitivity of various human leukemia cell lines to paclitaxel has been demonstrated to be directly related to the propensity of the cells to form irreversible microtubule bundles following in vitro treatment. Whereas cancer cell lines that are relatively sensitive to paclitaxel form irreversible bundles and are critically affected during interphase, most relatively resistant cells are unaffected during traverse through G_0/G_1 and S phases and accumulate in G_2/M, with subsequent formation of multiple abnormal asters and polyploidal DNA content. In a phase I trial of paclitaxel in leukemia, the sensitivity of leukemic blasts to form microtubule bundles ex vivo was directly related to the magnitude of clinical antitumor activity (7). These results suggest that microtubule bundles and DNA polyploidization may be useful indices of lethal drug effects that could be performed on clinical material. This morphological assay is currently being studied prospectively in clinical trials in hematological malignancies (42).

VI. PHARMACOLOGICAL IMPLICATIONS OF POLYOXYETHYLATED CASTOR OIL

Two mechanisms of acquired resistance to paclitaxel in vitro have been well characterized following prolonged exposure to low drug concentrations. Both mechanisms, including alterations in alpha- and beta-tubulin resulting in an impaired ability to polymerize tubulin dimers into microtubules and the multidrug resistance (*mdr*) phenotype involving the amplification of membrane *p*-glycoproteins that function as drug efflux pumps, are discussed in Chapter 3 (Mechanisms of Resistance). The ability of many diverse classes of drugs—including calcium channel blockers, tamoxifen, cyclosporin A, and antiarrhythmic agents—to

modulate drug resistance conferred by *mdr* is well known. Recently, polyoxyethylated castor oil, the principal constituent of paclitaxel's clinical formulation
vehicle, has also been demonstrated to be a potent modulator of *mdr* (43,44).
Therefore, the polyoxyethylated castor oil vehicle may be contributing in part to
some of the clinical activity observed with paclitaxel, especially in breast cancer
and lymphoma patients who are clearly resistant to the vinca alkaloids and
anthracyclines, presumably on the basis of *mdr*. The potential clinical role that
polyoxyethylated castor oil may play in reversing resistance to paclitaxel is further
highlighted by studies in which plasma levels of polyoxyethylated castor oil were
readily measured using a flow cytometric bioassay that quantitates intracellular
increases in daunorubicin in *mdr* human T-cell leukemia cells (45). After 3-hr
infusions of paclitaxel 135 to 175 mg/m^2, plasma concentrations of polyoxyethylated castor oil were capable of inhibiting P-glycoprotein activity in vitro (45).
Based on these observations, it is reasonable to propose that any modification of
paclitaxel's clinical formulation should require studies documenting that there is
also no loss of efficacy.

VII. PHARMACODYNAMICS: TOXICITY

During the early clinical development of paclitaxel, only limited analyses that
sought to identify relationships between paclitaxel-induced toxicities and pharmacological parameters were performed. In phase I studies of paclitaxel administered as a 6-hr infusion at University of Texas, San Antonio (UTSA), and JHOC,
the severity of leukopenia roughly correlated with paclitaxel AUCs using a linear
model (3,8). A more detailed analysis of the JHOC data from the original report
revealed that the relationship between the percent decrease in the white blood cell
(WBC) count, paclitaxel's principal dose-limiting toxicity, and AUC is well
characterized by a sigmoidal maximal effect (E_{max}) model in which the maximal
effect is a 100% fall in the WBC count (46). The E_{max} model is a more appropriate
model for describing biological processes with saturable end points than a linear
model. The percentage decreases in the WBC counts were related to AUC by the
following formula:

Percent change in WBC $= 100 \times AUC^{1.04}/(1372 + AUC^{1.04})$

Similarly, the percentage change in absolute neutrophil count (ANC) in untreated
and minimally pretreated patients receiving paclitaxel 135 to 350 mg/m^2 (24-hr
infusion) before cisplatin 75 to 100 mg/m^2 and granulocyte colony stimulating
factor (G-CSF) has also been well characterized by an E_{max} model (19). The
percentage change in the ANC was related to paclitaxel C_{ss} by the following
formula:

Percent change in ANC $= 100 \times C_{ss}/(0.36 + C_{ss})$

Data from the NCIC CTG trial, in which previously treated patients with ovarian cancer were randomized to treatment with paclitaxel given over 3 or 24 hr and then randomized to treatment with either 135 mg/m^2 or 175 mg/m^2, have indicated that both AUC and C_{max} is substantially higher when identical doses of paclitaxel are given over short (3-hr) compared with prolonged (24-hr) infusions, but neutropenia is more severe in patients receiving paclitaxel over 24 hr (12). Furthermore, relationships between relevant pharmacological parameters (e.g., AUC, C_{max}, and clearance) and the severity of neutropenia were not able to be adequately described by either linear or nonlinear models. Instead, the percentage decreases in both the WBC and ANC were well characterized by an E_{max} model that relates these parameters to the duration that plasma paclitaxel concentrations are maintained above 0.1 μmol/L. With that model, 11.2 and 15.2 hr of exposure above the plasma concentration threshold of 0.1 μmol/L were predicted to yield 50% decreases in ANCs and WBCs, respectively. The Hill constants were 2.7 and 2.2, respectively. Other investigators have optimally modeled this relationship using lower threshold values (0.05 μM) since more prolonged infusions with lower C_{ss} also induce neutropenia (30). Relationships between various pharmacological parameters and neurotoxicity have also been sought. In an early phase I trial of paclitaxel at UTSA, neurotoxicity grade was also demonstrated to roughly correlate with AUC (8). In this study, patients were found to be more prone to develop a symptomatic peripheral neuropathy if their AUC exceeded 20 μg-hr/mL. The grade of neurotoxicity was also demonstrated to be related to paclitaxel C_{ss} ($r = 0.54$, $p < 0.01$) in a phase I trial of paclitaxel 135 to 350 mg/m^2 combined with cisplatin, 75 to 100 mg/m^2, and G-CSF and JHOC; however, the correlation between the grade of neurotoxicity and paclitaxel dose was nearly identical ($r = 0.56$, $p < 0.01$), suggesting that the predictive value of C_{ss} was not superior to the value of administered dose in predicting for the development of neurotoxicity (19). In addition, a POG phase I trial in which peripheral neurotoxicity precluded dose escalation of paclitaxel above 420 mg/m^2 on a 24-hr infusion schedule, the development of paresthesias occurred principally in children with paclitaxel systemic exposures above the median (AUC > 62 μmol-h/L) (28).

Both neutropenia and mucositis have also been found to be related to paclitaxel C_{ss} in a phase I study of paclitaxel administered as a 96-hr continuous infusion at the National Cancer Institute (20,21). Patients with grade 4 neutropenia had significantly higher paclitaxel C_{ss} compared with patients with $\leqslant$ grade 3 ($p = 0.011$). Similarly, patients with severe mucositis had a significantly higher paclitaxel C_{ss} compared with those with no or mild mucositis ($p_2 = 0.0043$). Both mucosal and neutrophil toxicity were significantly more severe in patients with C_{ss} above a threshold of 0.07 μmol/L. Of 11 patients with paclitaxel C_{ss} above 0.07 μmol/L, 10 (91%) had grade 4 neutropenia and eight (73%) had $\geqslant$ grade 3 mucosal toxicity. By comparison, only five of 14 (36%) patients with paclitaxel C_{ss} $\leqslant$ 0.07 μmol/L had grade 4 neutropenia ($p = 0.012$) and none had grade 3 or 4 mucositis (p_2 = 0.0002) (21). These investigators also demonstrated that the extent of liver involvement with metastatic breast cancer was directly related to paclitaxel C_{ss} and therefore indirectly related to paclitaxel clearance (see Section XI in this chapter). Relationships between toxicities and pertinent pharmacological parameters are also being sought in ongoing, prospectively randomized, major cooperative group studies of paclitaxel.

VIII. INTRAPERITONEAL PHARMACOKINETICS

At first glance, paclitaxel appears to be an attractive agent for intraperitoneal (IP) administration, especially in ovarian cancer, which is generally confined to the peritoneal cavity even in advanced stages. These attractive characteristics are its high molecular weight, bulky chemical structure, and hepatic metabolism. Additionally, the induction of pertinent microtubule and cytotoxic effects in vitro also appears to be dependent on both concentration and exposure duration, factors which may be optimized by regional drug delivery.

The feasibility of paclitaxel administration via the IP route was initially studied by the Gynecological Oncology Group (GOG) using single IP doses of paclitaxel (25 to 200 mg/m^2) every 3 weeks (47). Dose escalation above 125 mg/m^2 was precluded by severe abdominal pain; systemic toxicities were mild at doses below 175 mg/m^2.

From a pharmacological perspective, this initial IP study demonstrated that paclitaxel may be an ideal drug for IP use. The correlation between administered IP dose and peak IP concentration, as well as the low apparent V_d that resulted (mean ± SE, 1.9 ± 0.3 L/m^2; range 0.5 to 5.0 L/m^2), suggested that initial drug distribution is primarily confined to the peritoneal cavity. The C_{max} of IP paclitaxel ranged from 19 to 324 μmol/L at doses of 25 to 175 mg/m^2 IP. Paclitaxel's C_{max} at the recommended phase II dose, 125 mg/m^2 (mean, 198 μmol/L), ranged several orders of magnitude higher than levels required to induce pertinent microtubule and cytotoxic effects in vitro (37–39). In addition, paclitaxel concentrations of this magnitude were maintained for several days, indicating that IP clearance is extremely slow. The mean clearance of paclitaxel from the peritoneal cavity was 0.42 ± 0.09 L/m^2/day (range, 0.13 to 0.91 L/m^2/day). Of considerable importance, biologically relevant paclitaxel concentrations (> 0.1 μmol/L) were readily obtained and sustained in the plasma after IP administration for the entire sampling period of 48 hr. These concentrations generally exceeded minimal concentrations required to induce pertinent effects in vitro and are encouraging, since the achievement of relevant systemic concentrations appears to be an important in order for a drug to be advantageous when given by the IP route. Peak plasma levels were typically achieved by 1 hr and ranged from < 0.05 μmol/L (lower limits of detection) to 0.86 μmol/L. Mean peak plasma concentrations also correlated roughly with administered dose (r = 0.66, p > 0.2). A profound IP exposure advantage for paclitaxel was demonstrated, with IP/systemic AUC ratios ranging from 336 to 2890 times (mean ± SE, 996 ± 93). Given the dose-limiting toxicity as well as the extremely high paclitaxel concentrations and AUCs achieved with this schedule, the administration of lower IP doses on a weekly schedules is currently being evaluated. Thus far, weekly doses up to 60 mg/m² have been well tolerated, with minimal abdominal pain and systemic toxicity (48). The preliminary results of pharmacological studies also demonstrated the achievement of IP paclitaxel levels > 100 μmol/L in some patients, with a similar magnitude of high concentrations persisting at 7 days in some patients. Similarly, plasma paclitaxel concentrations exceeding 0.1 μmol/L have been documented in some patients.

IX. COMBINATION CHEMOTHERAPY: SEQUENCE-DEPENDENT DRUG INTERACTIONS

When paclitaxel began to be combined with other chemotherapy agents, such as cisplatin, there was a recognition of the fact that the optimal exploration of these combinations would require a detailed knowledge of drug-drug interactions and possible effects of sequence of administration on both toxic and therapeutic effects. Therefore, studies were designed to address the possibility that sequence-dependent pharmacological and toxicological interactions between paclitaxel and other chemotherapy agents may occur.

The most vivid example of the potential for sequence-dependent pharmacological and toxicological effects between paclitaxel and other cytotoxic agents is given by results of phase I studies of the paclitaxel-cisplatin combination. In the first study, patients with no or minimal prior therapy received alternating sequences of paclitaxel (24-hr schedule) and cisplatin to determine if drug sequencing influenced the toxicity patterns and pharmacological behavior of either agent (9). Neutropenia was the dose-limiting toxicity of the paclitaxel-cisplatin combination without G-CSF; however, the severity of neutropenia was demonstrated to be sequence-dependent. Mean ANC nadirs were significantly lower and the percentage of courses associated with ANCs ≤ 500/μL was significantly higher when patients received cisplatin before paclitaxel. To determine if drug sequencing affected the pharmacological disposition of paclitaxel, clearance rates for paclitaxel were calculated during courses in which paclitaxel was given before cisplatin ($Cl_{t/c}$) and courses in which cisplatin was given before paclitaxel ($Cl_{c/t}$). Mean paclitaxel clearance rates were significantly lower when paclitaxel followed cisplatin, 321 ± 44 mL/min/m² (range, 99–844 mL/min/m²) compared to 405 ± 65 mL/min/m² (range, 141–1097 mL/min/m²) for the alternate sequence, paclitaxel followed by cisplatin ($p = 0.013$ by paired t-test). Correlation analysis of the paired clearance data revealed a linear relationship ($R = 0.93, p < 0.001$), and regression analysis demonstrated that the clearance rate values for alternate sequences were defined by the following relationship:

$$Cl_{c/t} = 0.75 \ Cl_{t/c}$$

The sequence of cisplatin followed by paclitaxel induced more profound neutropenia than the reverse drug sequence in phase I studies and was also demonstrated to be the suboptimal sequence with respect to cytotoxic activity against L1210 leukemia and ovarian cancer cell lines in concurrent in vitro studies compared with both the reverse sequence and simultaneous drug treatment (49,50). In contrast, the sequence in which paclitaxel is followed by cisplatin, which was associated with less neutropenia in vivo, was the sequence that produced maximal cytotoxicity against L1210 leukemia cells. The mechanisms for these sequence-dependent effects in vitro are not entirely clear; however, paclitaxel has been demonstrated to increase the net numbers of cisplatin induced DNA adducts, possibly by inhibiting DNA repair mechanisms (51). Other investigators have not been able to demonstrate that paclitaxel augments the net formation of DNA interstrand crosslinks (49). Another possible explanation is that treatment with cisplatin before paclitaxel produces antagonistic effects, since cisplatin may inhibit cell cycle progression in the G_2 phase, thereby preventing progression into and through mitosis, which may be the optimal period of cell sensitivity to paclitaxel. Regardless of the mechanism, these clinical and in vitro observations formed the rationale for the selection of the sequence of paclitaxel (24-hr schedule) followed by cisplatin as the treatment sequence to be used in subsequent phase II/III trials of the paclitaxel-cisplatin doublet. These have included the pivotal phase III GOG study of paclitaxel (24-hr schedule) plus cisplatin versus cyclophosphamide plus cisplatin in untreated patients with suboptimally debulked ovarian epithelial neoplasms (52), as well as Eastern Cooperative Oncology Group (ECOG) studies of paclitaxel and cisplatin in head/neck and lung cancers.

Although the mechanisms for sequence-dependent pharmacological interactions between paclitaxel and cisplatin are not known, one potential mechanism is the modulation of cytochrome P450-dependent paclitaxel-metabolizing enzymes by cisplatin (see Section X, Drug Disposition, below) since platinum compounds may modulate the activities of specific cytochrome P450 enzymes (53). Interestingly, the ability to modulate cytochrome P450 enzymes is not shared by all the platinum compounds. For example, carboplatin does not appear to be capable of modulating P450 enzyme systems (53). The potential for sequence-dependent effects with shorter paclitaxel infusions and cisplatin is currently being evaluated.

The potential for sequence-dependent interactions has also been studied in conjunction with developmental studies of paclitaxel-doxorubicin and paclitaxel-cyclophosphamide combinations for breast cancer. In the first study of the paclitaxel-doxorubicin doublet at M.D. Anderson Cancer Center, Holmes et al. reported that severe stomatitis was dose-limiting at the first dose level when paclitaxel (125 mg/m^2 as a 24-hr infusion on day 1) preceded doxorubicin (60 mg/m^2

as a 48-hr infusion on days 2 and 3) and G-CSF (5 μg/kg/day days 4–9) (54,55). The maximum tolerated doses were paclitaxel 125 mg/m^2 and doxorubicin 48 mg/ m^2; however, a substantial proportion of patients required dose reductions with subsequent courses. To evaluate the effects of drug sequencing on toxicity, these investigators initiated another phase I trial in which sequencing was reversed in another group of patients. In this study, doxorubicin was administered on days 1 and 2 (48-hr infusion) and paclitaxel (24-hr infusion) was begun on day 3. The latter sequence has been much better tolerated, and dose escalation has safely proceeded to paclitaxel 150 mg/m^2 and doxorubicin 60 mg/m^2 with G-CSF. Sledge et al. have also reported similar sequence-dependent effects in an ECOG pilot study of paclitaxel administered as a 24-hr infusion combined with doxorubicin given as a bolus injection and G-CSF (56). Mucositis was significantly more prominent when paclitaxel was administered before doxorubicin; the recommended schedule and doses for subsequent ECOG phase II/III trials were doxorubicin 50 mg/m^2 before paclitaxel 150 mg/m^2 with G-CSF (5 μg/kg/day beginning on day 3). Preliminary pharmacological data once again indicates that the increased toxicity appears to be related to decreased clearance (32%) of doxorubicin when it is administered after paclitaxel (57).

Similar sequence-dependent toxicological effects have been noted in a JHOC phase I study of paclitaxel (24-hr infusion) and cyclophosphamide (1-hr infusion) with G-CSF in patients with anthracycline-resistant metastatic breast cancer (58). Similar to the initial phase I study of paclitaxel and cisplatin at JHOC, the sequence of drug administration has been alternated with each new patient as well as with each subsequent course in the same subject. Severe neutropenia has been the principal toxicity with paclitaxel 135 to 250 mg/m^2 combined with cyclophosphamide 750 to 2000 mg/m^2. The percentages of courses associated with ANCs $< 500/\mu l$ ($p < 0.001$) and platelet counts $< 75,000/\mu l$ ($p < 0.05$) are significantly higher with the treatment sequence of cyclophosphamide before paclitaxel. The mechanism for the differential toxicological effects between sequences is not clear at this time. A preliminary analysis of paired pharmacokinetic data from patients receiving both sequences has failed to demonstrate significant pharmacological differences with respect to both paclitaxel and cyclophosphamide between the two sequences to account for the toxicological differences. In addition, significant cytotoxic differences between the sequences have not been demonstrated in preclinical studies. In breast cancer cell lines, similar IC$_{90}$s for paclitaxel and 4-hydroperoxycyclophosphamide have been demonstrated for both sequences (58).

X. DRUG DISPOSITION

The principal mechanisms of systemic clearance were never determined during early clinical investigations of paclitaxel. In early phase I and pharmacological studies, the systemic clearance of paclitaxel was demonstrated to range from 100 to 833 mL/min/m^2 (cumulative mean, 344 mL/min/m^2) (Table 1). Although the parent compound was found in urine collected in the peritreatment period, total urinary excretion of unmetabolized paclitaxel was low (cumulative mean, 5.5%; range, 1.4–8.2%) (Table 1). These early data indicated that renal clearance contributes minimally to systemic clearance and that metabolism, biliary excretion, and/or extensive tissue binding are probably responsible for the bulk of the disposition of an administered dose of paclitaxel. In early phase I trials, metabolites were identified in neither plasma nor urine of patients receiving paclitaxel on 6- and 24-hr infusion schedules. More recently, several metabolites have been detected and identified using very sensitive HPLC assays in the plasma of patients receiving 3-hr infusions of paclitaxel (12,30).

Monsarrat and colleagues at the National Center for Scientific Research (NCSR) in Toulouse, France, were the first to firmly identify the structures of paclitaxel metabolites (59). Initially, these investigators reported on the identification of high concentrations of paclitaxel and several hydroxylated metabolites in the bile of rats. In subsequent studies performed at NCSR and JHOC, high concentrations of paclitaxel and several hydroxylated metabolites were also identified in the human bile of patients with indwelling biliary catheters (60,61). Monsarrat et al. reported that renal excretion of the parent compound accounts for the disposition of only 10% of a dose of paclitaxel administered to rats, and urinary metabolites were not detected (59–61). However, approximately 40% of the administered paclitaxel dose was recovered as both parent compound and metabolites from rat bile collected for 24 hr posttreatment. Similarly, approximately 20% of the dose of paclitaxel administered to a patient with a biliary drainage catheter was recovered as both parent compound and metabolites from bile collected for 24 hr after treatment (60,61). Since paclitaxel is widely distributed to peripheral compartments and biliary collections were not carried out for a relatively long period after treatment, it is also possible that hepatic metabolism and biliary excretion account for a much greater share of paclitaxel's disposition and that other, as yet unidentified metabolites may be metabolized and excreted into bile. Furthermore, animal studies were performed by Gaver et al. in which 98% of total radioactivity was recovered from the feces of rats collected for 6 days following the administration of ^{14}C-paclitaxel, while < 10% of the radioactivity was recovered from urine (62).

Detection and identification of both human and rat metabolites in bile was reported by collaborators at NSCR and JHOC using analytical HPLC, mass spectrometry, and NMR spectroscopy (59–61). Neither glucuronidated nor sulfated metabolites were identified; however, nine and five metabolite peaks were detected in rat and human bile, respectively (Fig. 1). To date, all human metabolites identified have had intact side chains at positions C-2 and C-13 of the taxane ring. In contrast, very low concentrations of baccatin III, which lacks the side chain at position C-13 of the taxane ring, have been identified as a minor metabolite in rats.

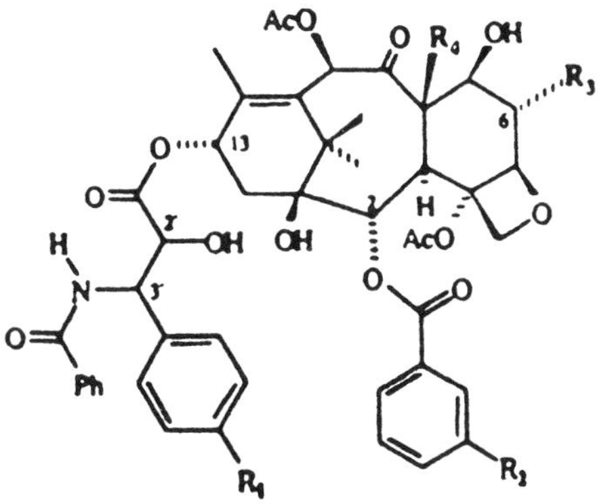

	R_1	R_2	R_3	R_4
Paclitaxel	H	H	H	CH_3
Baccatin (Rat)	13-OH	H	H	CH_3
Rat and Human	OH	H	H	CH_3
Rat	H	OH	H	CH_3
Rat	H	H	H	CH_2OH
Human	OH	H	OH	CH_3

Figure 1   Chemical structures of paclitaxel and biliary metabolites identified to date in rat and humans (59–61).

With the exception of baccatin III, which has only been found in rat bile, all biliary metabolites identified to date have been hydroxylated derivatives. These metabolites are hydroxylated on the side chains at position C-2 and C-13 of the taxane ring as well as on the taxane ring itself. Four of the nine metabolites in rat bile have been spectroscopically identified as monohydroxylated derivatives and one metabolite as a dihydroxylated derivative. These rat metabolites are substantially less active against L1210 leukemia than paclitaxel, but some are as active as paclitaxel in stabilizing microtubules against disassembly in cell-free tubulin preparations (59). One possible explanation for this discrepancy is that these hydroxylated metabolites, which are relatively more polar than paclitaxel, may not be transported into the cell as readily as the less polar parent compound. Similarly, among the five metabolites detected in human bile, two have been identified as monohydroxylated derivatives and one as a dihydroxylated derivative. Interestingly, the major metabolite of paclitaxel in human bile, a monohydroxylated derivative with a single hydroxyl group on position C-6 of the taxane ring, was not identified in rat bile, whereas the major metabolite in rat bile, a monohydroxylated metabolite with a single hydroxylated group on the side chain at position C-13, was only a minor metabolite in human bile. The major metabolite in human bile has also been identified in the plasma of patients receiving 3-hr paclitaxel infusions (12,30). As anticipated from previous studies of hydroxylated metabolites in rats (59), the major hydroxylated human metabolite was 30-fold less active than paclitaxel in inhibiting the growth of L1210 and P388 leukemias (Wright M., unpublished results, September 1993).

The hydroxylated nature of the majority of metabolites of paclitaxel suggests that hepatic P450 mixed-function oxidases, which are generally involved in hepatic hydroxylation reactions, play a major role in paclitaxel metabolism. Interspecies differences in the sites of hydroxylation suggest that different P450 enzymes may be involved in drug metabolism in humans and rodents. In an elegant series of in vitro metabolic studies using human microsomes and other methologies, Creistil et al. have demonstrated that at least two subfamilies of these enzymes are involved in the formation of the two major hydroxylated paclitaxel metabolites in humans (63). They have shown that cytochrome P450 enzymes of the CYP2C subfamily are responsible for the formation of the major human metabolite that is hydroxylated on the taxane ring, whereas cytochrome P450 enzymes of the CYP3A subfamily are responsible for the formation of the minor human metabolite that is hydroxylated on the side chain at position C13. In contrast, elegant studies by Harris et al. have shown that there was good correlation between the formation of one minor metabolite and CYP3A but the correlation of the major metabolite's (6α-hydroxypaclitaxel) formation with markers for several P450 subfamilies, including CYP2C, was poor (64). Interestingly, a variety of P450 inducers, as well as both selective and nonselective inhibitors have been demonstrated by both Creistil et al. and Harris et al. to significantly affect the formation of paclitaxel metabolites in human hepatic microsomal studies (63,64). However, the overall excretion of unmetabolized paclitaxel and metabolites has not been demonstrated to be affected by pretreatment of rats with various inducers of cytochrome P450 enzymes, including benzopyrene, troleandomycine, and phenobarbital, but the percentage of minor metabolites increased after pretreatment with phenobarbital (61). Interestingly, preliminary clinical observations have also suggested possible drug interactions between paclitaxel and pharmacological inducers of hepatic metabolism. For example, in a phase I study of paclitaxel in children, rapid drug clearance was associated with the use of anticonvulsant agents (27). Similarly, plasma paclitaxel concentrations and toxicity were much lower than predicted in patients with glioblastome multiforme receiving 96-hr infusions of paclitaxel in a phase II study, possibly due to the induction of metabolism by anticonvulsant agents that are coadministered with paclitaxel (18). In addition, several in vitro, animal, and human studies have indicated that several classes of pharmacological agents may alter the metabolism and biliary excretion of paclitaxel (63–67) (see Section XII, Conclusion: Current Pharmacological Issues, below).

This metabolic profile may also be useful in explaining the sequence-dependent interactions that have been observed between paclitaxel and cisplatin and perhaps paclitaxel and doxorubicin (see Section IX, Combination Chemotherapy: Sequence-Dependent Drug Interactions, above). To evaluate this possibility, Monsarrat et al. pretreated rats with cisplatin before paclitaxel treatment (61). In both male and female rats pretreated with cisplatin, biliary metabolites were qualitatively similar compared with rats that were not pretreated. In contrast, total biliary excretion of unmetabolized paclitaxel determined over a 6-hr period following treatment was increased in rats that were pretreated with cisplatin. This increase was primarily observed in female rats, in which total biliary excretion of paclitaxel and metabolites accounted for 23% $\pm$ 3% of total drug disposition and increased to 34% $\pm$ 3% after cisplatin pretreatment; respective values in males were 30% $\pm$ 3% and 23% $\pm$ 3%. In both males and females, pretreatment with cisplatin modified the biliary excretion of neither major nor minor metabolites. Instead, the increase in total biliary excretion was due to the enhanced biliary excretion of unmetabolized paclitaxel. These results do not explain the sequence-dependent interactions noted in patients receiving cisplatin prior to paclitaxel. It is possible that cisplatin modulates alternate pathways of paclitaxel metabolism that have not yet been identified, thereby accounting for a reduction in the clearance of paclitaxel in patients pretreated with cisplatin.

Investigators at UTSA also identified another potential new metabolite peak on reverse-phase HPLC that eluted before paclitaxel in the plasma of a single patient receiving paclitaxel over 6 hr (68). Although the spontaneous conversion of paclitaxel to 7-*epi*paclitaxel has been demonstrated to occur in normal saline solution at 37°C after 48 hr and in the tissue culture medium of J774.2 murine macrophage cells, with approximately 50% of parent drug converted to 7-*epi*paclitaxel after 72 hr of drug treatment (8,69), the new peak was not felt to be due to 7-*epi*paclitaxel, since this epimer elutes after the parent compound. In addition, the epimerization of paclitaxel is reversible and 7-*epi*paclitaxel is also partially converted to paclitaxel under the same conditions.

XI. PHARMACOLOGY IN PATIENTS WITH ALTERED PHYSIOLOGY

Since patients with abnormal renal and hepatic excretory functions were not eligible to participate in early phase I, II, and III studies of paclitaxel, only limited information is available pertaining to the pharmacological behavior and toxicity of paclitaxel in patients with abnormal excretory organ function, especially in patients with moderate to severe hepatic dysfunction. Since the renal excretion of paclitaxel has been consistently demonstrated to be negligible and urinary metabolites have not been identified to date, dose modifications would not be anticipated to be necessary for patients with mild to moderate renal dysfunction. Preliminary clinical observations to date support this even in patients with severe renal insufficiency (70; Rowinsky ER; unpublished results). In contrast, since available evidence indicates that the magnitude of excretion of both paclitaxel and metabolites into bile in the 24-hr period after dosing in humans and rats is similar to that of other anticancer agents, such as the vinca alkaloids, in which dose modifications are required for hepatic excretory dysfunction, it is possible that hepatic dysfunction may significantly affect the clearance of paclitaxel. A retrospective analysis of 385 patients with and without mild to moderate elevations in liver function tests (predominantly elevations in hepatocellular enzymes) or renal function abnormalities participating in early phase II and III trials revealed no differences in the severity of both hematological and nonhematological toxicities in these abnormal groups (Bristol-Myers Squibb; data on file). However, Wilson et al. reported that patients with abnormal liver function tests (ALT $> 2 \times$ normal) had significantly reduced paclitaxel clearance rates in a phase I study of paclitaxel administered as a continuous 96-hr infusion (20,21). They also determined that the extent of the liver metastases was strongly associated with decreased paclitaxel clearance. Thirteen patients with no liver involvement had a mean paclitaxel clearance of 471 ml/min/ m^2, compared with nine patients with extensive disease who had a clearance of 336 ml/min/m^2 ($p_2 = 0.0022$). Seven of the nine patients with extensive liver involvement had a ≥ 1.5-fold ALT elevation, compared with 0 of 16 with modest or no liver involvement ($p_2 < 0.0001$). Reduced clearance and hepatic abnormalities were also associated with more severe mucositis requiring dose reductions. Preliminary data from a prospective Cancer and Leukemia Group B (CALGB) phase I and pharmacological study of paclitaxel in patients with hepatic dysfunction also indicates that patients with chemical evidence of hepatic dysfunction are more prone to the principal toxicities of the agent administered on a prolonged 24-hr schedule, specifically prolonged severe myelosuppression (71). Compared to patients without chemical evidence of hepatic dysfunction, there was a higher rate of dose-limiting myelosuppression defined as platelets $< 25,000/\mu L$ for greater than 3 days or ANC $< 500/\mu L$ for greater than 3 days in each of three groups of patients with the following liver chemistry profiles: 1) aspartate aminotransferase $> 2\times$ normal and normal bilirubin; 2) bilirubin ranging from 1.6 to 3.0 mg/dL; and 3) bilirubin > 3.0 mg/dL. Although formal recommendations for dose reductions have not been formulated, it seems prudent to reduce paclitaxel doses by at least 50% in patients with moderate and severe hepatic excretory dysfunction (hyperbilirubinemia) and/or significant hepatocellular enzyme elevations.

The severity of both hematologic and nonhematologic toxicities does not appear to be affected by age. Elderly patients (age > 65 years) who participated in early phase II studies were more likely to develop similar myelosuppressive and non-hematologic effects compared with younger patients (Bristol-Myers Squibb; data on file). Similar retrospective review of toxicity in the elderly have been performed by other investigators (72,73). In patients with recurrent or refractory ovarian cancer who participated in a phase II study of high doses of paclitaxel (250 mg/m^2 over 24 hr) and G-CSF indicated that age does not influence the ability to deliver paclitaxel on a dose-intensive schedule (72). However, the pharmacologic behavior of paclitaxel in elderly patients has not been evaluated in a rigorous prospective manner.

XII. CONCLUSION: CURRENT PHARMACOLOGICAL ISSUES

Although several biliary metabolites have been identified, the pharmacological disposition of the bulk of an administered dose of paclitaxel has not yet been determined. One possibility is that a substantial proportion is not metabolized immediately and avidly binds to tubulin and/or other proteins for relatively long durations. A planned study involving the JHOC, Research Triangle Institute, National Cancer Institute, and Bristol-Myers Squibb will determine the complete metabolic fate of paclitaxel using ^{14}C-labeled paclitaxel. These metabolic studies are important supplements to phase I studies that are establishing optimal dosing schemes for patients with excretory organ dysfunction. It is also anticipated that an understanding of paclitaxel's metabolic pathways will lead to an improved comprehension of the mechanisms for the nonlinear pharmacological behavior that is currently being observed, especially when paclitaxel is administered on brief infusion schedules. Such knowledge may lead to improved dose modification schemes, which are especially important in view of the potential unpredictability of paclitaxel due to its nonlinear pharmacokinetic behavior. This information may also lead to a further understanding of the relationships between pharmacological parameters, toxicity, and drug activity. The optimal use of paclitaxel in combination with other antineoplastic agents—such as carboplatin, topotecan, and cyclophosphamide—as well as potential interactions with other unrelated classes of agents are also currently being evaluated.

The extent of paclitaxel's hepatic metabolism may be significant enough to account for substantial interactions between it and other classes of antineoplastic agents, particularly agents that may modulate or be metabolized by cytochrome P450 enzymes. Although the mechanism for sequence-dependent interactions between paclitaxel and cisplatin are unknown, similar types of interactions may occur when paclitaxel is combined with other antineoplastic agents that either differentially inhibit P450 enzyme functions or are metabolized by P450 enzyme systems. The steps taken to develop the paclitaxel-cisplatin doublet, which involved an extensive evaluation of toxicological and pharmacological differences between drug sequences during phase I testing and the effects of drug sequencing on cytotoxicity in vitro, could be used as a model to develop other paclitaxel-based chemotherapy combinations. Similar analyses of sequence dependence are currently being incorporated into developmental studies of paclitaxel combined with cyclophosphamide, topotecan, and doxorubicin at JHOC.

Another potentially important source of drug interactions and variable pharmacological and toxicological results may be the differential effects of various H_2-

histamine antagonist premedications on the hepatic metabolism and biliary excretion of paclitaxel. H_2-histamine antagonists have been successfully incorporated into the premedication regimen used for prophylaxis against HSRs. Although cimetidine has been the most commonly administered H_2-antagonist in clinical trials of paclitaxel to date, ranitidine and famotidine have also been used, and the availability of these agents often differs significantly among practitioners. These H_2-histamine antagonists may have variable modulatory effects on the activities of many hepatic P450 enzyme systems, which may be involved in critical steps in the metabolism of paclitaxel (63–65). Of the commonly used H_2-histamine antagonists, cimetidine, has been implicated as being the most potent modulator of P450 enzymes, whereas famoditine and ranitidine have little or no modulating capability (74,75). Since it was perceived that the use of different H_2-histamine antagonists in clinical trials may portend variable effects on drug metabolism and may differentially affect pharmacological, toxicological, and antitumor profiles, both animal and human studies were begun to assess these potentially important concerns. In a study at JHOC, patients participating in the National Cancer Institute Treatment Referral Center ovarian cancer study were randomized to receive either famotidine 20 mg IV or cimetidine 300 mg IV before one course of paclitaxel and then crossed over to the alternate H_2-histamine antagonist before the next course. This effort has failed to demonstrate either substantial pharmacological or toxicological differences (67). Similar to this study, several other in vitro and clinical studies failed to demonstrate that cimetidine affects the metabolic and pharmacological behavior of paclitaxel. In a study in which ^{3}H-paclitaxel was incubated with human liver microsomes in vitro, cimetidine did not inhibit the metabolism of ^{3}H-paclitaxel, whereas other modulators of P450 enzymes—such as ketoconazole and fluconazole but not erythromycin—were inhibitory (65). In addition, investigators also failed to demonstrate that cimetidine alters the metabolism and biliary excretion of ^{3}H-paclitaxel in rats (34) and that large increases in the dose of cimetidine do not alter paclitaxel clearance rates (66). Other pharmacologic inhibitors of specific P450 isozymes have been demonstrated to inhibit specific metabolic pathways in human microsomal systems in vitro. For example, diazepam, an inhibitor of CYP3A isozymes, inhibits the formation of paclitaxel's major metabolite in vitro, whereas inhibitors of CYP2C, such as orphenadrine, erythromycin, testosterone, and troleandomycin, are potent inhibitors of the metabolism of paclitaxel to a minor metabolite with a hydroxyl group substitution on the phenyl group on the C13 side chain (63). Similar, modulatory effects have also been demonstrated with a diverse list of P450 inhibitors (64). Conversely, both in vitro and preliminary clinical studies indicate that inducers of P450 enzymes, such as phenytoin and phenobarbital, may induce metabolism (18,27,63).

Thus far, few clinical studies have attempted to study the population pharmacokinetics and pharmacodynamics of paclitaxel, particularly with respect to the influence of several critical pharmacological parameters, including the effect of paclitaxel C_{ss} and AUC, on response and toxicity. Several randomized GOG and ECOG phase II and III trials, which are evaluating dose response and scheduling, are incorporating limited pharmacological studies to address critical pharmacological issues prospectively.

REFERENCES

1. Hamel E, Lin CM, Johns DG. Tubulin-dependent biochemical assay for the antineoplastic agent taxol and applications to measurements of the drug in the serum. Cancer Treat Rep 1982;66:1381–1386.
2. Ohnuma T, Zimet AS, Coffey VA, et al. Phase I study of taxol in a 24-hr infusion schedule. Proc Am Soc Clin Oncol 1985;26:662.
3. Longnecker SM, Donehower RC, Cates AE, et al. High performance liquid chromatographic assay for taxol (NSC 125973) in human plasma and urine pharmacokinetics in a phase I trial. Cancer Treat Rep 1986;71:53–59.
4. Grem JL, Tutsch KD, Simon KJ, et al. Phase I study of taxol administered as a short IV infusion daily for 5 days. Cancer Treat Rep 1987;71:1179–1184.
5. Wiernik PH, Schwartz EL, Strauman JJ, et al. Phase I clinical and pharmacokinetic study of taxol. Cancer Res 1987;47:2486–2493.
6. Wiernik PH, Schwartz EL, Einzig A, et al. Phase I trial of taxol given as a 24-hour infusion every 21 days: Responses observed in metastatic melanoma. J Clin Oncol 1987;5:1232–1239.
7. Rowinsky EK, Burke PJ, Karp JE, et al. Phase I study of taxol in refractory adult acute leukemia. Cancer Res 1989;49:4640–4647.
8. Brown T, Havlin K, Weiss G, et al. A phase trial of taxol given by 6-hour intravenous infusion. J Clin Oncol 1991;9:1261–1267.
9. Rowinsky EK, Gilbert M, McGuire WP, et al. Sequences of taxol and cisplatin: A phase I and pharmacologic study. J Clin Oncol 1991;9:1692–1703.
10. Wall ME, Wani MC, Abreo MJ, et al. Determination of taxol in human plasma, urine, and bile (abstract). Second NCI Workshop on Taxol and Taxus. Alexandria, VA: National Cancer Institute, 1992.
11. Beijnen JH. Bio-analysis, pharmacokinetics and metabolism of taxol. European Cancer Center Newsletter. 1993;1:46–48.
12. Huizing MT, Keung ACF, Rosing H, et al. Pharmacokinetics of paclitaxel and metabolites in a randomized comparative study in platinum-pretreated ovarian cancer patients. J Clin Oncol 1993;11:2127–2135.
13. Bitsch F, Ma W, Macdonald F, et al. Analysis of taxol and related diterpenoids from cell culture by liquid chromatography-electrospray mass spectrometry. J Chromatogr 1993;615:273–280.
14. Grothaus PG, Bignami GS, Lazo CB, et al. Analysis and purification of taxol and taxanes using monoclonal antibodies (abstract). Second NCI Workshop on Taxol and Taxus. Alexandria, VA: National Cancer Institute, 1992.
15. Grothaus PG, Raybould TJG, Bignami GS, et al. An enzyme immunoassay for the determination of taxol and taxanes in Taxus sp. tissues and human plasma. J Immunol Methods 1993;158:5–15.

16. Leu J-G, Jech KS, Wheeler NC, et al. Immunoassay of taxol and taxol-like compounds in plant extracts. Life Sci 1993;53:183–187.

17. Leu J-G, Chen B-X, Schiff PB, et al. Characterization of polyclonal and monoclonal anti-taxol antibodies and measurement of taxol in serum. Cancer Res 1993;53:1388–1391.

18. Fettel MR, Grossman SA, Balmaceda C, et al. Clinical and pharmacological study of preirradiation taxol administered as a 96-hour infusion in adults with newly diagnosed glioblastoma multiforme (abstract). Proc Am Soc Clin Oncol 1994;13:179.

19. Rowinsky EK, Chaudhry V, Forastiere AA, et al. A phase I and pharmacologic study of taxol and cisplatin with granulocyte colony-stimulating factor: Neuromuscular toxicity is dose-limiting. J Clin Oncol 1993;11:2010–2020.

20. Wilson WH, Berg S, Kang Y-K, et al. Phase I/II study of taxol 96-hour infusion in refractory lymphoma and breast cancer: Pharmacodynamics and analysis of multidrug resistance (mdr-1) (abstract). Proc Am Soc Clin Oncol 1993;12:134.

21. Wilson WH, Berg S, Bryant G, et al. Paclitaxel in doxorubicin-refractory or mitoxantrene refractory breast cancer: A phase I/II trial of 96-hour infusion J Clin Oncol 1994;12:1621–1629.

22. Tamura T, Sasaki Y, Shinkai K, et al. Phase I and pharmacologic study of taxol by a 24 hour intravenous infusion (abstract). Proc Am Soc Clin Oncol 1993;12:143.

23. Horikoshi N, Ogawa M, Inoue K, et al. Pharmacokinetics of a 24 hour infusion of taxol (abstract). Proc Am Soc Clin Oncol 1993;12:146.

24. Eisenhauer E, ten Bokkel Huinink W, Swenerton KD, et al. European–Canadian randomized trial of taxol in relapsed ovarian cancer: high versus low dose and long versus short infusion. J Clin Oncol 1994;12:2654–66.

25. Kearns C, Gianni L, Vigano L, et al. Non-linear pharmacokinetics of taxol in humans (abstract). Proc Am Soc Clin Oncol 1993;12:135.

26. Schiller JH, Tutsch K, Arzoomanian R, et al. Phase I trial of a 3 hour taxol infusion plus or minus granulocyte colony stimulating factor (G-CSF) (abstract). Proc Am Soc Clin Oncol 1993;12:166.

27. Hurwitz CA, Relling MV, Weitman SD, et al. Phase I trial of paclitaxel in children with refractory solid tumors: A Pediatric Oncology Group study. J Clin Oncol 1993;11:2324–2329.

28. Sonnichsen D, Hurwitz C, Pratt C, Shuster J, Relling M. Saturable pharmacokinetics and paclitaxel pharmacodynamics in children with solid tumors. J Clin Oncol 1994;12:532–538.

29. Seibel N, Ames M, Ivy P, et al. Phase I and pharmacokinetic trial of taxol as a continuous 24 hour infusion in refractory leukemia in children (abstract). Proc Am Soc Clin Oncol 1993;12:145.

30. Gianni L, Kerns CM, Giani A, et al. Nonlinear pharmacokinetics, metabolism, and pharmacodynamics of paclitaxel in adult patients with solid tumors. J Clin Oncol 1995; In press.

31. Kumar GN, Walle UK, Bhalla KN, et al. Binding of taxol to human plasma, albumin, and alpha 1-acid glycoprotein. Res Commun Chem Pathol Pharm 1993;80:337–344.

32. Helmans JJ, Beijnen JH, Eeltink CM, et al. Paclitaxel (TAXOL) concentrations in glioma. Proc 8th NCI-EORTC Symposium. Amsterdam, Netherlands March 15–18, 1994, page 199 (abstract).

33. Lesser GJ, Grossman SA, Eller S, et al. Distribution of ^{3}H-taxol in the nervous system of rats (abstract). Proc Am Soc Clin Oncol 1993;12:160.

34. Klecker RW, Jamis-Dow CA, Egorin MJ, et al. Distribution and metabolism of ^{3}H-taxol in the rat (abstract). Proc Am Assoc Cancer Res 1993;34:380.

35. Gaver RC, Cheng T, Puhl RJ, Knupp CA. Tissue distribution of 14C-paclitaxel in the rat. Proc Am Assoc Cancer Res 1994;35:426.

36. Eiseman JL, Eddington N, Leslie J, et al. Pharmacokinetics and tissue distribution of paclitaxel in CD2F1 mice. Cancer Chemother Pharmacol 1994;34:465–471.

37. Rowinsky EK, Donehower RC, Jones RJ, et al. Microtubule changes and cytotoxicity in leukemic cell lines treated with taxol. Cancer Res 1988;48:4093–4100.

38. Roberts JR, Rowinsky EK, Donehower RC, et al. Demonstration of the cell cycle positions for taxol-induced "asters" and "bundles" by measurement of fluorescence, Feulgen-DNA content, and autoradiographic labeling of the same cells. J Histochem Cytochem 1989;37:1659–1665.

39. Roberts JR, Allison DC, Dooley WC, et al. Effects of taxol on cell cycle traverse: Taxol-induced polyploidization as a marker for drug resistance. Cancer Res 1990; 50:710–716.

40. Tishler RB, Schiff PB, Geard CR, et al. Taxol: A novel radiation sensitizer. Int J Radiat Oncol Biol Phys 1992;22:613–617.

41. Tishler RB, Geard CR, Hall EJ, et al. Taxol sensitizes human astrocytoma cells to radiation. Cancer Res 1992;52:3495–3497.

42. Dimopoulos M, Arbuck S, Weber M, et al. Primary paclitaxel (TAXOL) therapy for previously untreated multiple myeloma (abstract). Proc Am Soc Clin Oncol 1994;13:409.

43. Woodcock DM, Jefferson S, Linsenmeyer ME. Reversal of the multidrug resistance phenotype with Cremophor EL, a common vehicle for water-insoluble vitamins and drugs. Cancer Res 1990;50:4199–4203.

44. Chervinsky DS, Brecher ML, Hoelcle MJ. Cremophor-EL enhances taxol efficacy in a multi-drug resistant C1300 neuroblastoma cell line. Anticancer Res 1993;13:93–96.

45. Webster L, Linenmyer M, Millward M, et al. Measurement of Cremophor EL following taxol: Plasma levels sufficient to reverse drug exclusion mediated by the multidrug-resistant phenotype. J Natl Cancer Inst 1993;85:1685–1690.

46. Rowinsky EK. The pharmacology of taxol. J Natl Can Inst Monograph, 1993;15:25–37.

47. Markman M, Rowinsky E, Hakes T, et al. Phase I trial of taxol administered by the intraperitoneal route: A Gynecologic Oncology Group study. J Clin Oncol 1992;10: 1485–1491.

48. Francis P, Rowinsky E, Hakes T, et al. Phase I trial of weekly intraperitoneal (ip) taxol in patients with residual ovarian carcinoma (oc): A GOG study (abstract). Proc Am Soc Clin Oncol 1993;12:257.

49. Rowinsky EK, Citardi M, Noe DA, Donehower RC. Sequence-dependent cytotoxicity between cisplatin and the antimicrotubule agents taxol and vincristine. J Cancer Res Clin Oncol 1993;119:737–743.

50. Parker RJ, Dabholkar MD, Lee KB, et al. Taxol effect on cisplatin sensitivity and cisplatin accumulation in human ovarian cells. Monograph J Nat Can Inst 1993;15: 83–88.

51. Reed E, Parker RJ, Dabholkar M, et al. Taxol effect on cisplatin-DNA adduct repair in human ovarian cancer cells (abstract). Second NCI Workshop on Taxol and Taxus. Alexandria, VA: National Cancer Institute, 1992.

52. McGuire WP, Hoskins WJ, Brady MR, et al. A phase III trial comparing cisplatin/ cytoxan (pc) and cisplatin/taxol (pc) in advanced ovarian cancer (aoc) (abstract). Proc Am Soc Clin Oncol 1993;12:255.

53. LeBlanc GA, Sundseth SS, Weber GF, et al. Platinum anticancer drugs modulate P-450 mRNA levels and differentially alter hepatic drug and steroid hormone metabolism in male and female rats. Cancer Res 1992;5:540–547.

54. Holmes FA, Frye D, Valero V, et al. Phase I study of taxol and doxorubicin with G-CSF in patients without prior chemotherapy for metastatic breast cancer (abstract). Proc Am Soc Clin Oncol 1992;11:60.

55. Holmes FA, Walters R, Valero V, et al. The M.D. Anderson Experience with taxol in metastatic breast cancer (abstract). Second NCI Workshop on Taxol and Taxus. Alexandria, VA: National Cancer Institute, 1992.

56. Sledge GW, Robert N, Goldstein LJ, et al. Phase I trial of Adriamycin and Taxol in metastic breast cancer (abstract). Eur J Cancer 1993;29A(suppl 6):S81.

57. Holmes FA, Newman RA, Madden V, et al. Schedule dependent pharmacokinetics in a phase I trial of taxol and doxorubicin as initial chemotherapy for metastatic breast cancer (abstract). Proc 8th NCI-EORTC symposium on new drugs in cancer therapy. Amsterdam, March 15–18, 1994, p.197.

58. Kennedy MJ, Armstrong D, Donehower R, et al. The hematologic toxicity of the taxol/ cytoxan doublet is sequence-dependent (abstract). Proc Am Soc Clin Oncol 1994;13:137.

59. Monsarrat B, Mariel E, Crois S, et al. Taxol metabolism: Isolation and identification of three major metabolites in rat bile. Drug Metab Dispos 1990;18:895–901.

60. Monsarrat B, Alvinerie P, Gares M, et al. Hepatic metabolism and biliary excretion of taxol. Cell Pharmacol 1993;1(suppl 1):S77–S81.

61. Monsarrat B, Alvinerie P, Dubois J, et al. Hepatic metabolism and biliary clearance of taxol in rats and humans. Monograph. J Natl Can Inst 1993;15:39–46.

62. Gaver RC, Deeb G, Willey T, et al. The disposition of paclitaxel (taxol) in the rat (abstract). Proc Am Assoc Cancer Res 1993;34:390.

63. Cresteil T, Monsarrat B, Alvinerie P, et al. Taxol metabolism by human hepatic microsomes: identification of cytochrome P450 isozymes involved in its biotransformation. Cancer Res 1994;54:386–392.

64. Harris JW, Rahman A, Kim B-R, et al. Metabolism of taxol by human hepatic microsomes and liver slices: Participation of cytochrome P450 3A4 and an unknown P450 enzyme. Cancer Res 1994;54:4026–4035.

65. Klecker RW, Jamis-Dow CA, Egorin MJ, et al. Effect of cimetidine, probenecid, and ketoconazole on the distribution, biliary secretion, and metabolism of ^{3}H-taxol in the Sprague-Dawley rat. Drug Metab Dispos 1994;22:254–262.

66. Reed E, Sarosy G, Jamis-Dow C, et al. Cimetidine does not influence taxol steady-state levels (abstract). Proc Am Assoc Cancer Res 1993;34:395.

67. Slichenmyer W, McGuire W, Donehower R, et al. Pretreatment H$_2$ receptor antagonists that differ in P450 modulating activity; comparative effects on paclitaxel clearance. Cancer Chemother Pharm 1995; In Press.

68. Rizzo J, Riley C, Von Hoff D, et al. Analysis of anticancer drugs in biological fluids: Determination of taxol with application to clinical pharmacokinetics. J Pharm Biomed Anal 1990;8:159–164.
69. Ringel I, Horwitz SB. Taxol is converted to 7-epitaxol, a biologically active isomer in cell culture medium. J Pharmacol Exp Ther 1987;242:692.
70. Schilder LE, Egorin ME, Zuhowski EG, et al. The pharmacokinetics of taxol in a dialysis patient (abstract). Proc Am Soc Clin Oncol 1994;13:136.
71. Venock AP, Egorin M, Braun TD, et al. Paclitaxel (TAXOL) in patients with liver dysfunction (CAL6B 9264). Proc Am Soc Clin Oncol (abstract) 1994;13:139.
72. Bicher A, Sarosy G, Kohn E, et al. Age does not influence taxol dose intensity in recurrent carcinoma of the ovary. Cancer 1993;71(2 suppl):594–600.
73. Zaheer W, Lichtman SM, DeMarco L, et al. The use of taxol in elderly patients. Proc Am Soc Clin Oncol (abstract) 1994;13:441.
74. Somogyi A, Muirhead M. Pharmacokinetic interactions of cimetidine. Clin Pharmacol 1987;12:321–366.
75. Klotz U, Kroemer HK. The drug interaction potential of ranitidine: An update. Pharmacol Ther 1991;50:233–244.

7

Safety Profile

NICOLE ONETTO, MARCIA DOUGAN, SUSAN HELLMANN,
NANCY GUSTAFSON, JAMES BURROUGHS,
ALEXANDER FLORCZYK, RENZO CANETTA,
and MARCEL ROZENCWEIG
Pharmaceutical Research Institute
Bristol-Myers Squibb Company
Wallingford, Connecticut

I. INTRODUCTION

The taxanes represent a novel class of antineoplastic agents with broad antitumor activity (1). It is apparent that these new agents will play an important role in the treatment of patients with solid tumors. Paclitaxel was the first taxane in clinical development and has been administered to more than 10,000 patients worldwide. A variety of doses and schedules have been studied in an effort to optimize the antitumor activity of this new agent (2,3). New treatments for cancer must not only be effective but also have a favorable therapeutic index, especially in the palliative setting. Therefore, a careful analysis of paclitaxel-related adverse events is warranted to define the safety profile for the many doses and schedules which have been tested in clinical studies.

In the first clinical trials, safety concerns were raised because of the occurrence of severe hypersensitivity reactions and troublesome cardiac rhythm disturbances (4–6). As experience with paclitaxel increased, it became evident that severe hypersensitivity reactions could be prevented by administering a premedication regimen and that the cardiac disturbances associated with paclitaxel treatment consisted mainly of asymptomatic bradycardia or hypotension. The safety profile of paclitaxel has now been extensively studied, with myelosuppression and peripheral neuropathy being the major dose-limiting toxicities. Tolerance to paclitaxel treatment as well as its antitumor activity are affected to a great extent

121

by the regimen of administration. A clear understanding of the respective roles of the dose and schedule in the severity and frequency of paclitaxel-related adverse events is necessary in order to define the optimal therapeutic regimen and also to appropriately manage patients treated with various regimens.

II. CLINICAL TRIALS DATABASE

Most of the analyses presented in this chapter have been carried out on a clinical trials database containing information on 812 patients treated with single-agent paclitaxel in eight phase II and two phase III studies (Table 1) (7–16). Two hundred seventy-five patients were treated in eight phase II trials sponsored by the National Cancer Institute (NCI): 192 patients with ovarian carcinoma and 83 patients with breast carcinoma. Five hundred thirty-seven patients were treated in two randomized phase III trials sponsored by Bristol-Myers Squibb (BMS): 301 patients with ovarian carcinoma and 236 with breast carcinoma. All the data included in this database have been audited by BMS personnel. A wide range of doses and schedules were utilized in these 10 trials; thus, the effects of dose and schedule on the toxicity profile of paclitaxel could be characterized.

Table 1 Clinical Trials Included in the Clinical Database

	Institution	Patients treated[a]	Dose (mg/m^2)	Schedule (hours)	# Courses per patient	G-CSF
Ovarian carcinoma						
Phase II	NCI-MB[b]	15	170–300	24	1–12	+
	Albert Einstein	34	200 or 250	24	1–34	−
	Johns Hopkins	47	135–250	24	1–21	−
	GOG[c]	46	170 or 135	24	1–32	−
	NCI-MB	50	250	24	1–13	+
Phase III	Multinational	301	135 or 175	3 or 24	1–17	−
Breast carcinoma						
Phase II	MD Anderson	25	200 or 250	24	2–21	−
	MSK[d]	28	250	24	1–12	+
	MSK[d]	30	200	24	1–12	+·
Phase III	Multinational	236	135 or 175	3	1–10	−

[a]Corresponds to the number of patients included in this safety analysis.
[b]National Cancer Institute—Medicine Branch.
[c]Gynecologic Oncology Group.
[d]Memorial Sloan-Kettering.

The starting doses of paclitaxel in the 10 studies ranged from 135 to 300 mg/m^2. Prior to each paclitaxel infusion, a premedication regimen consisting of an oral steroid, a parenteral H$_2$ blocker, and a parenteral antihistamine was administered to prevent hypersensitivity reactions. Of the 10 trials, 4 utilized a lower starting dose for patients with poor pretreatment characteristics, such as extensive exposure to chemotherapeutic agents or radiation therapy. The range of doses tested in phase II studies was greater (135 to 300 mg/m^2) than that tested in the phase III trials (135 to 175 mg/m^2). In all protocols, courses were to be repeated every 3 weeks, providing adequate hematological counts and recovery from any non-hematological toxicity. In all of the phase II studies, paclitaxel was administered as a 24-hr continuous infusion. In the phase III ovarian study, patients were randomized to receive either a 3- or a 24-hr infusion, and all patients treated in the phase III breast study received paclitaxel as a 3-hr infusion. Granulocyte colony stimulating factor (G-CSF) was administered in four of the eight phase II studies but was not used in the phase III studies.

Eligibility criteria, dose and schedule of paclitaxel, and use of G-CSF varied from study to study. Consequently, some patients were at greater risk than others of developing adverse events. In general, patients in the phase II studies were at higher risk because of exposure to multiple prior regimens of chemotherapy and utilization of larger doses of paclitaxel administered by the 24-hr schedule. Finally, cardiac monitoring was more rigorous in the phase II studies, which led to increased reporting of cardiac events in these patients.

III. HEMATOLOGICAL TOXICITY

A. Leukopenia and Neutropenia

Leukopenia, specifically neutropenia, is the principal hematological toxicity associated with paclitaxel administration. The dose dependency and the rapid reversibility of paclitaxel-induced leukopenia and neutropenia were clearly established in the early clinical trials. More recent data from the phase III experience also demonstrated that leukopenia and neutropenia are greatly affected by the schedule of administration (12).

In the clinical database, 90% of patients experienced leukopenia or neutropenia (Table 2). Grade IV neutropenia (absolute neutrophil count < 500/mm^3) occurred in 52% of all patients, but the frequency of severe neutropenia varied greatly among studies (13% to 81% of the patients). The effects of dose and schedule were further clarified in the phase III ovarian trial. Grade IV neutropenia was more frequent with the high than with the low dose, irrespective of the duration of infusion. Among patients treated with a 3-hr infusion, 27% experienced grade IV neutropenia with a dose of 175 mg/m^2 compared to 13% at a dose of 135 mg/m^2 ($p = 0.05$). The infusion duration had an even greater impact than dose on

Table 2 Worst Myelosuppression

	Phase II Ovary	Phase II Breast	Phase III Ovary				Phase III Breast		Total
Infusion duration (hr)	24	24	24	24	3	3	3	3	
Dose (mg/m²)	135–250	200–250	175	135	175	135	175	135	
Total patients	$n = 192$	$n = 82$	$n = 84$	$n = 82$	$n = 62$	$n = 73$	$n = 118$	$n = 117$	$n = 810$[a]
Neutropenia (% pts)									
Any	94	94	99	98	79	79	91	84	90
WHO grade IV	79	76	81	70	27	13	27	21	52
Nadir (10³/mm³)									
Median	0.1	0.1	0.2	0.3	1.0	1.3	0.8	1.0	0.4
Range	0–6.4	0–10.9	0–6.6	0–7.0	0–11.8	0–6.3	0–13.4	0–8.1	0–13.4
Thrombocytopenia (% pts)									
Any	40	40	18	7	3	10	8	9	20
WHO grade IV	6	10	5	1	—	—	—	—	3
Nadir (10³/mm³)									
Median	128	124.5	146	108	212.5	230	195	190	166
Range	0–638	12–308	9–384	23–710	26–688	25–667	25–493	34–411	0–710

[a]Data not available for two patients.

the severity of neutropenia in this trial. At 175 mg/m^2, grade IV neutropenia was observed in 81% of the patients treated with the 24-hr infusion versus 27% of those receiving the 3-hr infusion (p <0.001). A similar difference in the frequency of neutropenia was observed for the patients treated at 135 mg/m^2, confirming that longer infusions were associated with more myelosuppression than shorter infusions irrespective of dose.

In order to determine whether paclitaxel-induced myelosuppression was cumulative, the impact of treatment duration on the severity of neutropenia was assessed by calculating the worst nadirs in the subset of patients receiving more than six courses of therapy (Table 3). For these patients, the worst neutrophil nadir documented during the first six courses of treatment was compared to the worst neutrophil nadir observed during the remaining courses. The median nadir counts were found to be comparable for the early and late periods, with a slightly higher median count in the later treatment period. This analysis demonstrates that neutropenia did not worsen with cumulative exposure to paclitaxel.

Analyses were also conducted to determine whether some specific pretreatment characteristics placed the patients at higher risk of developing severe myelosuppression. First, the number of prior chemotherapy regimens was considered. In both phase III trials, the frequency of grade IV neutropenia was comparable for patients previously treated with one prior regimen of chemotherapy, and those who received more than one prior regimen (ovarian study, 47% versus 53%; breast study, 24% versus 23%; respectively). The type of prior antineoplastic agent administered appeared to have little effect on the hematological safety profile of paclitaxel. Among ovarian carcinoma patients treated in the phase III trial, the frequency of grade IV neutropenia was comparable among patients who had previously received carboplatin and those who had not (53% versus 46%). In the randomized breast study, the frequency of myelosuppression was not affected by prior doxorubicin treatment. Finally, the effect of prior radiation therapy on the severity of paclitaxel-induced myelosuppression was examined. In the phase III breast trial, the frequency of grade IV neutropenia was similar among patients previously irradiated and those who were never exposed to radiation therapy (68% versus 65% at 175 mg/m^2). These observations made for patients treated with the 3-hr infusion may, however, not be generalizable to other schedules of administration associated with more severe myelosuppression.

Recent publications have further established the importance of the infusion duration on paclitaxel-induced myelotoxicity. With the 3-hr infusion, dose-limiting myelotoxicity does not occur with doses up to 210 mg/m^2 (17). Similarly, when administered over 1 hr, doses of 200 mg/m^2 can be administered without hematopoietic growth factors (18). In contrast, when paclitaxel is administered as a 96-hr infusion, the maximum tolerated dose is 140 mg/m^2 and hematopoietic support with G-CSF is necessary (19). In summary, the findings of the phase III ovarian study, which established the safety advantage of short infusions in

Table 3 Worst Neutrophil Nadir Counts by Treatment Duration (Patients Treated for Six Courses or More)

	Phase II Ovary	Phase II Breast		Phase III Ovary		Phase III Breast			Total
Infusion duration (hr)	24	24	24	24	24	3	3	3	3
Dose (mg/m²)	135–250	200–250	175	135	175	135	175	135	135
No. of pts with > 6 courses	$n = 63$	$n = 44$	$n = 35$	$n = 15$	$n = 24$	$n = 24$	$n = 24$	$n = 30$	$n = 259$
Neutrophil Nadir ($10^3/mm^3$)									
• Worst nadir up to 6 courses									
Median[a]	0.6	0.5	0.5	0.5	1.1	1.7	1.1	1.1	0.8
Range	0–10.5	0–12.6	0–2.8	0–1.5	0.2–2.6	0.7–4.6	0.3–2.6	0.3–3.3	0–12.6
• Worst nadir after 6 courses									
Median[a]	0.8	0.4	0.6	0.7	1.2	1.9	1.2	1.1	1.0
Range	0.1–8.2	0.1–5.0	0.1–3.1	0–6.5	0–3.6	0.4–5.0	0.2–2.8	0.1–3.5	0–8.2

[a]Median of the worst nadirs for patients over all courses per treatment period.

avoiding myelosuppression, have been confirmed by several investigators in different clinical settings.

B. Febrile Neutropenia/Infection

Paclitaxel-induced neutropenia, though frequent, is generally well tolerated. Only 13% of all treatment courses (590/4670) were associated with febrile episodes, which in about one-quarter of the cases were accompanied by a documented grade IV neutropenia (Table 4). This corresponds to an overall incidence of febrile neutropenia in 3% of courses (146/4670). Of interest, in the phase III ovarian study, febrile neutropenia was documented only in patients receiving the 24-hr infusion, further illustrating the safety advantage of the reduced myelosuppression associated with short infusions.

In the clinical database, infectious episodes were observed in 30% of patients and in 9% of all courses, but severe infections were rare. Nine patients (1%) died of infection; six of the fatal infections were septic episodes. For seven of the nine deaths, leukopenia or neutropenia was documented at the time of the infectious episode. Overall, the urinary and respiratory tracts were the most common sites of infection. The frequency of infection was higher in the phase II studies, in which all patients were treated with a 24-hr infusion. In the phase III trials, the rate of infection remained fairly constant throughout the treatment period (6% to 19% per course). However, a slight increase in the frequency of infection was noted after course six for the patients receiving extended therapy (data not shown).

Additional information available in the literature and in the BMS worldwide drug surveillance database on adverse events occurring with marketed use of paclitaxel confirms that severe infections are rare with paclitaxel treatment. It should, however, be emphasized that most of the patients treated with high doses (≥ 200 mg/m^2) and long infusions (≥ 24 hr) usually received G-CSF support, which probably reduces the frequency of both infectious episodes and febrile neutropenia (3).

C. Thrombocytopenia

Thrombocytopenia is rare and almost never severe. Eighty percent of the 812 patients included in the database maintained a platelet count $\geq 100 \times 10^3$/mm^3 while on therapy (Table 2). Thrombocytopenia occurred more frequently and was more pronounced in patients treated with higher doses and longer infusions. The phase III ovarian study confirms, in a randomized setting, the dose- and schedule-dependency of thrombocytopenia, but the magnitude of these effects was less marked than for neutropenia. Importantly, for the patients who remained on treatment for six courses or more, no increase in the frequency or severity of thrombocytopenia was noted (data not shown).

As expected, given the low incidence of thrombocytopenia, bleeding episodes

Table 4 Febrile Neutropenia and Infections

	Phase II Ovary	Phase II Breast	Phase III Ovary			Phase III Ovary		Phase III Breast		Total
Infusion duration (hr)	24	24	24	24	3	24	3	3	3	
Dose (mg/m^2)	135–250	200–250	175	135	175	135	175	175	135	
Total courses	$n = 1127$	$n = 652$	$n = 547$	$n = 400$	$n = 370$	$n = 433$	$n = 587$	$n = 554$		$n = 4670$
% Courses with fever	21	20	11	10	6	9	5	5		13
% Courses with febrile neutropenia	6	7	3	3	—	—	1	1		3
% Courses with infection	15	15	6	4	4	7	5	3		9

were uncommon and were only reported in 4% of all courses and in 14% of patients. Most hemorrhages were localized and minor. In the phase III studies, bleeding episodes were reported at similar frequencies irrespective of paclitaxel dose or infusion duration (4% to 10% of patients). Only six patients had an abnormal platelet count ($< 100 \times 10^3/mm^3$) at the time of a bleeding event, suggesting that most of the hemorrhagic episodes were more closely related to disease than to therapy. In addition, a minimal number of patients (18/812, or 2%) required platelet transfusions during paclitaxel therapy. The low incidence of bleeding and platelet transfusions confirms that paclitaxel does not usually induce clinically relevant thrombocytopenia.

D. Anemia

Anemia was observed in 78% of the patients and was severe (Hb < 8 g/dL) in 16% of the cases (Table 5). At the phase III doses (175 and 135 mg/m^2), anemia was more frequent and of greater severity in patients with ovarian carcinoma than in those with breast carcinoma, and no clear dose or schedule dependency was observed.

To better delineate the respective roles of underlying disease and paclitaxel therapy in the etiology of anemia observed on study, only patients with normal baseline hemoglobin were considered. In this subset, 69% became anemic on study and 7% had severe anemia (Table 5). A higher incidence of anemia was observed in the phase II studies, suggesting an increase in the incidence of paclitaxel-related anemia with doses ≥ 200 mg/m^2 given as a 24-hr infusion. However, no clear evidence of a dose-effect relationship was found in the phase III studies, in which lower doses were tested. The impact of treatment duration on the severity of anemia was evaluated by assessing the worst nadir according to treatment duration. For the subset of patients who had normal baseline hemo-globin values and received more than six courses of therapy, the median nadir hemoglobin value was 11 g/dL in the first six courses; this value did not change for the later courses, indicating the lack of cumulative toxicity on the erythroid lineage in the absence of preexisting anemia.

Twenty-five percent of all patients and 12% of those with normal baseline hemoglobin had red cell transfusions. No consistent relationship between pacli-taxel dose or schedule and red cell transfusions was observed in the randomized studies.

IV. HYPERSENSITIVITY REACTIONS

Hypersensitivity reactions were identified as one of paclitaxel's principal toxicities in early clinical trials. The current data confirm that a standard premedication regimen containing dexamethasone, an antihistamine, and an H$_2$ blocker largely prevents severe hypersensitivity reactions; minor hypersensitivity reactions remain common but are of little clinical significance. More importantly, phase III

Table 5 Worst Anemia

	Phase II Ovary	Phase II Breast	Phase III Ovary			Phase III Breast		Total
Infusion duration (hr)	24	24	24	3	3	3	3	
Dose (mg/m²)	135–250	200–250	135	175	135	175	135	
All Patients (% pts)								
Any	n = 192	n = 82	n = 84	n = 62	n = 73	n = 118	n = 117	n = 810[a]
	96	93	88	84	73	51	50	78
Hb < 8g/dL	35	27	12	13	8	3	2	16
Nadir (g/dL)								
Median	8.5	8.8	9.4	9.8	9.9	10.9	11.0	9.7
Range	3.6–12.7	3.2–12.4	6.4–12.1	6.6–12.9	5.2–13.2	5.9–12.8	5.8–14.3	3.2–14.7
Normal baseline (% pts)								
Any	n = 94	n = 57	n = 57	n = 38	n = 46	n = 106	n = 102	n = 552
	93	89	84	76	59	47	44	69
Hb < 8g/dL	24	16	4	3	2	—	—	7
Nadir (g/dL)								
Median	9.1	9.1	9.7	10.5	10.6	11.0	11.1	10.4
Range	6.6–12.7	3.2–12.4	6.4–12.1	7.8–12.9	7.1–13.2	8.0–12.8	8.0–14.3	3.2–14.7

[a]Data not available for two patients.

data demonstrate that with premedication, the risk of hypersensitivity reactions is not higher for short infusions (3 hr) as compared to long infusions (24 hr) (12). In the clinical database, severe hypersensitivity reactions were observed in 13 of 812 patients (2%) and they always occurred early in the treatment period (course 1, 2 or 3; Table 6). The most frequent symptoms encountered in these severe reactions were dyspnea, flushing, chest pain, and tachycardia. Of these 13 patients, 12 had the infusion interrupted and 10 required symptomatic therapy generally consisting of bronchodilators or intravenous fluids. Seven of the patients were rechallenged with paclitaxel without incident, using a reinforced premedication regimen as recommended by Peereboom et al. (20). Among these seven "rechallenged" patients, all paclitaxel infusions given following the severe hypersensitivity reaction were administered over 24 hours or more. No data are currently available to support the safety of a rechallenge using a 3-hr infusion. Minor hypersensitivity reactions are frequent (39% of all patients) and consist almost exclusively of flushing or rashes. Symptomatic treatment is usually not required. Minor reactions may occur at any course of therapy; the severity of these reactions does not increase with repeated administration of paclitaxel.

The phase III trials have addressed concerns regarding hypersensitivity reactions in patients receiving paclitaxel as a 3-hr infusion. The phase III ovary study demonstrated that short infusions were not associated with a higher frequency of severe hypersensitivity reactions than long infusions. This observation was confirmed in the randomized breast carcinoma trial, where all patients received a 3-hr infusion and no significant hypersensitivity reactions were reported. Similarly, minor hypersensitivity reactions were observed at comparable rates for short and long infusions: 45% of patients treated with the 175 mg/m^2 dose given over 24 hours had hypersensitivity reactions, as compared with 44% of patients treated over 3 hr. Additional data have become available in the literature on other schedules of administration. Hainsworth et al. (18) did not observe any severe hypersensitivity reactions in 88 patients receiving paclitaxel over 1 hr with premedication. Preliminary data suggest that the clinical premedication regimen may be simplified. Uziely et al. reported that 22 patients receiving more than 109 courses of paclitaxel with a reduced dose of dexamethasone did not develop severe hypersensitivity reactions (21). Interestingly also, at the National Cancer Institute (NCI), investigators conducting a phase I study with a 96-hr infusion decided not to administer the standard premedication regimen; their rationale was that the risk of developing severe hypersensitivity reactions was related to the rate of infusion. This phase I study was completed without incident despite the lack of premedication (19). Additional patients are receiving paclitaxel over 96 hours without premedication in various clinical trials conducted at several institutions in the United States. These trials should establish whether the omission of the premedication regimen is safe with such prolonged infusions. Currently, however, the administration of paclitaxel using a simplified premedication regimen or without premedication cannot be recommended.

Table 6 Hypersensitivity Reactions

	Phase II Ovary	Phase II Breast	Phase III Ovary				Phase III Breast		Total
Infusion duration (hr)	24	24	24	24	3	3	3	3	
Dose (mg/m²)	135–250	200–250	175	135	175	135	175	135	Total
Total patients	$n = 192$	$n = 83$	$n = 84$	$n = 82$	$n = 62$	$n = 73$	$n = 119$	$n = 117$	$n = 812$
% Patients with minor	39	46	45	46	44	36	37	29	39
% Patients with severe	4	—	—	1	3	3	—	—	2
Courses 1–3	$n = 498$	$n = 236$	$n = 233$	$n = 218$	$n = 168$	$n = 202$	$n = 332$	$n = 314$	$n = 2201$
% Courses with minor	18	21	23	32	21	19	22	14	21
% Courses with severe	2	—	—	<1	1	—	—	—	1
Courses 4–6	$n = 300$	$n = 175$	$n = 187$	$n = 133$	$n = 118$	$n = 133$	$n = 214$	$n = 182$	$n = 1442$
% Courses with minor	12	17	24	28	24	23	17	19	19
% Courses with severe	—	—	—	—	—	—	—	—	—
Courses > 6	$n = 329$	$n = 241$	$n = 127$	$n = 49$	$n = 84$	$n = 98$	$n = 41$	$n = 58$	$n = 1027$
% Courses with minor	10	16	30	31	27	21	7	16	18
% Courses with severe	—	—	—	—	—	—	—	—	—

V. CARDIOVASCULAR TOXICITY

The occurrence of severe hypersensitivity reactions led to extensive monitoring of vital signs and even to continuous electrocardiogram recording in most of the early clinical trials (6). This intense monitoring allowed for a detailed analysis of cardiac parameters during paclitaxel treatment and demonstrated that sinus bradycardia and asymptomatic declines in blood pressure were the most frequent observations. As experience with the drug increased, it became apparent that most of the reported events were not associated with clinically significant symptoms and that some of the cardiac disturbances were related to preexisting conditions rather than to paclitaxel therapy. However, high-level cardiac monitoring was usually restricted to the first courses of therapy and no data are available to study the impact of treatment duration on the frequency of cardiac adverse events.

In the clinical database, hypotension (a drop in systolic blood pressure by more than 30 mm Hg, as compared to baseline) and bradycardia (heart rate < 50 bpm) were common but generally did not occur simultaneously. Hypotension was reported in 26% of the patients and 7% of the courses. Bradycardia occurred in 10% of the patients and 3% of the courses. A decrease in blood pressure and/or heart rate was observed more frequently in patients treated with longer infusions; this may be related to the longer observation period. Importantly, most of the episodes of bradycardia or hypotension did not require any therapeutic intervention.

Significant cardiovascular events are rare during paclitaxel therapy. Among the 812 patients, 9 experienced severe cardiovascular disturbances that could be attributed to paclitaxel (Table 7). Five patients developed rhythm abnormalities during the infusion. Three of the patients continued therapy after the occurrence of dysrhythmia, but in two cases, a pacemaker was placed prior to any additional paclitaxel administration. Three patients had syncopal episodes after discontinuation of the infusion. One of these patients with a postinfusion syncopal episode had a history of coronary disease and died due to persistent hypotension despite pressor therapy. Finally, one patient developed a transient rise in blood pressure (maximum BP: 198/116), which resolved spontaneously after interruption of the infusion.

Other cardiac events occurred in 15% of the patients; these events often could not be clearly attributed to paclitaxel and did not require immediate therapeutic intervention. Special attention was given to the patients previously treated with doxorubicin to better define the cardiac tolerance of paclitaxel in this subset of patients. Interestingly, the frequency of cardiac events and vital sign alterations (i.e., bradycardia and hypotension) was not affected by prior exposure to anthracycline (Table 7).

In addition to the clinical database, information collected on more than 4000 patients participating in other NCI-sponsored trials confirms that most cardiac events do not appear to be clinically significant (22). This large compilation of data

Table 7 Cardiovascular Events

	Phase II Ovary	Phase II Breast		Phase III Ovary			Phase III Breast		Total
Infusion Duration (hr)	24	24	24	24	3	3	3	3	
Dose (mg/m²)	135–250	200–250	175	135	175	135	175	135	
Total patients	$n = 192$	$n = 83$	$n = 84$	$n = 82$	$n = 62$	$n = 73$	$n = 119$	$n = 117$	$n = 812$
% Pts with significant cardiac events	2	1	2	1	2	—	1	—	1
Type of event (% pts)									
Rhythm abnormality	1	1	—	1	—	—	1	—	1
Syncope	1	—	2	—	—	—	—	—	<1
Hypertension	—	—	—	—	2	—	—	—	<1
% Pts with other cardiac events	26	22	10	15	11	11	8	6	15
Type of event[a] (% pts)									
Tachycardia	7	10	—	4	3	—	3	2	4
Ventricular extrasystole	11	1	1	1	—	3	1	—	3
Palpitation	5	5	1	5	—	1	2	3	3
Extrasystole	9	1	—	—	6	—	—	—	2
Hypertension	3	—	2	2	—	1	2	2	2
Arrhythmia	4	6	1	—	—	4	—	—	2
Prior anthracycline									
Patients with anthracycline	$n = 73$	$n = 60$	$n = 16$	$n = 12$	$n = 6$	$n = 11$	$n = 86$	$n = 81$	$n = 345$
% Pts with cardiac events	30	22	13	33	—	—	9	7	16

[a]Events affecting 2% or more of the total patient population.

is certainly sufficient to indicate that routine cardiac monitoring is not required during paclitaxel administration in patients who do not suffer from preexisting cardiac problems. These conclusions, however, may not apply to patients with cardiac risk factors, such as unstable coronary disease or altered cardiac conduction; careful monitoring is still warranted for such patients.

VI. NEUROLOGICAL TOXICITY

Peripheral neuropathy is well recognized as the most important nonhematological side effect associated with paclitaxel therapy. Neurological symptoms often become dose-limiting when the severity of paclitaxel-induced myelosuppression is minimized by the utilization of short infusions or the administration of hematopoietic growth factors (11,17,23).

At the dose ranges tested in the database, 60% of all patients and 52% of patients without preexisting neuropathy experienced peripheral neurological symptoms consisting chiefly of numbness, tingling, and burning pains in the extremities (Table 8). These symptoms are clearly dose-dependent; in the two randomized studies, the incidence of neuropathy was significantly higher at 175 mg/m^2 than at 135 mg/m^2. On the other hand, at the doses tested in the randomized studies, infusion duration did not seem to have an impact on neurological symptoms. Despite their frequency, neurological manifestations were rarely severe, in particular in the two phase III trials ($< 5\%$).

The incidence and the severity of neurological symptoms are clearly affected by cumulative exposure to paclitaxel (Table 9). In both randomized studies, the median number of courses to first occurrence of neuropathy was determined for the subset of patients with no neurological symptoms at study entry. Among the patients treated with a 3-hr infusion in the ovarian study, the median number of courses to first symptoms was four in the 175 mg/m^2 arm and ten in the 135 mg/m^2 arm ($p < 0.01$). In the breast study, the corresponding number of cycles was three at 175 mg/m^2 and seven at 135 mg/m^2 ($p < 0.01$). Furthermore, in both trials, the median cumulative dose to first neurological symptoms was similar for the treatment arms using equivalent doses. Despite the increased incidence of neurological symptoms with cumulative dose, neurological toxicity did not usually require discontinuation of treatment in these two studies. Discontinuation of treatment is undoubtedly more common in studies using higher doses ($\geqslant 200$ mg/m^2), but it can generally be avoided if appropriate dose reductions are rapidly implemented upon development of severe neurological toxicity.

Neurological adverse events other than peripheral neuropathy are uncommon in patients receiving paclitaxel therapy. Two episodes of grand mal seizures have been reported in adult patients during the early single-agent trials (9,24). In a pediatric phase I study, one patient receiving 420 mg/m^2 over 24 hr developed a generalized seizure within 24 hours of completion of the infusion (25). Since these initial reports, some sporadic cases of convulsions have been reported to BMS

Table 8 Worst Peripheral Neuropathy

	Phase II Ovary	Phase II Breast	Phase III Ovary				Phase III Breast		Total
Infusion Duration (hr)	24	24	24	24	3	3	3	3	
Dose (mg/m²)	135–250	200–250	175	135	175	135	175	135	
Total patients	$n = 192$	$n = 83$	$n = 84$	$n = 82$	$n = 62$	$n = 73$	$n = 119$	$n = 117$	$n = 812$
% Pts with									
Any symptoms	64	89	65	39	65	55	63	44	60
Severe symptoms	5	7	2	—	2	—	6	3	3
Pts with no baseline neuropathy	$n = 133$	$n = 66$	$n = 63$	$n = 65$	$n = 51$	$n = 50$	$n = 110$	$n = 111$	$n = 649$
Any symptoms	53	86	56	23	59	36	60	42	52
Severe symptoms	2	5	2	—	2	—	5	2	2

Table 9 Number of Courses and Cumulative Dose to First Neuropathy (Patients with Normal Baseline)

	Phase III Ovary				Phase III Breast	
Infusion Duration (hr)	24	24	3	3	3	3
Dose (mg/m²)	175	135	175	135	175	135
No of pts asymptomatic at baseline	$n = 63$	$n = 65$	$n = 51$	$n = 50$	$n = 110$	$n = 111$
% Pts developing neuropathy	56	23	59	36	60	42
No. of courses to first neuropathy						
Median	4	N/R	4	10	3	7
95% CI	3–10	N/R	2–5	6–13	2–5	5–9
Cumulative dose to first neuropathy symptoms (mg/m²)						
Median	695	N/R	679	1323	521	940
95% CI	457–1223	N/R	354–719	807–1840	351–704	542–1071

drug surveillance, but in most cases the presence of brain metastases or the concomitant utilization of other chemotherapeutic agents confounded the causality analysis. The pathophysiology of these events is difficult to evaluate, since the penetration of paclitaxel into the central nervous system is nil or negligible (26,27).

Most recently, Capri et al. reported reversible visual disturbances consisting of scintillating scotomata and loss of visual acuity in patients with breast cancer treated with paclitaxel at a dose of 175 mg/m^2 or 225 mg/m^2 by 3-hr infusion (28). The decline of visual acuity occurred in 3 patients, all of whom were treated at the 225 mg/m^2 dose; visual evoked potential studies suggested a toxicity of paclitaxel to the optic nerve.

VII. MUSCULOSKELETAL SYMPTOMS

Transient arthralgia and myalgia without signs or laboratory indicators of inflammation have commonly been observed in patients receiving paclitaxel. These symptoms generally begin 2 to 3 days after completion of the paclitaxel infusion and resolve spontaneously within 5 or 6 days. Several factors have confounded the evaluation of the relationship between these musculoskeletal symptoms and paclitaxel administration: the wide range of doses tested, the concomitant administration of G-CSF, and the frequency of disease-related musculoskeletal pains, especially in patients with breast cancer.

In the clinical database, musculoskeletal symptoms were reported by 60% of the patients and were severe in 8%. Arthralgia-myalgia was more frequent in the phase II breast studies than in the other trials (90%, any symptoms; 17%, severe symptoms). This may be partially related to the use of higher doses of paclitaxel and the administration of G-CSF in two of the three trials (Table 10). No consistent dose- or schedule-dependency was observed in the randomized studies; however, the doses administered were moderate and the range tested in these trials was quite narrow (135 to 175 mg/m^2). Of interest, no increase in the severity or frequency of the musculoskeletal symptoms was observed following repeated courses of therapy, suggesting that these manifestations, unlike peripheral neuropathy, are unrelated to cumulative dosing. These mild musculoskeletal symptoms do not interfere with continued therapy and can be improved by nonsteroidal anti-inflammatory agents or other minor analgesics, if necessary (26,29).

The literature experience confirms that arthralgia-myalgia is more prevalent with higher doses ($\geqslant$ 200 mg/m^2). These symptoms may even become dose-limiting at doses higher than 250 mg/m^2 and occasionally require dose reductions and/or narcotics for palliation. In a phase I study using a 3-hr infusion with G-CSF, 44% and 66% of the patients treated with doses of 250 and 300 mg/m^2 developed severe arthralgia-myalgia requiring narcotic administration in the first course of treatment (17). Despite the limited number of patients enrolled in this trial, these

Table 10 Worst Arthralgia—Myalgia

	Phase II Ovary	Phase II Breast	Phase III Ovary				Phase III Breast		Total
Infusion duration (hr)	24	24	24	24	3	3	3	3	
Dose (mg/m²)	135–250	200–250	175	135	175	135	175	135	
Total patients	n = 192	n = 83	n = 84	n = 82	n = 62	n = 73	n = 119	n = 117	n = 812
% Pts with									
Any symptoms	58	90	67	46	60	58	51	56	60
Severe symptoms	3	17	10	5	10	1	13	10	8

results suggest that when very high doses are administered, musculoskeletal symptoms may be worse with shorter infusions.

VIII. GASTROINTESTINAL TOXICITY

Digestive symptoms generally do not interfere with paclitaxel therapy. Emesis occurs in approximately half of the patients, is generally of mild or moderate intensity, and is slightly more frequent at doses higher than 200 mg/m^2. Digestive symptoms usually do not justify the administration of prophylactic antiemetics other than the dexamethasone which is included in the routine premedication regimen for paclitaxel. Mucositis is also mild and was reported by 31% of the patients included in the database. Dose and schedule definitely affected the frequency of mucositis. In the phase III ovarian study, mucositis occurred in 31% of all patients who were treated with a 24-hr infusion as compared to 19% of those who received paclitaxel over 3 hours ($p = 0.02$). In both randomized studies, patients treated with 175 mg/m^2 were slightly more likely to experience mucositis than those treated with 135 mg/m^2, and mucositis was more common in the phase II high-dose trials (67% in the phase II breast studies and 41% in the phase II ovarian trials).

In addition to mucositis, rare cases of typhlitis have been reported as dose-limiting when paclitaxel is administered over 72 hours in combination with doxorubicin and G-CSF (30). The respective role of each of the antineoplastic agents in the genesis of this toxicity remains to be elucidated.

IX. ALTERATIONS IN LIVER FUNCTION

Since hepatic metabolism and biliary excretion play a major role in the elimination of paclitaxel (31), a careful analysis of liver test modifications during paclitaxel therapy was conducted in the clinical database. Overall, abnormal bilirubin, alkaline phosphatase, and SGOT values were reported in 8%, 38%, and 29% of the patients respectively. In order to more accurately evaluate the effect of paclitaxel on liver function and to avoid the bias introduced by preexisting abnormalities, an analysis restricted to the patients with normal liver function at study entry was performed (Table 11). In this subset of patients, abnormal values were documented for 7% (bilirubin), 22% (alkaline phosphatase), and 19% (SGOT) of the patients. In the randomized trials, no clear effect of dose or schedule on liver function alterations was documented. However, alterations in liver tests were more frequent with the higher doses administered in the phase II trials, suggesting a dose-response relationship (32). The frequency of liver function alterations was also analyzed by treatment duration for the patients with normal baseline values. Prolonged exposure to paclitaxel did not result in any cumulative hepatic toxicity; the frequency of bilirubin and SGOT alterations did not vary with time on

Table 11 Worst Liver Function Test (Patients with Normal Baseline)

	Phase II Ovary	Phase II Breast	Phase III Ovary				Phase III Breast		Total
Infusion duration (hr)	24	24	24	24	3	3	3	3	
Dose (mg/m²)	135–250	200–250	175	135	175	135	175	135	
Bilirubin (% pts)	n = 172	n = 79	n = 80	n = 77	n = 60	n = 71	n = 112	n = 114	n = 765
WHO grade I/II	11	6	5	3	3	3	4	4	6
WHO grade III/IV	3	—	3	—	—	—	1	—	1
Alkaline phosphatase (% pts)	n = 140	n = 52	n = 62	n = 64	n = 47	n = 60	n = 81	n = 69	n = 575
WHO grade I/II	31	35	15	13	17	8	17	17	20
WHO grade III/IV	2	4	—	—	2	2	—	—	1
SGOT (% pts)	n = 156	n = 42	n = 66	n = 65	n = 48	n = 59	n = 77	n = 78	n = 591
WHO grade I/II	24	17	11	9	13	8	21	31	18
WHO grade III/IV	1	—	3	—	—	2	—	—	1

treatment. Finally, no difference was observed in the safety profile of paclitaxel in patients with mildly abnormal liver function at baseline as compared to patients entering the studies with normal liver function (data not shown).

These observations, made in patients with normal or minimally altered liver function, are not necessarily generalizable to patients with severe liver dysfunction. A study has recently been completed in patients with more severe hepatic alterations. In this trial, the maximum tolerated dose of paclitaxel decreased with the severity of the liver impairment (33). Patients with bilirubin > 4 mg/dL did not seem to tolerate doses higher than 75 mg/m^2 administered over 24 hours. However, the criteria used in this study to define dose-limiting toxicity were conservative in comparison to most paclitaxel studies, especially for myelosuppression. Nevertheless, these data indicate that careful monitoring and appropriate dosage reductions are required for patients with preexisting liver dysfunction during paclitaxel therapy. More information is needed to develop guidelines for dose reduction in these high-risk patients, and further studies are also needed to determine the tolerance of other infusion schedules, particularly the 3-hr infusion.

X. OTHER SIGNS AND SYMPTOMS

A. Edema/Weight Gain

A fluid retention syndrome characterized by progressive peripheral edema, pleural effusion, and ascites has been reported with docetaxel, another taxane in clinical development. This syndrome has been described in patients receiving multiple courses of therapy and has led to treatment discontinuation after a median of five courses of docetaxel (1,34,35). Clinical manifestations of cumulative fluid retention have not been reported by investigators using paclitaxel in clinical studies. In order to carefully investigate the possibility of fluid retention associated with paclitaxel administration, the database was reviewed for any adverse events related to edema or other indicators that may be indicative of fluid accumulation, such as weight gain.

Edema in any location was reported in 21% of all patients (Table 12) and in 17% of the subset of patients who had no edema prior to paclitaxel therapy. Seven patients (1%) had severe symptoms (grade III). In six of these seven patients, edema was clearly related to disease. In the seventh patient, edema appeared after large volumes of fluids were administered. No patient had to discontinue therapy for fluid retention. Peripheral edema was the most common site of fluid accumulation (16% of patients). Upper extremity edema was reported more frequently in patients with breast carcinoma and may have been related to prior axillary node surgery. Ovarian cancer patients more frequently experienced lower extremity edema, which could be secondary to intraabdominal disease. Facial edema and generalized edema were each reported in 2% of patients. In summary, most of

Table 12 Worst Edema

	Phase II Ovary	Phase II Breast	Phase III Ovary				Phase III Breast		
Infusion duration (hr)	24	24	24	24	3	3	3	3	
Dose (mg/m^2)	135–250	200–250	175	135	175	135	175	135	Total
Total patients	$n = 192$	$n = 83$	$n = 84$	$n = 82$	$n = 62$	$n = 73$	$n = 119$	$n = 117$	$n = 812$
Grade (% pts)									
Any	30	37	25	13	16	12	13	13	21
Grade III[a]	1	1	—	1	—	3	1	1	1
% Pts with									
Peripheral edema	21	30	18	12	13	11	8	10	16
Facial edema	1	2	2	1	3	—	5	1	2
General edema	2	5	—	1	2	—	3	1	2
Unspecified	9	10	5	2	5	1	3	1	5
Patients with normal baseline	$n = 170$	$n = 73$	$n = 71$	$n = 79$	$n = 58$	$n = 69$	$n = 112$	$n = 112$	$n = 744$
Grade (% pts)									
Any	26	34	15	10	14	9	11	10	17
Grade III[a]	—	1	—	1	—	1	1	1	1

[a]No grade IV reported.

these manifestations could be attributed at least in part to the underlying disease and did not interfere with the delivery of paclitaxel therapy.

Since on-study weight gain could be a symptom of fluid accumulation, an analysis was performed in patients for whom weight gain and edema were reported in the same course. Among the 39 patients who gained 10% of body weight on-study, only 4 (2 with ovarian cancer and 2 with breast cancer) had concomitant edema, which was always mild or moderate. The lack of association between weight gain and edema suggests that reasons other than drug-related fluid retention, such as concurrent medical problems or even improvement in the patient's general condition, accounted for the observed weight gain.

B. Alopecia, Skin and Nail Changes, and Injection Site Reactions

Alopecia is almost universal after paclitaxel administration, especially in patients previously exposed to other chemotherapeutic agents (87% of the patients in the database). Paclitaxel-related alopecia is characterized by its abrupt onset and reversibility after drug discontinuation as well as by its completeness. In addition to scalp hair, axillary and pubic hair, eyebrows, and eyelashes are also lost.

Other skin events are rare and generally mild. A careful review of skin symptoms reported in the database was undertaken to rule out the existence of any peculiar dermatological toxicity associated with paclitaxel administration, since both skin and nail changes, sometimes dose-limiting, have been reported with docetaxel therapy. Excluding the transient rashes which were attributed to hypersensitivity reactions, rash and erythema were reported in 9% and 5% of the patients, respectively. Rashes were usually focal, and the upper body (i.e., neck, face, back, and chest) was often affected. Erythema was most frequently noted at previously traumatized areas such as radiation fields, surgical scars, and ostomy sites. Additional disorders reported in at least 2% of patients included itching (7%), skin ulcers (3%), and dry skin (2%). Onycholysis was reported in seven patients (1%) and was never severe. Onycholysis was associated with pain in only one patient and did not cause any functional limitations. Nailbed discoloration was observed in five patients. These minor skin and nail changes were never dose-limiting and, in most cases, not clearly attributable to paclitaxel therapy.

One type of dermatological toxicity that has been associated with paclitaxel therapy is the occurrence of radiation recall reaction. Three cases have been published in the literature. In two cases, the reactions were described as transient, localized, and rapidly reversible; both patients were treated with a combination of paclitaxel and cisplatin (36). The third case was more serious and consisted of extensive desquamation and necrosis of the chest wall in a patient who presented with superficial desquamation and brisk erythema in the irradiated field prior to paclitaxel therapy (37). In addition, six cases of minor radiation recall reactions have been reported through the BMS drug surveillance program. The underlying mechanism of these adverse skin reactions could be related to the ability of paclitaxel to potentiate radiation effects (1,36–38).

Injection site reactions have occurred at a low rate after paclitaxel administration (13% of patients), but the frequency might have been underestimated by the utilization of central lines in many patients. These local reactions tended to be more frequent with the 24-hr schedule than with the 3-hr infusion: in the randomized phase III ovarian study, 20% of the patients developed mild or moderate reactions at the injection site with the 24-hr infusion as compared to 7% with the 3-hr infusion. All injection reactions reported in the clinical database were managed successfully with noninvasive measures and did not result in any long-term sequelae. However, a recent report on three patients treated with 250 mg/m^2 of paclitaxel over 24 hours suggested that paclitaxel may be a vesicant and may cause delayed soft tissue reactions similar to those reported with vinblastine (39). In these three patients, the morbidity was modest and paclitaxel therapy was continued. At this time, the standard preadministration precautions for vesicant agents are not recommended, but careful monitoring should continue, especially when paclitaxel is administered in longer infusions (24 to 96 hr) via percutaneous intravenous lines.

XI. DISCUSSION

The large number of clinical trials performed with paclitaxel has enabled researchers to define the safety profile of this novel antineoplastic agent precisely. The specific toxicities related to paclitaxel as well as their respective incidence rates and dose/schedule relationships have been clearly established. Toxicities initially identified as potential threats to the clinical development of paclitaxel are now controlled: severe hypersensitivity reactions can be prevented effectively with premedication and cardiac toxicity was found to be a minor issue in patients with no cardiac risk factors. Furthermore, no new clinically significant toxicities attributable to paclitaxel therapy have emerged since the completion of the phase I program.

Myelosuppression remains the principal dose-limiting adverse event. Neutropenia is frequent, dose-dependent, and generally well tolerated. A peculiar characteristic of paclitaxel-induced neutropenia is the schedule-dependency, which confers a clear safety advantage to short infusions. The absence of febrile neutropenia in the patients treated with a 3-hr infusion in the randomized phase III ovarian cancer study underlines the clinical benefit associated with short infusions. In clinical settings where comparable efficacies of short and long infusions have been demonstrated, such as recurrent ovarian carcinoma (12), short infusions may represent a better therapeutic option. This is likely to be true for any patient receiving palliative rather than curative treatment. The reduced myelosuppression associated with short infusions presents some additional advantages. The administration of high doses of paclitaxel (200 to 250 mg/m^2) is feasible without growth factor support (17), and the reduced myelosuppression of short infusions facilitates the combination of paclitaxel with other antineoplastic agents. The lack of cumulative myelosuppression associated with paclitaxel administration is also important, especially in clinical settings where extended therapy might be beneficial, as in recurrent ovarian or breast carcinoma (9,10,13). Anemia and thrombocytopenia have not been dose-limiting with paclitaxel therapy, and transfusion requirements for patients receiving paclitaxel are minimal.

Peripheral neuropathy continues to be the second most important dose-limiting toxicity related to paclitaxel administration. It is clearly dose-dependent and not influenced by schedule, at least when moderate doses are administered. In contrast to myelotoxicity, neurological symptoms clearly increase in frequency and severity with cumulative exposure. However, a review of the clinical database has shown that with doses of paclitaxel less than 200 mg/m^2, peripheral neuropathy rarely requires discontinuation of treatment if appropriate dose adjustments are made. Peripheral neuropathy can be a troublesome adverse effect for combination therapy with other neurotoxic antineoplastic agents such as cisplatin and for the treatment of patients with predisposing medical disorders such as diabetes mellitus (1,4,23). The most successful therapeutic approach for relieving painful paresthesias remains the utilization of analgesics. Some experimental approaches with neuroprotectors or nerve growth factor are currently being tested and may be effective in preventing or minimizing the neurotoxicity (23).

With a larger number of patients treated, the low incidence of severe hypersensitivity reactions and cardiovascular events has become evident. The frequency of hypersensitivity and cardiac events is not affected by dose. The phase I experience suggested that the risk of hypersensitivity was increased when short infusions were administered without premedication (1,4,5). Therefore, before the completion of the phase III trials, the standard method of delivery was a 24-hr infusion with careful recording of the vital signs throughout. Sufficient data are now available to confirm the safety of a 3-hr infusion with premedication and to limit the monitoring of the vital signs to the beginning of the infusion in order to identify the rare patient who will develop a significant hypersensitivity reaction (12,16). Preliminary data even suggest that with premedication, paclitaxel can be administered safely as a 1-hr infusion (18). Similarly, with increasing experience, it appears that routine cardiac monitoring is not necessary. These recent observations have greatly simplified paclitaxel administration and have allowed for outpatient treatment. Still, the existing data may not be generalizable to patients with preexisting cardiac conditions, for whom careful monitoring should be recommended until additional data become available (22).

Of interest, emesis is mild during paclitaxel treatment; this represents a quality-of-life advantage, particularly for patients previously exposed to chemotherapeutic agents such as cisplatin or other highly emetic chemotypes. Transient and generally mild musculoskeletal symptoms are dose-dependent adverse events usually not reported with other cytotoxic agents. These symptoms may require analgesic therapy when high doses of paclitaxel (250 mg/m^2) are administered. Symptoms of arthralgia and/or myalgia do not worsen with prolonged treatment duration; if appropriately managed with symptomatic therapy and dose reductions, they do not limit the duration of paclitaxel therapy. Additional analyses are warranted to better define the effect of paclitaxel on liver function. In patients with normal hepatic tests, sufficient data are available to demonstrate that paclitaxel is well tolerated and that monitoring of liver function is not necessary, especially when doses of 200 mg/m^2 or less are used. The safety of paclitaxel in patients with impaired liver function remains to be defined. Preliminary data in patients treated with 24-hr infusion suggest that doses of paclitaxel should be considerably reduced in this patient population (33). The pharmacokinetics of paclitaxel in patients with liver impairment must be studied and might provide useful information for dose adjustments. Currently, the risk/benefit ratio should be carefully assessed before prescribing paclitaxel to patients with impaired liver function, and careful monitoring of laboratory tests should be instituted. In contrast to alterations in liver function, impairment in kidney function does not seem to interfere with the metabolism of paclitaxel or to change individual tolerance.

Fluid accumulation and dermatological adverse events have been dose-limiting with docetaxel. The extensive analysis of the clinical database presented in this review has established that paclitaxel therapy is not associated with edema or fluid retention even after multiple courses of treatment and that treatment was never discontinued for fluid accumulation, even in patients treated with high doses. Similarly, the skin and nail modifications reported in the clinical database were mild and nonspecific. Therefore, the types of limiting toxicities seem to differ between the two taxanes in clinical development.

The safety profile of paclitaxel has been carefully defined with experience in a large number of patients treated with various doses and schedules. This information should allow the treating physician to select the therapeutic regimen associated with the most favorable therapeutic index in accordance with the clinical context. The extent of monitoring should take into account the dose/schedule of administration and individual risk factors, such as prior cardiac abnormalities or hepatic dysfunction. Overall, the most important adverse events associated with paclitaxel are predictable, and paclitaxel-related toxicities are easily manageable, especially when moderate doses and short infusions are used.

ACKNOWLEDGMENT

We wish to extend our thanks to Mary Dion for her enthusiasm and good humor during the completion of this project, in spite of the time constraints.

148

Onetto et al.

REFERENCES

1. Pazdur R, Kudelka A, Kavanagh J, et al. The taxoids: paclitaxel (Taxol®) and docetaxel (Taxotere®). Cancer Treat Rev 1993; 19:351–386.
2. Arbuck S. Paclitaxel: What schedule? What dose? J Clin Oncol 1994; 12:233–236.
3. Arbuck S, Canetta R, Onetto N, et al. Current dosage and schedule issues in the development of paclitaxel (Taxol). Semin Oncol 1993; 20(4):31–39.
4. Donehower R, Rowinsky E. An overview of experience with Taxol (paclitaxel) in the USA. Cancer Treat Rev 1993; 19(suppl C):63–78.
5. Weiss R, Donehower R, Wiernik P, et al. Hypersensitivity reactions from Taxol. J Clin Oncol 1990; 8:1263–1268.
6. Rowinsky E, McGuire W, Guarnieri T, et al. Cardiac disturbances during the administration of Taxol. J Clin Oncol 1991; 9:1704–1712.
7. Sarosy G, Kohn E, Stone D, et al. Phase I study of Taxol and granulocyte colony-stimulating factor in patients with refractory ovarian cancer. J Clin Oncol 1992; 10:1165–1170.
8. Einzig A, Wiernik P, Sasloff J, et al. Phase II study and long term follow-up of patients treated with Taxol for advanced ovarian adenocarcinoma. J Clin Oncol 1992; 10:1748–1753.
9. McGuire W, Rowinsky E, Rosenshein E. Taxol, a unique antineoplastic agent with significant activity in advanced ovarian epithelial neoplasms. Ann Intern Med 1989; 111:273–279.
10. Thigpen T, Blessing J, Ball H, et al. Phase II trial of Taxol as second-line therapy for ovarian carcinoma: A gynecologic oncology group study (abstr 604). Proc ASCO 1990; 9:156.
11. Sarosy G, Bicher A, Kohn E, et al. Patterns of G-CSF usage in ovarian cancer patients receiving dose-intense Taxol (abstr 1331). Proc Am Assoc Cancer Res 1992; 33:222.
12. Eisenhauer E, ten Bokkel Huinink W, Swenerton K, et al. A European-Canadian randomized trial of Taxol in relapsed ovarian cancer: High vs low dose and short vs long infusion. J Clin Oncol. In press.
13. Holmes F, Walters R, Theriault R, et al. Phase II trial of Taxol, an active drug in the treatment of metastatic breast cancer. JNCI 1991; 83:1797.
14. Reichman B, Seidman A, Crown J, et al. Paclitaxel and recombinant human granulocyte colony-stimulating factor as initial chemotherapy for metastatic breast cancer. J Clin Oncol 1993; 11:1943–1951.
15. Seidman A, Norton L, Reichman B, et al. Preliminary experience with paclitaxel (Taxol) plus recombinant human granulocyte colony-stimulating factor in the treatment of breast cancer. Semin Oncol 1993; 20(4):40–45.
16. Nabholtz J, Gelmon K, Bontenbal M, et al. Randomized trial in two doses of Taxol in metastatic breast cancer: An interim analysis (abstr 42). Proc ASCO 1993; 12:60.
17. Schiller J, Storer B, Tutsch K, et al. Phase I trial of 3-hour infusion of paclitaxel with or without granulocyte colony-stimulating factor in patients with advanced cancer. J Clin Oncol 1994; 12:241–248.
18. Hainsworth J, Hopkins L, Thomas M, et al. Taxol administration by one-hour infusion: Preliminary results of a phase I/II study comparing two dose schedules (abstr 413). Proc ASCO 1994; 13:155.

19. Wilson W, Berg S, Kang Y, et al. Phase I/II study of Taxol 96-hour infusion in refractory lymphoma and breast cancer: Pharmacodynamics and analysis of multidrug resistance (mdr-1) (abstr 335). Proc ASCO 1993; 12:134.

20. Peereboom D, Donehower R, Eisenhauer E, et al. Successful re-treatment with Taxol after major hypersensitivity reactions. J Clin Oncol 1993; 11:885–890.

21. Uziely B, Jeffers S, Muggia F. Low doses of dexamethasone protect against paclitaxel (Taxol)-related hypersensitivity reactions following cycle 1. Ann Oncol 1994; 5:474.

22. Arbuck S, Strauss H, Rowinsky E, et al. A reassessment of cardiac toxicity associated with Taxol. Natl Cancer Inst Monogr 1993; 15:117–130.

23. Rowinsky E, Chaudhry V, Cornblath D, et al. Neurotoxicity of Taxol. Natl Cancer Inst Monogr 1993; 15:107–115.

24. Brown T, Havlin K, Weiss G, et al. A phase I trial of Taxol given by a 6-hour intravenous infusion. J Clin Oncol 1991; 9:1261–1267.

25. Hurwitz C, Reilling M, Ragab Y, et al. Phase I trials of Taxol in children with refractory solid tumors: A pediatric oncology group study (abstr 1410). Proc ASCO 1993; 12:412.

26. Rowinsky E, McGuire W, Donehower R. The current status of Taxol. Prin Pract Gynecol Oncol Updates 1993; 1(1):1–16.

27. Rowinsky E, Burke P, Karp J, et al. Phase I and pharmacodynamic study of Taxol in refractory adult leukemia. Cancer Res 1989; 49:4640–4647.

28. Capri G, Munzone E, Tarenzi E, et al. Optic nerve disturbances: A new form of paclitaxel neurotoxicity. JNCI 1994; 86:1099–1101.

29. Martoni A, Zamigani C, Aspasia G, et al. Antihistamines in the treatment of Taxol-induced paroxystic pain syndrome. JNCI 1993; 85:676.

30. Pestalozzi B, Sotos G, Choyke P, et al. Typhlitis resulting from treatment with Taxol and doxorubicin in patients with metastatic breast cancer. Cancer 1993; 71:1797–1800.

31. Rowinsky E, Donehower R. The clinical pharmacology of paclitaxel (Taxol). Semin Oncol 1993; 20(4,suppl 3):16–25.

32. Onetto N, Canetta R, Winograd B, et al. Overview of Taxol safety. Natl Cancer Inst Monogr 1993; 15:131–139.

33. Venook A, Egorin M, Brown T, et al. Paclitaxel (Taxol) in patients with liver dysfunction (CALGB 9264) (abstr 350). Proc ASCO 1994; 13:139.

34. Fumoleau P, Chevallier B, Kerbrat P, et al. First line chemotherapy with Taxotere (T) in advanced breast cancer (ABC): A phase II study of the EORTC Clinical Screening Group (CSG) (abstr 27). Proc ASCO 1993; 12:56.

35. Eisenhauer E, Lu F, Maldal A, et al. Predictors and treatment of docetaxel (D) toxic effects (abstr 506). Proceedings of the 8th NCI-EORTC Symposium on New Drugs in Cancer Therapy 1994:202.

36. Shenkier T, Gelmon K. Paclitaxel and radiation-recall dermatitis. J Clin Oncol 1994; 12:439.

37. Raghavan V, Bloomer W, Merkel D. Taxol and radiation recall dermatitis. Lancet 1993; 341:1354.

38. Tischler R, Schiff P, Gerard C, et al. Taxol: A novel radiation sensitizer. Int J Radiat Oncol Biol Phys 1992; 22:613–617.

39. Ajani J, Dodd L, Dougherty K. Taxol-induced soft-tissue injury secondary to extravasation: Characterization by histopathology and clinical course. JNCI 1994; 86:51–53.

8

Dose and Schedule Issues

SUSAN G. ARBUCK
National Cancer Institute
National Institutes of Health
Bethesda, Maryland

BARBARA A. BLAYLOCK
ADP/National BioSystems, Inc.
Rockville, Maryland

I. INTRODUCTION

Accumulating laboratory and clinical data suggest that it *may* be possible to enhance paclitaxel's effectiveness by increasing the dose, adding granulocyte colony stimulating factor (G-CSF), and/or prolonging the duration of infusion. Since all of these approaches alter toxicity, it is imperative to establish with certainty whether they improve efficacy. Laboratory experiments evaluating the effects of different paclitaxel concentrations and exposure durations provide helpful information, but randomized phase III clinical trials are required to identify the paclitaxel regimen with the optimal therapeutic index. This chapter summarizes available laboratory and clinical data, ongoing clinical trials, and some additional questions regarding dose and schedule that require investigation.

II. PRECLINICAL IN VITRO STUDIES

A. In Vitro Biological Effects

Biological effects of paclitaxel, including microtubule binding (1), microtubule bundling (2), promotion of microtubule assembly (3), and resistance to depolymerization (3) are concentration-related, and microtubule binding correlates with cell growth inhibitory effects in vitro (1).

Recent studies suggest that paclitaxel's mechanism of action may differ depending upon drug concentration (4). Half-maximal inhibition of HeLa cell proliferation and mitosis occurred at 0.008 μM paclitaxel, but there was no increase in microtubule polymer mass until concentrations of 0.01 μM or greater were reached. At high concentrations, the unique effects of paclitaxel in increasing microtubule polymer mass and microtubule bundles may contribute to its antiproliferative action. However, since these effects were not observed at the lowest effective concentrations, they could not account for the inhibition of proliferation observed at low concentrations. Instead, growth inhibition was associated with an abnormal organization of chromosomes and spindle microtubules similar to that observed with low concentrations of vinblastine and other antimitotic drugs that depolymerize microtubules (4). The microtubule mass increased half-maximally at 0.08 μM paclitaxel and attained maximal levels (five times normal) at 0.33 μM paclitaxel.

At high concentrations, paclitaxel binds stoichiometrically to tubulin in a 1:1 ratio (5). However, paclitaxel alters the process of shortening and lengthening bovine brain microtubules at paclitaxel/tubulin ratios as low as 1:150 (4). Under conditions with maximal mitotic block (0.003 to 0.010 μM paclitaxel) and no increase in microtubule polymer formation, the intracellular paclitaxel concentration was 40% to 70% less than the concentration of tubulin in microtubule polymer. Although the mechanism of inhibition of microtubule dynamics by paclitaxel is not understood, these in vitro results suggest that inhibition of microtubule dynamics and mitosis may result from binding of small numbers of paclitaxel molecules per microtubule and that low paclitaxel doses might effectively inhibit tumor cell growth.

The antifungal (6) and bacteriostatic (7) effects of paclitaxel are also dose-dependent. In a dose-dependent manner, paclitaxel decreased tumor necrosis factor-α (TNF-α) receptors in murine macrophages (range, 0.1 to 3 μM) (8), stimulated production of TNF-α in murine macrophages (range, 1 to 100 μM) (9), and activated the tumoricidal activity of murine macrophages in the presence of interferon-γ (5 to 35 μM) (10). Paclitaxel impaired the cytotoxicity of unstimulated peripheral blood mononuclear cells and natural killer (NK) cells against the NK-sensitive cell line K-562 and against an ovarian cancer cell line, OV-2774, also in a concentration-dependent fashion (11). Maximal effect was observed with 10 μg/mL. In addition, paclitaxel (10 μg/mL) interfered with induction of lymphokine-activated cytotoxicity and with lymphocyte growth in interleukin-2 (IL-2) cultures when paclitaxel followed IL-2.

Other paclitaxel-induced biological effects in human cancer cells are also dose-related. These include apoptosis in myeloid leukemia cells (range, 0.1 to 10 μM) (12) and in MCF-7 breast cancer cells (0 to 0.020 μg/mL) (13), chemotaxis in PC-3 ML prostatic cancer cells (range, 0.05 to 1μM) (14), and radiosensitization of astrocytoma cells (range, 0.001 to 0.1 μM) (15,16).

B. In Vitro Cytotoxicity

Although there is a clearly established relationship between paclitaxel concentration and a variety of biological effects, a number of investigators using a variety of cell lines and different assays reported plateaus on paclitaxel dose-response cytotoxicity curves (17–20). No additional benefit was achieved by increasing paclitaxel concentration above the plateau concentration, which differed for each cell line. These results suggest that it may be possible to identify a clinical dose above which toxicity but not efficacy increases. However, they also suggest that this dose will vary for different tumors.

In contrast to exponentially growing cells, cells in plateau growth phase are relatively resistant to paclitaxel, with an increase in IC_{50} (20,21). Several investigators have suggested that cytotoxic effects can be increased by prolonging the period of drug application and increasing the number of cells exposed while they are progressing through the cell cycle (17,20).

There is also evidence that prolonging duration of exposure to paclitaxel increases its effectiveness in multi-drug-resistant (mdr) cells (18,22). Some other natural product anticancer drugs applied for longer duration have similar effects in cells with the mdr phenotype (23). In many cell lines, even those without the mdr phenotype, paclitaxel IC_{50} or IC_{90} decreases when exposure duration increases (24–26).

Differences in a cell's ability to accumulate paclitaxel may contribute to the drug's relative effectiveness, even in cells without the mdr phenotype. Paclitaxel was 15- to 25-fold more toxic to A2780 human ovarian carcinoma cells than to CHO hamster cells (17). The difference in sensitivity correlated with a higher intracellular paclitaxel concentration.

Rowinsky was the first to report that prolonging paclitaxel exposure time produced greater cytotoxic effects than increasing concentration (27,28). Rowinsky's studies demonstrate that in some cell lines, for the same concentration $\times$ time ($c \times t$) product, exposure time was more important than concentration (Table 1). For example, in LC8A leukemia cells, an 11-fold increase in exposure duration was more effective than a 100-fold increase in concentration. Others reported similar results for a variety of cell lines using clonogenic assays, but conflicting data have also been reported, most often from studies using growth-inhibition assays (Table 2) (12,18,24,29).

A superior increase in effectiveness with prolongation of drug exposure is not observed in some cells that are very sensitive to paclitaxel (18,28). When the drug is very effective even with short exposure time, additional benefit with prolonged drug application time might be difficult to achieve.

Paclitaxel potentiates the effects of radiotherapy in a variety of cell lines in vitro. When astrocytoma cells were incubated with 0.01 μM paclitaxel for 2, 8, or 24 hr before radiotherapy (6 Gy), radiosensitization was achieved only with the 24-

Table 1 Concentration/Exposure Effects in the Clonogenic Assay of Paclitaxel

Human cell line	Concentration[a]	Exposure (hr)	% Survival	Reference
	μg/mL			
Lymphoblastic	0.1	2, 4, 22	88.1, 64.9, 6.5	28
leukemia	1.0	2, 4, 22	43.6, 49.6, 2.7	
LC8A	10.0	2, 4, 22	20.8, 1.1, 1.5	
Promyelocytic	0.1	2, 4, 22	34.2, 34.8, 3.4	
leukemia	1.0	2, 4, 22	12.5, 9.7, 1.2	
HL-60	10.0	2, 4, 22	0.05, 0.04, 0.05	
Lymphoblastic	0.1	2, 4, 22	60.2, 51.4, 51.2	
leukemia	1.0	2, 4, 22	33.4, 40.7, 23.1	
Daudi	10.0	2, 4, 22	35.4, 29.5, 0.02	
Myeloblastic	0.1	2, 4, 22	68.9, 66.7, 23.4	
leukemia	1.0	2, 4, 22	58.9, 63.0, 19.5	
K562	10.0	2, 4, 22	44.3, 51.0, 16.9	
Ovarian	0.01	2, 7, 18	NA, ≈80%, 2%	17
carcinoma	0.1	2, 7, 18	≈90%, ≈40%, 1%	
A2780	1.0	2, 7, 18	≈90%, ≈40%, 3%	
	μM			
Breast	0.01	24, 48, 72	6, 5, 4	20
adenocarcinoma	0.05	6, 12, 24, 48, 72	100, 54, 4.4, 3, 1	
MCF7	1.00	24, 48, 72	6, 1.5, 0.8	
	10	24, 48, 72	14, 14, 8	
Lung	0.01	24, 48, 72	4.5, 1.5, 0.7	
adenocarcinoma	0.05	6, 12, 24, 48, 72	88, 40, 3.6, 0.3, 0.05	
A549	1.00	24, 48, 72	6, 0.2, 0.02	
	10	24, 48, 72	44, 25, 16	
Myeloid leukemia	0.01	4, 24	<20, >60	12
HL-60	0.1	4, 24	<30, >80	
	1.0	4, 24	<60, ≈90	

[a]$1 \mu M = 0.854 \mu g/mL$.

hr exposure to the drug (15). Although paclitaxel administration for 90 min, 48 hr prior to radiation, had a radiosensitizing effect on ovarian cancer cells (30), Chang et al. (31) could not demonstrate a radiosensitizing effect of paclitaxel on lung adenocarcinoma cells for exposures of less than 6 hr at any paclitaxel concentration tested.

Preliminary reports from two in vitro studies performed with fresh human tumor specimens suggest that the paclitaxel concentration at which cytotoxicity (32) or microtubule bundling (33) is observed is highly variable. Still unresolved

Table 2 Concentration/Exposure Effects in Growth Inhibition Assays of Paclitaxel

Human cell line	Concentration[a]	Exposure (hr)	% Growth inhibition	Assay	Reference
	μg/mL				
Neuroblastoma	0.01	1, 4, 24	15, 25, 50	MTT	18
SK-N-AS	0.1	1, 4, 24	65, 67, 81		
	1.0	1, 4, 24	87, 82, 89		
Neuroblastoma	0.1	1, 4, 24	0, 0, 14		
SK-N-FI	1.0	1, 4, 24	0, 58, 76		
Neuroblastoma	0.1	1, 4, 24	61, 66, 68		
VA-N-BR	1.0	1, 4, 24	87, 84, 83		
Neuroectodermal	0.01	1, 4, 24	0, 0, 17		
tumor	0.1	1, 4, 24	43, 56, 47		
SK-N-LO	1.0	1, 4, 24	54, 58, 57		
Glioblastoma	0.1	1, 4, 24	56–58		
multiforme	1.0	1, 4, 24	86–90		
VA-MG-SL					
Glioblastoma	0.1	1, 4, 24	46–57		
multiforme	1.0	1, 4, 24	74–79		
U-373-MG					
	μM				
Myeloid	0.01	4, 24	≈20[b], ≈80	Cell density	12
leukemia	0.1	4, 24	<90, ≈95	(suspension	
HL-60	1.0	4, 24	≈95, ≈95	culture)	

[a] $1 \mu M = .854\ \mu g/ml$
[b] Approximate values ≈, greater than > and less than < values are estimated from graphs in cited reference.

are the therapeutic effects of polyoxyethylated castor oil, which in vitro appears to act as an mdr reverser and also to antagonize cytotoxicity at high polyoxyethylated castor oil concentrations (20).

III. PRECLINICAL IN VIVO STUDIES

In early studies performed by the National Cancer Institute (NCI), paclitaxel was administered as a suspension and antitumor effects were limited to intra-peritoneally (IP) implanted tumors treated with IP administration of paclitaxel or to human xenografts implanted in the subrenal capsule and treated subcutaneously (34). Later, optimization of the vehicle allowed a clear establishment of dose-effect curves in vivo in murine and human tumor xenograft models.

In mice bearing IP implanted P388 leukemia, paclitaxel administration every 3 hr for 8 doses (simulating a 24-hr infusion) was more effective than other schedules evaluated, including multiple treatments on days 1, 5, and 9 or for 9 consecutive days (34). However, the solubility of paclitaxel was not optimal and the maximally tolerated dose was not identified or evaluated for the single-daily-dose schedule (34). Thus, proper comparisons of 24-hr infusion and single dose were not done.

When studies to evaluate different schedules were performed by the Bristol-Myers Squibb (BMS) Company in the M109 lung cancer model with polyoxyethylated castor oil- or Tween 80-based formulations, no schedule differences were observed (35). However, the apparent best schedule from the P388 leukemia experiments was not evaluated. Neither a q3hr × 8 nor a 24-hr infusion schedule was tested.

Experiments performed in the M109 model did suggest that a daily × 5 or a daily × 7 (36) schedule was better than multiple dosing with longer intervals (2 or 3 days) between injections. Notably, maximal antitumor effect was achieved at dose levels that were only a fraction of the maximum tolerated dose (MTD). With a daily × 7 dosing schedule, administration of the MTD did not result in any therapeutic advantage over an equally effective but less toxic lower dose (36). These results are consistent with the plateau reported for dose-response curves from a variety of cell lines studied in vitro.

A dose effect was also seen with reduction of the number of metastases to lumbar vertebrae of severe combined immunodeficient mice following injection of PC-3 ML prostatic cancer cells that were previously incubated with paclitaxel at 0.1, 0.5, or 1 μM concentrations (14). The higher concentrations prevented the formation of metastases. A dose effect with decreased bladder tumor weight was also demonstrated when C3H mice were treated with paclitaxel administered directly into the bladder (37).

Dose-related toxicities were observed in preclinical paclitaxel toxicology studies in mice, rats, and dogs (38). They were most evident in tissues with rapid cell turnover and particularly in myeloid and lymphoid elements. Lethality was dose-related in rodents. Dose-dependent toxic effects on the peripheral nervous system were observed in mice treated with IP paclitaxel (changes in behavior, biochemistry, and electrophysiology) (39). Paclitaxel injections into the sciatic nerve of rats produced morphological degeneration, with abnormalities decreasing with distance from the injection, suggesting a concentration-gradient effect (40).

Preclinical toxicology studies indicated that a higher total dose was needed to induce death in rats when a daily × 5 schedule was compared with a single-dose schedule (34). For example, the LD_{50} (lethal dose for 50% of rats) was 255 mg/m² and 206 mg/m² for the daily × 5 versus single-dose schedules, respectively. With the exception of more severe gastrointestinal side effects in dogs receiving five daily doses, the type and frequency of toxicity observed did not vary with schedule. In contrast, when polyoxyethylated castor oil alone was administered to dogs, multiple smaller doses were better tolerated than single doses (34).

IV. CLINICAL TRIALS

A. Phase I Trials

The clinical development of paclitaxel almost ended during phase I evaluation because of an unacceptably high incidence of life-threatening hypersensitivity reactions and one fatality (41). These reactions are probably due to the polyoxyethylated castor oil required to formulate this poorly soluble compound; however, hypersensitivity to some component of the taxane itself cannot be excluded (42). Serious hypersensitivity reactions were observed more frequently when patients received the drug on shorter infusion schedules (Table 3) (42–54). Consequently, the 24-hr infusion schedule, with which objective responses were observed in phase I trials (53), was adopted for broad phase II evaluation. All subsequent patients also received a three-drug regimen (dexamethasone, diphenhydramine, and an H_2 histamine antagonist) prior to paclitaxel administration in an effort to prevent or ameliorate hypersensitivity reactions. With the adoption of both the 24-hr schedule and the three-drug prophylactic regimen, the incidence of severe hypersensitivity reactions decreased from approximately 18% on the 1- and 3-hr schedules (43–47) to 3% or less (53–56). Thus, the optimal schedule can now be chosen based on efficacy and not hypersensitivity concerns.

Paclitaxel 250 mg/m² can be administered over 24 hr with G-CSF support (54), and this dose can also be given by 3-hr infusion (55,57). A recent report documents that breast cancer patients who have had no more than prior adjuvant therapy tolerate a 3-hr infusion of 250 mg/m² without growth-factor support (57). Patients who have had more extensive prior therapy or extensive radiotherapy to

Table 3 Effect of Schedule and Premedication on the Incidence of Severe Hypersensitivity Reactions During Paclitaxel Phase I Clinical Trials

Duration of infusion (hr)	Without premedication			With premedication		
	No. of patients	% Severe hypersensitivity reaction	Reference	No. of patients	% Severe hypersensitivity reaction	Reference
1	49	16	43,44, 45,46	—		
3	17	18	47	20	None	55
6	31	3	(48)	51	2	44,45,46
24	42	2	49,50	70	3	53,54,56
96	20	None	51	—		
120	7	None	52	13	None	52

Source: Ref. 2.

bone marrow require either a reduction in starting dose (210 mg/m^2) or the addition of G-CSF (55). On either the 3- or the 24-hr schedules, however, 250 mg/ m^2 is the highest starting dose that can be recommended for adults. Neurotoxicity is dose-limiting, even with growth-factor support.

Although the 24-hr schedule of administration has been extensively studied, it may not represent the optimal duration of exposure. Longer administration schedules are under evaluation in phase I trials, alone or in combination with radiotherapy.

A preliminary report also documents that a shorter 1-hr infusion of paclitaxel can be administered safely with premedications (58). Its relative clinical efficacy is unknown.

B. Phase II Trials

Most initial phase II clinical trials were sponsored by the National Cancer Institute (NCI) and performed with a paclitaxel dose of 250 mg/m^2. Until recently, most were also performed with the 24-hr infusion schedule. Therefore, for many tumor types, neither lower doses nor shorter infusion durations have been studied.

A phase II trial was performed in platinum-pretreated ovarian cancer patients who received paclitaxel 250 mg/m^2 in a 24-hr infusion, with G-CSF (59). A higher than usual dose intensity (mg/m^2/week) resulted in a response rate of 48%; this was the highest response rate reported in phase II ovarian cancer trials (60). However, apparent differences in single-institution phase II response rates with large confidence intervals (often overlapping) are frequently related to factors other than treatment, including differences in characteristics of treated patients.

Table 4 summarizes response rates for breast cancer trials performed in patients with varying amounts of prior therapy and with varying paclitaxel doses and schedules of administration (51,61–69). The highest response rates were obtained in studies of less heavily pretreated patients who received higher doses administered over 24 hr. The response rate of 23% in patients with two or more prior therapies for metastatic disease (66% had received three or more prior regimens for metastatic disease), 87% of whom had anthracycline-resistant disease, is also notable when reviewed in conjunction with results of 3-hr infusions in generally more favorable patient populations. Again, one cannot compare results among phase II trials, but they can be used to generate testable hypotheses in randomized trials.

A 48% response rate was reported in anthracycline-resistant breast cancer patients who received paclitaxel administered by 96-hr infusion (51). Recently, this regimen was evaluated in patients whose breast cancers had already progressed during paclitaxel administered at 175 to 250 mg/m^2 over 3 hr or docetaxel 100 mg/ m^2 administered over 1 hr (70). Partial responses were reported in 6 of 16 evaluable patients (4 had previously received paclitaxel and 2 had received docetaxel). These very interesting results mandate additional study.

Table 4 Response Rates for Paclitaxel in Metastatic Breast Cancer

Institution	Dose (mg/m²)[a]	Schedule (hr)	Number of regimens for metastatic disease	% with prior anthracycline (% resistant)	No. evaluable	% CR + PR (95% CI)	Reference
Phase III							
Bristol-Myers Squibb Study Group[p]	135 / 175	3 / 3	0 or 1	67% (23%)	229 / 225	23 (17–29) / 29 (23–25)	61
Phase II							
Instituto Nazionale Tumori and Bristol-Myers Squibb[p]	175	3	≥1	100% 53% adjuvant 47% metastatic	15	46 (21–73)	62
European Cancer Center and Bristol-Myers Squibb[p]	250 + G-CSF	3	≥1	100% 53% doxorubicin 47% epirubicin	14	7 (2–34)	63
Univ. Southern Calif.[p]	135	24	≥1	NA	34	18 (7–35)	64
MD Anderson[p]	150 (135)	24	≥3	86%	18	33 (13–59)	65
NCI Treatment Referral Center[p]	175 (135)	24	≥2 (66% ≥3)	100% (87%)	156	23 (17–31)	66
Memorial Sloan-Kettering Cancer Center[p]	200 + G-CSF	24	≥2	≥96%	51	26 (14–40)	68
MD Anderson	250 (200)	24	≤1	92% (24%)	25	56 (35–76)	67
Memorial Sloan-Kettering Cancer Center	250 + G-CSF	24	0	—	26	62 (41–80)	69
NCI Medicine Branch[p]	140 + G-CSF	96	≥1	85% doxorubicin 21% mitoxantrone (73%)	33	48 (31–66)	51

[a]Lower dose in parentheses for poor-risk patients

[p]Preliminary report

Abbreviations: CR, complete response; PR, partial response; NA, not available

159

Paclitaxel was the first investigational drug with dose-limiting neutropenia for which the NCI Cancer Therapy Evaluation Program incorporated routine administration of G-CSF in phase II screening. It was also the first investigational cytotoxic agent that underwent phase II development without routine dose reduction for grades 3 and 4 neutropenia. Instead, doses were modified for prolonged or febrile neutropenia due to the observation that G-CSF affects the duration more than the depth of neutropenia. Several issues pertaining to G-CSF require resolution. With the addition of G-CSF, can higher paclitaxel doses be administered? If higher doses can be administered, is there evidence that G-CSF with these doses improves clinical results either by increasing response rate or decreasing toxicity? If the only benefit is decreased toxicity (without increased efficacy), could comparable benefit be achieved by the standard clinical oncology approach to dose-limiting toxicity—that is, by decreasing administered drug dose?

Recently, the NCI sent a warning letter describing the rare but sometimes lethal occurrence of neutropenic enterocolitis (typhlitis), which is not dissimilar to that seen in myelosuppressed leukemic patients undergoing induction therapy. Even rarer reports of gastrointestinal ischemia were reported (data on file, Cancer Therapy Evaluation Program, NCI). These adverse events occurred in patients receiving paclitaxel at higher doses, over 24 hr, with G-CSF and sometimes with other anticancer drugs. They may be the result of a more aggressive definition of dose-limiting neutropenia. If so, since this approach appears to be extending to the development of other drugs, the incidence of these serious toxicities may increase. It is imperative, for many reasons, that the true value of higher-dose paclitaxel therapy in conjunction with G-CSF be determined.

C. Phase III Trials

At the present time, data comparing different durations of paclitaxel infusion are available from only one trial (71). In it, NCI Canada/European investigators randomized patients with platinum-pretreated ovarian cancer in a 2×2 factorial design to one of two infusion durations, 3 or 24 hr, and one of two doses of paclitaxel, 135 or 175 mg/m^2. The higher dose was associated with a 5-week prolongation in time to progression. Neither response rates (17% versus 20%) nor survival differed for patients on the 3- and 24-hr arms.. However, more patients on the 24-hr arm had grade 4 neutropenia (74% versus 17%) and febrile neutropenia (12% versus 0%). Consequently, only 76% of patients in the 24-hr group received at least 90% of the planned dose, as compared with 92% in the 3-hr arm ($p < 0.0001$, personal communication, Elizabeth Eisenhauer). The incidence of severe hypersensitivity reactions was similar for the 3- and 24-hr schedules (2.2% and 1.2%, respectively).

The size of this trial, with its bifactorial design, precludes effective comparison of any single cell with another. Nevertheless, it is useful to consider the two higher-dose cells, 175 mg/m^2, which together appear superior because of their association with a 5-week increase in time to progression. There is a modest suggestion that the longer infusion schedule could be better than the shorter one when response rates are compared. These data suggest the need for an adequately powered trial comparing high doses on the 3- and 24-hr schedules, and such a trial is ongoing.

Data are now available from two randomized trials that compared paclitaxel administered at lower doses: 135 or 175 mg/m^2. The first trial, already described, was performed in women with ovarian cancer, and the other in women with breast cancer (61). In the latter trial, 471 patients with metastatic breast cancer (73% with visceral involvement) were randomized to receive paclitaxel 135 or 175 mg/m^2 administered by 3-hr infusion. All patients had previously received chemotherapy. Thirty percent had received only adjuvant chemotherapy, 39% had received only one prior chemotherapy regimen for metastatic disease, and only 31% had received two prior regimens, one for adjuvant therapy and one for metastatic disease. Sixty-seven percent of patients had received anthracycline-containing therapy, but only 23% were considered resistant to anthracyclines. A total of 454 patients were evaluable for response; response rates were 29% on the high-dose arm and 22% on the low-dose arm ($p = 0.16$). In patients who were resistant to anthracyclines, response rates were 29% and 13% with the high and low doses, respectively ($p = 0.15$). In this trial, although there were no statistically significant differences in overall response rate, response rate for anthracycline-resistant patients, or in median survival (11.7 versus 10.5 months), there was also a 5-week increase in time to progression for patients on the high-dose arm ($p = 0.02$). Thus, two phase III trials comparing doses lower than those maximally tolerated have demonstrated a 5-week increase in time to progression with 175 mg/m^2 as compared with 135 mg/m^2.

Although one cannot compare response rates from the phase III multicenter BMS trial with those reported in smaller, single-institution phase II trials, the 29% response rate obtained with 175 mg/m^2 administered on the 3-hr schedule, in a relatively favorable patient population with metastatic disease, is somewhat disappointing. It may be that this larger multicenter experience response rate is closer to that which would be expected in the community for similar patients. Alternatively, higher doses, which were evaluated in many of the other studies, the longer infusion schedule, or both may be important determinants of clinical efficacy.

D. Ongoing Phase III Trials

Several clinical trials were designed to address the schedule question (Table 5). Bristol-Myers Squibb has completed accrual of women with metastatic breast cancer to a trial that compares 175 mg/m^2 administered over 3 or 24 hr. Because

Table 5 Clinical Trials Addressing Dose and/or Schedule Issues with Paclitaxel

Ovarian cancer			Breast cancer			Lung cancer		
Dose mg/m²	Schedule (hr)	Others	Dose mg/m²	Schedule (hr)	Others	Dose mg/m²	Schedule (hr)	Others
BMS 016[a]			*BMS048*			*ECOG 5592*		
135	24		175	3		250	24	CDDP[b] + G-CSF
135	3		135	3		135	24	CDDP
175	24		*BMS 071*			—	—	CDDP + VP16[c]
175	3		175	24				
GOG 134			175	3				
250	24	G-CSF	*NSABP B26*					
175	24	—[d]	250	3	—[d]			
			250	24	G-CSF			
			T93-0165					
			250	3	—[d]			
			140	96	—[d]			
			CALGB 9342					
			250	3	—[d]			
			210	3				
			175	3				

[a]Bifactorial design 175 versus 135; 24 hr versus 3 hr.
[b]CDDP = cisplatin, 75 mg/m² dl.
[c]VP16 = etoposide, 100 mg/m², d × 3.
[d]G-CSF is administered on subsequent cycles only if dose-limiting neutropenia develops.

the degree of neutrophil toxicity varies on these two schedules, dose escalations were permitted in an attempt to achieve equitoxic doses on the two arms. Results from this trial are not yet available.

Another study was designed to compare the highest doses that can be administered on each schedule in an effort to establish the optimal schedule for adjuvant therapy. Paclitaxel, 250 mg/m^2, is administered over 3 or 24 hr to women receiving first-line therapy for metastatic breast cancer. In addition, G-CSF is administered in order to maintain dose intensity on the 24-hr arm; it is used on the 3-hr arm only if necessary.

The 48% response rate reported in anthracycline-refractory breast cancer patients receiving 96-hr infusion (51) in conjunction with objective responses with this schedule in breast cancer patients who had previously progressed during treatment with short taxane infusions (70) and the preclinical data reviewed previously, together provide the rationale for an ongoing study comparing 3- versus 96-hr infusions in breast cancer patients.

Important questions regarding dose and G-CSF are also under investigation in phase III trials (Table 5). Based upon encouraging phase II results with high-dose paclitaxel and G-CSF (59), the Gynecologic Oncology Group (GOG) initiated a trial comparing doses of 135, 175, and 250 mg/m^2 administered over 24 hr to platinum-pretreated ovarian cancer patients. The high-dose arm includes prophylactic G-CSF. Since this study was designed to test the dose-response question, G-CSF is added in the lower-dose arms in an effort to maintain the dose if dose-limiting neutropenia develops without other dose-limiting toxicity. Unfortunately, when accrual declined precipitously following commercial availability of paclitaxel and the release of efficacy results from the NCIC/European ovarian cancer trial (71), the GOG discontinued the low-dose arm with only 77 of 200 patients accrued.

The Cancer and Leukemia Group B is evaluating 175, 210, and 250 mg/m^2 administered over 3 hr to patients receiving second-line therapy for metastatic breast cancer. Only if dose-limiting neutropenia occurs, G-CSF is administered to patients on the high-dose arm. No G-CSF will be administered to those patients receiving 210 mg/m^2. If this dose is not adequately tolerated, the arm will be dropped, using early-stopping-rule guidelines. This study was designed in an effort to identify the 3-hr dose with the optimal therapeutic index.

The Eastern Cooperative Oncology Group is performing a three-arm trial in non–small cell lung cancer in which all patients receive cisplatin 75 mg/m^2. Patients on two of the arms receive paclitaxel at one of two doses, either 250 mg/m^2 with G-CSF or 135 mg/m^2 without G-CSF. Patients who have dose-limiting neutropenia on the lower-dose arm subsequently receive a chemotherapy dose reduction and do not receive G-CSF. This trial will help determine whether there is clinical benefit from a higher paclitaxel dose with G-CSF compared with a lower dose without G-CSF.

V. PHARMACOKINETICS

Issues of paclitaxel dose and schedule cannot be addressed without some consideration of human pharmacokinetics and pharmacodynamics. Table 6 summarizes maximal plasma concentrations (C_{max}) and area-under-the-curve (AUC) data achieved with paclitaxel administered on a variety of schedules with a range of doses (46,51,53,55,72,73). In clinical trials with doses ranging from 135 to 250 mg/m^2, peak plasma concentrations of 2.5 to 14 μM were achieved with the 3-hr infusion (55,72,73) and plasma concentrations ranging from 0.23 to 0.94 μM were achieved with 24-hr infusions (53,72). With doses ranging from 120 to 140 mg/m^2 administered by 96-hr infusion, plasma concentrations ranged from 0.053 to 0.072 μM (51). The paclitaxel-beta half-life is approximately 4 to 8 hr (38).

Table 6   Plasma Concentrations of Paclitaxel with Intravenous Infusions[a]

	3 Hr		6 Hr		24 Hr		96 Hr	
Dose (mg/m^2)	AUC $\mu M \cdot$hr	C_{max} μM	AUC $\mu M \cdot$hr	C_{max} μM	AUC $\mu M \cdot$hr	C_{max} μM	AUC $\mu M \cdot$hr	C_{max} μM
120							NA	0.053 (51)
135	9.37; 10.8 (72); (73)	2.54; 3.3 (72); (73)			7.31 (72)	0.23 (72)		
140							NA	0.072 (51)
160							NA	0.077 (51)
175	16.8; 18.5 (72); (73)	4.27; 5.9 (72); (73)	26.3 (46)	3.19 (46)	9.30 (72)	0.43 (72)		
200			27.4 (46)	5.27 (46)	11.41 (53)	0.56 (53)		
210	22.4 (55)	6.0 (55)						
230			29.3 (46)	4.09 (46)				
250	37.3; 31.2 (73); (55)	10.0; 9.2 (73); (55)			14.87 (53)	0.88 (53)		
275			56.8 (46)	8.11 (46)	14.52 (53)	0.94 (53)		
300	47.6; 48.7 (73); (55)	12.9; 14.2 (73); (55)						

[a]Mean values. Figures in parentheses are reference numbers.

Abbreviations: NA, not available; AUC, area under concentration time curve; C_{max}, peak plasma concentration.

There is a disproportionate increase in C_{max} and AUC following administration of higher paclitaxel doses (Table 6). This nonlinear or saturable pharmacokinetic behavior was not appreciated in initial studies but has now been documented with both 3- and 24-hr paclitaxel schedules (55,72–74). Since nonlinearity is more apparent with the shorter infusion (72), dose adjustments on the shorter schedule are more likely to be associated with a disproportionate change in AUC and C_{max} (75). Such changes might be expected to have important clinical consequences. For example, a small dose increase may cause greater than expected toxicity. A small dose decrease may cause loss in anticancer efficacy. A lower incidence of neutropenia associated with the 3-hr schedule as compared with the 24-hr schedule, despite a higher AUC on the 3-hr schedule, is surprising (71,72). The percent decrease in neutrophil count was retrospectively associated with the time the plasma concentration exceeded a threshold concentration of 0.1 μM in one study (72) and 0.05 μM in another (76). When paclitaxel was administered on a 96-hr schedule, both neutropenia and mucositis appeared to correlate with a steady-state plasma concentration greater than 0.07 μM (51).

VI. DISCUSSION

Two phase III trials, one in ovarian (71) and one in breast (61) cancer, have demonstrated a dose effect. Although the 5-week improvement in median time to progression in patients who received 175 mg/m² compared with those who received 135 mg/m² was small, so was the dose increment (<30%). It is possible that comparisons with higher doses will demonstrate greater effectiveness.

Higher paclitaxel doses, however, result in added toxicity. Therefore, in an effort to ameliorate neutrophil toxicity and maximize dose intensity, G-CSF has been administered in combination with paclitaxel (54,59). Although G-CSF decreases the duration of severe neutropenia, it does not improve the neutrophil nadir (69). Nevertheless, when dose reductions were required by study protocol for prolonged or febrile neutropenia and not for a low nadir neutrophil count, one study suggested that G-CSF permitted maintenance of a higher paclitaxel dose intensity (59). This approach was used for many NCI-sponsored phase II paclitaxel trials. It is, however, accompanied by greater cumulative nonhematological toxicity, most often neurotoxicity, which may necessitate dose reduction (77). Other dose-related nonhematological toxicities—including myalgia, arthralgia, and mucositis—may also mandate a dose decrease (77).

When results of phase I studies with various paclitaxel doses are reviewed, it is apparent that the maximally tolerated dose decreases as infusion duration increases (60). Nevertheless, the lower incidence of neutropenia observed with the 3-hr as compared with the 24-hr administration schedule at the same dose was not predicted. Notably, no in vitro studies comparing cytotoxic effects of different paclitaxel exposure durations in human bone marrow and tumor cells have been reported. The lower incidence of neutropenia on the short infusion schedule, however, is consistent with in vitro studies demonstrating less tumor cell cytotoxicity with shorter periods of drug application. It provides additional support for testing the hypothesis that paclitaxel therapy has greater antitumor activity when it is administered by longer infusion. However, the relative therapeutic index of paclitaxel in relation to the duration of paclitaxel exposure remains to be determined.

In order to optimize the paclitaxel therapeutic index, the efficacy and toxicity of different paclitaxel doses and schedules must be established in carefully designed comparative trials. Studies that incorporate some evaluation of quality of life—for example, cancer- and toxicity-related symptoms—in addition to pharmacokinetic and pharmacodynamic evaluation would be most instructive. Such studies are ongoing in ovary, breast, and lung cancer.

The only completed randomized trial comparing schedules (3 and 24-hr) in pretreated ovarian cancer patients did not demonstrate schedule-related differences in efficacy (71). However, patients receiving the 24-hr infusion had more neutropenia, which resulted in more dose reductions and perhaps a lower effective dose intensity on that arm. In terms of $mg/m^2/week$ of paclitaxel, less was given with the 24-hr infusion, but the striking differences in both toxicity and AUC for the same dose administered on 3- or 24-hr schedules indicate that this traditional measure of dose intensity cannot be used to compare these schedules. The possible difference in administered dose intensity would be irrelevant if duration of severe neutropenia could not be shortened by the addition of G-CSF. Because of the low incidence of severe toxicity on the 3-hr arm, however, it is also apparent that a higher dose could have been administered on that arm. A randomized study comparing equitoxic paclitaxel doses might permit a clearer evaluation of the effects of schedule.

Perhaps more convincing support for the hypothesis that longer paclitaxel exposure is more effective is provided by the recent preliminary report demonstrating objective responses in patients with breast cancer whose tumors have already progressed on short taxane infusions administered at maximally tolerated doses (70). Responses occurred with 96-hr paclitaxel infusion in patients previously treated with paclitaxel or with docetaxel.

Available data suggest that a short infusion may be especially appropriate for sensitive tumors. However, tumors that are not exquisitely sensitive may require more prolonged paclitaxel exposure. This hypothesis is being addressed in a comparison of 3- versus 96-hr infusion in patients with breast cancer. The addition of a crossover at progression is under discussion. This study design, with an early-stopping rule for the crossover, would specifically address the relative merits of the two schedules (with differing C_{max} and AUC) upon initial exposure and at the time of tumor progression.

Although most patients were hospitalized for 24-hr infusions of paclitaxel in the past, increasing experience with outpatient administration of both 24- and 96-hr infusions is developing at several institutions. Infusion pumps with bags and tubing compatible with paclitaxel administration are now available (78). This development is facilitating randomized trials comparing 3-hr administration schedules with longer ones.

Although many studies with paclitaxel are focused on identifying the optimal dose and schedule of paclitaxel, additional work remains. Data obtained from palliative studies in heavily pretreated patients are usually not applicable to previously untreated patients where the objective is cure. Even a small improvement in cure rate resulting from alterations in paclitaxel dose and/or schedule would be an important achievement in women with early breast cancer, for example. The first generation of adjuvant paclitaxel trials in breast cancer uses the more convenient 3-hr schedule, which is associated with less neutropenia. However, if ongoing schedule comparisons show benefit of the 24- and 96-hr administration schedules, subsequent studies are expected to incorporate evaluation of a longer infusion.

Schedule comparisons should be carefully conducted using equitoxic and optimal doses that are appropriate for the target populations under consideration. With the 3-hr infusion, previously untreated patients tolerate doses higher than those administered on the completed phase III trials (135 and 175 mg/m^2), and these higher doses must be evaluated (225 to 250 mg/m^2).

Similarly, it is important to remember that clinical benefit (increased surgical response rate, time to progression, preliminary suggestion of increased survival) was reported in women with suboptimal ovarian cancer who received paclitaxel 135 mg/m^2 over 24 hr in combination with cisplatin, as compared with the standard cyclophosphamide/cisplatin regimen (79). A confirmatory study is planned; however, it does not precisely replicate the positive GOG study. In the planned European Organization for the Research and Treatment of Cancer (EORTC) study, paclitaxel will be administered over 3 hr to a population that includes earlier-stage disease (stages II to IV) and optimally debulked patients. If the GOG results are confirmed with the 3-hr schedule, this trial will provide support for adopting the 3-hr schedule. If, however, this trial does not appear to confirm the GOG results, it may be because an effective paclitaxel schedule was altered.

Docetaxel is a semisynthetic taxane produced from the needles of the European yew *Taxus baccata*. It differs chemically from paclitaxel at only two sites but is approximately twice as potent (80). Although fewer studies evaluating dose and schedule effects were done with this second-generation taxane, available data are similar to those reported with paclitaxel. Increased in vitro cytotoxicity with prolonged drug application was reported when six human ovarian carcinoma cell lines were treated with docetaxel over 2 and 96 hr (26). A preliminary communication summarizing results in 10 human cell lines exposed to a range of docetaxel concentrations over 24 hr stated that dose-response curves were plateau-shaped, and these curves were consistent with drugs where cytotoxicity depends more upon increased exposure duration than upon increased concentration after a certain cytotoxic concentration was reached (81). Also like paclitaxel, docetaxel was more cytotoxic to proliferating human small-cell lung cancer cells (N417) than to plateau-phase cells (21). Investigators reported that docetaxel did not show marked schedule-dependency in the advanced stage colon adenocarcinoma 38 model, but the highest nontoxic total doses on three different schedules did differ as much as twofold (82).

Phase I studies with docetaxel also demonstrated more frequent mucositis when the drug was administered by 24-hr infusion as compared with a shorter 1-hr infusion (83,84). Again, this finding of increased toxicity to normal host cells when duration of drug exposure is increased is consistent with paclitaxel results. These data suggest that schedule-dependency is a property of the taxanes. Although phases II and III docetaxel clinical trials have been limited to 1-hr infusions, mostly with 100 mg/m^2, further exploration to determine whether the therapeutic index can be modulated by dose and schedule is warranted.

In conclusion, paclitaxel, and perhaps other taxane derivatives, exhibits dose- and schedule-dependent effects. Paclitaxel produces striking schedule-dependent dose-limiting neutropenia. The apparent increased efficacy, albeit modest, with a small increase in dose is suggestive of the potential importance of dose intensity. Whether a higher dose or schedule manipulations will further enhance efficacy is under intense investigation. Well-designed randomized trials are under way to indicate how to optimize the use of paclitaxel through dose and schedule manipulations, with or without G-CSF. Studies of paclitaxel as a single agent and in combination chemotherapy are under way in different tumor types at both early and later disease stages.

REFERENCES

1. Manfredi JJ, Parness J, Horwitz SB. Taxol binds to cellular microtubules. J Cell Biol 1982; 94:688–696.
2. Schiff PB, Horwitz SB. Taxol stabilizes microtubules in mouse fibroblast cells. Proc Natl Acad Sci USA 1980; 77:1561–1565.
3. Schiff PB, Fant J, Horwitz SB. Promotion of microtubule assembly *in vitro* by Taxol. Nature 1979; 277:665–667.
4. Jordan MA, Toso RJ, Thrower D, Wilson L. Mechanism of mitotic block and inhibition of cell proliferation by Taxol at low concentrations. Proc Natl Acad Sci USA 1993; 90:9552–9556.
5. Parness J, Horwitz SB. Taxol binds to polymerized tubulin *in vitro*. J Cell Biol 1981; 91:479–487.
6. Young DH, Michelotti EL, Swindell CS, Krauss NE. Antifungal properties of taxol and various analogues. Experientia 1992; 48:882–885.
7. Vexler A, Levdansky L, Ringel I, et al. Taxol: Antiproliferating and radiomodifying

activity in eukaryotic and prokaryotic cells (abstr). 8th NCI-EORTC Symposium on New Drugs in Cancer Therapy, Amsterdam, March 15–18, 1994:195.

8. Ding AH, Porteu F, Sanchez E, Nathan CF. Shared actions of endotoxin and Taxol on TNF receptors and TNF release. Science 1990; 248:370–372.

9. Bogdan C, Ding A. Taxol, a microtubule-stabilizing antineoplastic agent, induces expression of tumor necrosis factor alpha and interleukin-1 in macrophages. J Leuk Biol 1992; 52:119–121.

10. Manthey CL, Perera P-Y, Salkowksi CA, Vogel SN. Taxol provides a second signal for murine macrophage tumoricidal activity. J Immunol 1994; 152:825–831.

11. Chuang LT, Lotzová E, Cook KR, et al. Effect of new investigational drug Taxol on oncolytic activity and stimulation of human lymphocytes. Gynecol Oncol 1993; 49: 291–298.

12. Bhalla K, Ibrado AM, Tourkina E, et al. Taxol induces internucleosomal DNA fragmentation associated with programmed cell death in human myeloid leukemia cells. Leukemia 1993; 7:563–568.

13. Saunders DE, Lawrence WD, Christensen C, et al. Taxol-induced apoptosis in MCF-7 breast cancer cell (abstr). Proc Am Assoc Cancer Res 1994; 35:317.

14. Stearns ME, Wang M. Taxol blocks processes essential for prostate tumor cell (PC-3 ML) invasion and metastases. Cancer Res 1992; 52:3776–3781.

15. Tishler RB, Schiff PB, Geard CR, Hall EJ. Taxol: A novel radiation sensitizer. Int J Radiat Oncol Biol Phys 1992; 22:613–617.

16. Tishler RB, Geard CR, Hall EF, Schiff PB. Taxol sensitizes human astrocytoma cells to radiation. Cancer Res 1992; 52:3495–3497.

17. Lopes NM, Adams EG, Pitts TW, Bhuyan BK. Cell kill kinetics and cell cycle effects of Taxol on human and hamster ovarian cell lines. Cancer Chemother Pharmacol 1993; 32:235–242.

18. Helson L, Helson C, Malik S, et al. A saturation threshold for Taxol cytotoxicity in human glial and neuroblastoma cells. Anti-Cancer Drugs 1993; 4:487–490.

19. Riccardi R, Servidei T, Spiridigliozzi A, et al. Cytotoxicity of taxol in neuroblastoma SH-SY5Y and medulloblastoma TE-671 cell lines *in vitro* (abstr). 8th NCI-EORTC Symposium on New Drugs in Cancer Therapy, Amsterdam, March 15–18, 1994:195.

20. Liebmann JE, Cook JA, Lipschultz C, et al. Cytotoxic studies of paclitaxel (Taxol) in human tumour cell lines. Br J Cancer 1993; 68:1104–1109.

21. Riou JF, Naudin A, Lavelle F. Effects of Taxotere on murine and human tumor cell lines. Biochem Biophys Res Commun 1992; 187:164–170.

22. Zhan Z, Kang Y-K, Regis J, et al. Taxol resistance: *In vitro* and *in vivo* studies in breast cancer and lymphoma (abstr). Proc Am Assoc Cancer Res 1993; 34:215.

23. Lai GM, Chen YN, Mickley LA, et al. P-glycoprotein expression and schedule dependence of Adriamycin cytotoxicity in human colon carcinoma cell lines. Int J Cancer 1991; 49:696–703.

24. Georgiadis MS, Russell E, Johnson BE. Prolonging the exposure of human lung cancer cell lines to paclitaxel improves the cytotoxicity (abstr). Proc Am Assoc Cancer Res 1994; 35:341.

25. Cahan MA, Walter KA, Colvin OM, Brem H. Cytotoxicity of Taxol *in vitro* against human and rat malignant brain tumors. Cancer Chemother Pharmacol 1994; 33:441–444.

26. Kelland LR, Abel G. Comparative *in vitro* cytotoxicity of Taxol and Taxotere against cisplatin-sensitive and -resistant human ovarian carcinoma cell lines. Cancer Chemother Pharmacol 1992; 30:444–450.

27. Rowinsky EK, Donehower RC, Tucker RW. Microtubule changes and cytotoxicity produced by Taxol in human ovarian cell lines (abstr). Proc Am Assoc Cancer Res 1987; 28:423.

28. Rowinsky EK, Donehower RC, Jones RJ, Tucker RW. Microtubule changes and cytotoxicity in leukemic cell lines treated with Taxol. Cancer Res 1988; 48:4093–4100.

29. Figg WD, Thibault A, McCall NA, et al. The *in vitro* activity of Taxol on three hormone refractory prostate cancer (HRPC) cell lines, PC3, DU145, and PC3M (abstr). Proc Am Assoc Cancer Res 1994; 35:431.

30. Steren A, Seven B-U, Perras J, et al. Taxol sensitizes human ovarian cancer cells to radiation. Gynecol Oncol 1993; 48:252–258.

31. Chang A, Keng P, Sobel S, Gu CZ. Interaction of radiation (XRT) and Taxol (abstr). Proc Am Assoc Cancer Res 1993; 34:364.

32. Au JL-S, Millenbaugh NE, Kalns JE, et al. Pharmacodynamics of Taxol in human solid tumors (abstr). Proc Am Assoc Cancer Res 1994; 35:426.

33. Huber MH, Hong WK, Hittelman WN. Microtubule changes in human tumor samples following *in vivo* and *ex vivo* paclitaxel exposure (abstr). Proc Am Assoc Cancer Res 1994; 35:212.

34. National Cancer Institute Clinical Brochure: Taxol (NSC 125973). Division of Cancer Treatment, NCI, Bethesda, MD, 1993.

35. Rose WC. Taxol: A review of its preclinical *in vivo* antitumor activity. Anticancer Drugs 1992; 3:311–321.

36. Rose WC. Taxol-based combination chemotherapy and other *in vivo* preclinical antitumor studies. Monogr Natl Cancer Inst 1993; 15:47–53.

37. Medalia O, Aronson M, Ringel I, Nativ O. Inhibition of mouse bladder tumor growth by intravesical instillation of Taxol (abstr). Proc Am Assoc Cancer Res 1994;35:325.

38. Rowinsky EK, Cazenave LA, Donehower RC. Taxol: A novel investigational antimicrotubule agent. JNCI 1990; 82:1247–1259.

39. Apfel SC, Lipton RB, Arezzo JC, Kessler JA. Nerve growth factor prevents toxic neuropathy in mice. Ann Neurol 1991; 29:87–90.

40. Röytta M, Horwitz SB, Raine CS. Taxol-induced neuropathy: Short-term effects of local injection. J Neurocytol 1984; 13:685–701.

41. Weiss R, Donehower RC, Wiernik PH, et al. Hypersensitivity reactions from Taxol. J Clin Oncol 1990; 8:1263–1268.

42. Arbuck SG, Canetta R, Onetto N, Christian MC. Current dosage and schedule issues in the development of paclitaxel (Taxol). Semin Oncol 1993; 20(3, suppl 3):31–39.

43. Legha SS, Tenney DM, Krakoff IR. Phase I study of Taxol using a 5-day intermittent schedule. J Clin Oncol 1986; 4:762–766.

44. Grem JL, Tutsch KD, Simon KJ, et al. Phase I study of Taxol administered as a short IV infusion daily for 5 days. Cancer Treat Rep 1987; 71:1179–1184.

45. Donehower RC, Rowinsky EK, Grochow LB, et al. Phase I trial of Taxol in patients with advanced cancer. Cancer Treat Rep 1987; 71:1171–1177.

46. Wiernik PH, Schwartz EL, Strauman JJ, et al. Phase I clinical and pharmacokinetic study of Taxol. Cancer Res 1987; 47:2486–2493.

47. Kris MG, O'Connell JP, Gralla RJ, et al. Phase I trial of Taxol given as a 3-hour infusion every 21 days. Cancer Treat Rep 1986; 70:605–607.

48. Brown T, Havlin K, Weiss G, et al. A phase I trial of Taxol given by a 6-hour intravenous infusion. J Clin Oncol 1991; 9:1261–1267.

49. Ohnuma T, Zimet AS, Coffey VA, et al. Phase I study of Taxol in a 24-hour infusion schedule (abstr). Proc Am Assoc Cancer Res 1985; 26:167.

50. Bristol-Myers Squibb. Pharmaceutical Research Institute, data on file.

51. Wilson WH, Berg SL, Bryant G, et al. Paclitaxel in doxorubicin-refractory or mitoxantrone-refractory breast cancer: A phase I/II trial of 96-hour infusion. J Clin Oncol 1994;12:1621–1629.

52. Spriggs DR, Tondini C. Taxol administered as a 120 hour infusion. Invest New Drugs 1992; 10:275–278.

53. Wiernik PH, Schwartz EL, Einzig A, et al. Phase I trial of taxol given as a 24-hour infusion every 21 days: Responses observed in metastatic melanoma. J Clin Oncol 1987; 5:1232–1239.

54. Rowinsky EK, Burke PH, Karp JE, et al. Phase I and pharmacodynamic study of Taxol in refractory acute leukemias. Cancer Res 1989; 49:4640–4647.

55. Schiller JH, Storer B, Tutsch K, et al. Phase I trial of 3-hour infusion of paclitaxel with or without granulocyte colony-stimulating factor in patients with advanced cancer. J Clin Oncol 1994; 12:241–248.

56. Sarosy G, Kohn E, Stone DA, et al. Phase I study of Taxol and granulocyte colony-stimulating factor in patients with refractory ovarian cancer. J Clin Oncol 1992; 10:1165–1170.

57. Seidman AD, Barrett S, Hudis C, et al. Three hour Taxol infusion as initial (I) and as salvage (S) chemotherapy of metastatic breast cancer (MBC) (abstr). Proc AMSCO 1994; 13:66.

58. Hainsworth JD, Hopkins L, Thomas M, Greco FA. Taxol administered by one-hour infusion: Preliminary results of a phase I/II study comparing two dose schedules (abstr). Proc AMSCO 1994; 13:155.

59. Kohn EC, Sarosy G, Bicher A, et al. Dose-intense Taxol: high response rate in patients with platinum-resistant recurrent ovarian cancer. JNCI 1994; 86:18–24.

60. Arbuck SG, Christian MC, Fisherman JS, et al. Clinical development of Taxol. Monogr Natl Cancer Inst 1993; 15:11–24.

61. Gelmon K, Nabholtz JM, Bontenbal M, et al. Randomized trial of two doses of paclitaxel in metastatic breast cancer after failure of standard therapy (abstr). 8th NCI-EORTC Symposium on New Drugs in Cancer Therapy, Amsterdam, March 15–18, 1994:198.

62. Munzone E, Capri G, Demicheli R, et al. Activity of Taxol (T) by 3 H infusion in breast cancer patients (PTS) with clinical resistance to anthracyclines (A) (abstr). Eur J Cancer 1993; 29A(suppl 6):S79.

63. Vermorken JB, Huizing MT, Leifting AJM, et al. High-dose Taxol (HDT) with G-CSF in patients with advanced breast cancer (ABC) refractory to anthracycline (ANT) therapy (abstr). Eur J Cancer 1993; 29A(suppl 6):S83.

64. Uziely G, Delaflor-Weiss E, Lenz HJ, et al. Paclitaxel (Taxol) in refractory breast cancer: Response correlates with low levels of MDR1 gene expression (abstr). Proc AMSCO 1994; 13:75.

65. Holmes FA, Valero V, Walters RS, et al. The M. D. Anderson Cancer Center experience with Taxol in metastatic breast cancer. Monogr Natl Cancer Inst 1993; 15:161–169.

66. Abrams JS, Vena DA, Baltz J, et al. Paclitaxel (Taxol) activity in heavily treated metastatic breast cancer (MBC) (abstr). 8th NCI-EORTC Symposium on New drugs in Cancer Therapy, Amsterdam, March 15–18, 1994:199.

67. Holmes FA, Walters RS, Theriault RL, et al. Phase II trial of Taxol: An active drug in the treatment of metastatic breast cancer. JNCI 1991; 83:1792–1805.

68. Seidman A, Crown J, Reichman B, et al. Lack of clinical cross-resistance of Taxol (T) with anthracycline (A) in the treatment of metastatic breast cancer (MBC) (abstr). Proc AMSCO 1993; 12:63.

69. Reichman BS, Seidman AD, Crown JPA, et al. Paclitaxel and recombinant human granulocyte colony-stimulating factor as initial chemotherapy for metastatic breast cancer. J Clin Oncol 1993; 11:1943–1951.

70. Hochhauser D, Seidman AD, Gollub M, et al. Efficacy of prolonged paclitaxel (P) infusion after failure of prior short taxane infusion: A phase II and pharmacologic study in metastatic breast cancer (MBC) (abstr). Proc 17th Annual San Antonio Breast Cancer Symposium. 1994. In press.

71. Swenerton K, Eisenhauer E, ten Bokkel Huinink W, et al. Taxol in relapsed ovarian cancer: High vs low dose and short vs long infusion: A European Canadian study coordinated by the NCI Canada Clinical Trials Group (abstr). Proc AMSCO 1993; 12:256.

72. Huizing MT, Keung ACF, Rosing H, et al. Pharmacokinetics of paclitaxel and metabolites in a randomized comparative study in platinum-pretreated ovarian cancer patients. J Clin Oncol 1993; 11:2127–2135.

73. Kearns C, Gianni L, Vigano L, et al. Non-linear pharmacokinetics of Taxol in humans (abstr). Proc AMSCO 1993; 12:135.

74. Sonnichsen DS, Hurwitz CA, Pratt CB, et al. Saturable pharmacokinetics and paclitaxel pharmacodynamics in children with solid tumors. J Clin Oncol 1994; 12:532–538.

75. Rowinsky E. Clinical pharmacology of Taxol. Monogr Natl Cancer Inst 1993; 15: 25–37.

76. Kearns CM, Gianni L, Egorin MJ. Paclitaxel pharmacokinetics and pharmaco-dynamics. Semin Oncol 1994; in press.

77. Rowinsky EK, Eisenhauer EA, Chaudhry V, et al. Clinical toxicities encountered with paclitaxel (Taxol). Semin Oncol 1993; 20:1–15.

78. Goldspiel BR, Kohler DR, Dousteni AG, et al. Paclitaxel administration using portable infusion pumps (letter). J Clin Oncol 1993; 11:2287–2288.

79. McGuire WP, Hoskins WJ, Brady MF, et al. A phase III trial comparing cisplatin/ cytoxan (PC) and cisplatin/Taxol (PT) in advanced ovarian cancer (AOC) (abstr). Proc AMSCO 1993; 12:255.

80. Ringel I, Horwitz SB. Studies with RP 56976 (Taxotere): A semi-synthetic analog of Taxol. JNCI 1991; 83:288–291.
81. Hill BT, Whelan RDH, Shellard SA, et al. Differential cytotoxic effects of Taxotere in a range of mammalian tumor cell lines *in vitro* (abstr). Ann Oncol 1992; 3(suppl 1):120.
82. Bissery MC, Guénard D, Guéritte-Voegelein F, Lavelle F. Experimental antitumor activity of Taxotere (RP 56976, NSC 628503), a Taxol analogue. Cancer Res 1991; 51:4845–4852.
83. Extra J-M, Rousseau F, Bruno R, et al. Phase I and pharmacokinetic study of taxotere (RP 56976; NSC 628503) given as a short intravenous infusion. Cancer Res 1993; 53: 1037–1042.
84. Bisset D, Setanoians A, Cassidy J, et al. Phase I and pharmacokinetic study of taxotere (RP 56976) administered as a 24-hour infusion. Cancer Res 1993; 53: 523–527.

9

Guidelines for Administration

BARRY R. GOLDSPIEL

National Institutes of Health Clinical Center
Bethesda, Maryland

I. INTRODUCTION

Paclitaxel is poorly water-soluble and is formulated as a concentrated solution containing paclitaxel 6 mg, polyoxyethylated castor oil 527 mg, and dehydrated alcohol, United States Pharmacopoeia (USP) 49.7% (v/v) per milliliter, which must be further diluted before administration (1,2). Surfactants such as polyoxyethylated castor oil are known to leach phthalate plasticizers [e.g. di(2-ethylhexyl)phthalate, DEHP] from polyvinylchloride (PVC) bags and intravenous (IV) administration set tubings (3–6). In addition, early observations with this formulation noted that particulate matter, within acceptable limits as established by the USP, formed in the solution over time, suggesting the need for in-line filtration during administration (2,7).

This chapter reviews plasticizer-leaching issues, paclitaxel preparation, administration, stability, and compatibility to allow physicians, nurses, and pharmacists to appreciate the unique pharmaceutical properties of this agent and to prepare and safely administer paclitaxel infusion solutions.

II. PLASTICIZER LEACHING ISSUES

A common plasticizer, DEHP is used to make PVC and other medical-grade plastics flexible (8). Depending on the specific material, DEHP-plasticized PVC can

175

contain up to 40% DEHP by weight (8). The degree of DEHP leaching depends on the initial amount of plasticizer in the bags and/or tubings, the polyoxyethylated castor oil concentration, the solution contact time with the plasticized surface, and storage temperature (3–6). Concern about DEHP administration to patients relates to the observation the DEHP can cause hepatic toxicity in animals and that it is carcinogenic in rodents given high doses over prolonged periods (9–12). This leads to the recommendation that patient exposure to DEHP be minimized (1–4,6). Because of this toxicity concern, alternative nonphthalate plasticizers, such as tris (2-ethylhexyl)trimellitate (trioctyl trimellitate, TOTM) have been used in PVC containers (8,12,13). Studies suggest that TOTM leaches to a much lesser extent with fat emulsion administration and is potentially less hepatotoxic than DEHP, making it a suitable alternative plasticizer for PVC products (14).

The extent of DEHP leaching from paclitaxel solutions prepared in 0.9% Sodium Chloride Injection, USP (NS) or 5% Dextrose Injection, USP (D5W) at clinically useful concentrations was examined using high-performance liquid chromatography (HPLC) analysis (4). No DEHP was detected after storage in glass or polyolefin containers. However, large amounts of DEHP were detected after storage in PVC bags, and the degree of DEHP leaching was dependent on the concentration of paclitaxel. These investigators also found the same amount of DEHP leaching when the polyoxyethylated castor oil/alcohol vehicle was tested alone, suggesting that future leaching studies can be conducted using only the paclitaxel vehicle.

In the same study, DEHP leaching from DEHP-plasticized PVC administration sets was also examined (4). Paclitaxel, 0.6 mg/mL, was passed through DEHP-plasticized PVC tubing sets or polyethylene-lined tubing sets (e.g., nitroglycerin-type sets) for 4 or 4.5 hr. The collection bottle from the DEHP-plasticized PVC set contained 9 mg DEHP while that from the polyethylene-lined tubing set contained only a trace of the plasticizer. The amount of DEHP leached was dependent on the duration of exposure, which is a function of the flow rate, rather than the volume of solution delivered.

Although the maximal acceptable amount of DEHP exposure has not been fully quantitated, comparisons have been made to the amount leached when blood products are stored in similar containers (15–17). However, since many transfusion medicine departments have changed their storage containers in response to this problem, it would seem prudent to limit patient exposure to DEHP. Thus, these observations suggest that most DEHP-plasticized PVC bags and intravenous administration sets should be avoided when preparing and delivering paclitaxel to patients. Leaching studies with other PVC plasticizers (e.g., TOTM) are ongoing.

III. TYPICAL PACLITAXEL ADMINISTRATION MATERIALS

The typical infusion apparatus for paclitaxel administration consists of the solution container, the intravenous administration set, an in-line filter, and the patient's

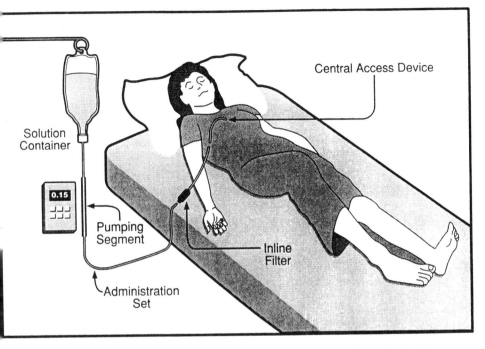

Figure 1 Typical administration material for paclitaxel infusions. The usual administration equipment for paclitaxel infusions consists of the solution container, the intravenous administration set, an in-line filter, and the vascular access device. This figure shows a central venous access device; peripheral access devices can also be used.

vascular access device (Fig. 1). In addition extension tubings may be needed to complete the administration setup.

A. Solution Containers

Many types of paclitaxel-compatible solution containers are available. These include glass bottles, semirigid polyolefin plastic bags, and polypropylene containers. Paclitaxel may be prepared in glass bottles because these containers do not contain DEHP. However, many institutions are avoiding glass bottles for drug administration, necessitating that an alternative solution container be selected. Polyolefin solution containers, frequently incorporating a polypropylene fluid contact surface, do not contain plasticizers and are therefore ideal for paclitaxel preparation. Ethylene vinyl acetate (EVA) bags, which are used for "3-in-1" parenteral nutrition administration containing fat emulsions, should also be suitable for paclitaxel solution preparation as this material does not contain plasticizers. Non-DEHP PVC bags made flexible with TOTM, also used for "3-in-1" parenteral nutrition administration, are currently being tested for paclitaxel compatibility. If it is decided to use a plastic container for paclitaxel preparation, there are clearly many good choices. Bags plasticized with DEHP should be avoided, as should PVC bags incorporating other plasticizers unless supporting compatibility information is available.

B. Intravenous Tubing Sets

Essentially every inpatient infusion pump manufacturer produces an administration set compatible with paclitaxel administration; these sets are usually labeled for use with nitroglycerin or fat emulsion administration and typically incorporate a plasticizer-free polyethylene lining (8). Particular attention should be given to the tubing segment (sometimes referred to as the pumping segment) that attaches to the pump mechanism. With sets suitable for paclitaxel administration, this pumping segment tubing is usually made of nonplasticized silicone rubber (Silastic) material. However, it should be noted that some administration sets labeled for use with nitroglycerin or fat emulsions incorporate a DEHP-plasticized pumping segment. Since this tubing is usually the most flexible portion of the administration set and can contain a large amount of plasticizer, a significant degree of DEHP leaching can occur (unpublished observations). Therefore administration sets incorporating DEHP-plasticized pumping segments should be used only after compatibility with paclitaxel solutions is confirmed. Indeed, Trissel et al. have demonstrated that some "NON-PVC" administration sets are not compatible with paclitaxel (18). Some manufacturers have produced administration sets that incorporate the necessary in-line filter (see below).

C. In-Line Filters

Paclitaxel should be administered with an in-line filter incorporating a membrane with a pore size no greater than 0.22 μm (1,2,7). Most of the initial paclitaxel studies used either the IVEX-2 (slip-lock end only) or IVEX-HP (available with a Secure Lock connector) in-line filter set (Abbott Laboratories, Chicago, IL), which incorporates a cellulose/Teflon filter membrane in a rigid housing. Although the short outlet extension tubing on this filter set is DEHP-plasticized PVC, studies have determined that this set does not leach a significant amount of DEHP over a 24-hr period (1). Several other in-line filters, both with and without non–DEHP plasticized extension tubings, have been tested for paclitaxel compatibility and are now available.

D. Extension Tubings

Sometimes it is necessary to introduce additional tubing into the administration setup—for example, an extension set attached to the needle entering an implanted subcutaneous central venous catheter. Most of the currently available extension sets incorporate DEHP-plasticized PVC, although a limited number of manufacturers produce a polyolefin material extension set. Recently, TOTM-plasticized PVC extension tubings and implanted port needles with integrated extension sets have become available; many of these sets have been demonstrated to be compatible with paclitaxel administration (18). At present, if it is necessary to introduce any extension tubing into the paclitaxel administration set, a polyolefin set, a non-DEHP set, or an extension tubing set that has been specifically tested for paclitaxel compatibility should be used.

E. Vascular Access Devices

Paclitaxel solutions are suitable for both peripheral and central administration (1,2). Most peripheral access catheters intended for short-term use ("hep locks") are made from nonplasticized Teflon material. Most central venous access devices including external lines, subcutaneous ports, and peripherally inserted central catheters (PICC lines) use tubing made from plasticizer-free silicone rubber or polyurethane and biocompatible metals (e.g., titanium). Therefore, the majority of these devices are acceptable for paclitaxel administration.

F. Approach to Selecting Administration Materials for Paclitaxel Infusions

Since the main restriction regarding product selection for paclitaxel infusions focuses on the need to avoid DEHP-plasticized material, the health care practitioner should ask the manufacturer whether any component in the product contains DEHP-plasticized material. In the absence of specific leaching quantitation and compatibility studies, products that contain DEHP-plasticized material should be avoided. Products incorporating other plasticizers (e.g., TOTM) should be used only after studies have demonstrated compatibility with paclitaxel solutions at clinically used concentrations and simulated actual infusion conditions.

Fortunately, intravenous product manufacturers have recognized these special considerations and have produced many solution containers, intravenous administration sets, in-line filters, and extension sets compatible with paclitaxel delivery.

IV. PACLITAXEL ADMINISTRATION USING PORTABLE INFUSION PUMPS

Questions frequently arise about paclitaxel administration using portable infusion pumps. Some portable infusion pump manufacturers have responded to the need for paclitaxel-compatible administration sets and have produced polyethylene-lined tubing sets with Silastic pumping segments while other manufacturers have produced TOTM-plasticized, paclitaxel compatible administration sets. Solution containers with portable infusion pumps must be purged of air before the infusion is started and therefore must be flexible. Polyolefin-lined containers and EVA-type bags currently meet this requirement. Several other collapsible, non-DEHP containers have been developed (e.g. TOTM-plasticized PVC) and are presently being tested for paclitaxel compatibility. The same in-line filters that are used for inpatient administration can be used with portable infusion devices.

We have delivered over 300 paclitaxel infusions using portable infusion pumps and have not observed any increase in infusion-related problems (19,20). As specialized tubing sets become available for all portable infusion pumps, clinicians will readily be able to consider this alternate delivery method for paclitaxel and other drugs with similar administration restrictions.

V. PACLITAXEL SOLUTION STABILITY

Paclitaxel concentrate for injection is stable until the expiration date if stored in the refrigerator ($2°–8°C$) (1). Freezing does not adversely affect the concentrated product (1).

The first stability study for paclitaxel concentrate further diluted in infusion solutions (NS or D5W) indicated that no loss of potency occurred over a 24-hr period when a 0.03 mg/mL concentration was passed through a 0.22-μm filter and stored at ambient room temperature (21).

Waugh et al. determined the stability of paclitaxel in various containers and infusion solutions (4). Paclitaxel was diluted in NS and D5W to clinically useful concentrations (0.3 mg/mL, 0.6 mg/mL, 0.9 mg/mL, or 1.2 mg/mL) and stored in PVC infusion bags, polyolefin plastic containers, and glass bottles. Solutions were maintained at 23 to 25°C for up to 26 hr and filtered through a 0.2-μm membrane. Using a stability-indicating reverse-phase HPLC assay, these authors concluded that paclitaxel was visually and chemically stable for at least 24 hr under the conditions of this study.

The Bristol-Myers Squibb Company sought to confirm these stability data (7,22). Paclitaxel was diluted in NS, D5W, 5% Dextrose in 0.9% Sodium Chloride Injection, USP, and 5% Dextrose in Ringer's Injection to concentrations ranging from 0.3 mg/mL to 1.2 mg/mL. It was then analyzed using HPLC. This study demonstrated that paclitaxel diluted in any of these vehicles is stable for up to 27 hr at ambient temperature (approximately 25°C) and normal room lighting conditions (1). These data allow pharmacies to prepare a single paclitaxel solution container for a 24-hr infusion with a 3-hr lead time for preparation.

As part of a pharmacokinetic and pharmacodynamic study, Brown et al. determined paclitaxel stability at concentrations resulting from diluting doses of 175 mg/m^2 to 275 mg/m^2 in a final volume of 1000 mL of D5W (approximately 0.25 mg/mL to 0.6 mg/mL) (23). Using reverse-phase HPLC analysis, they found no evidence of decomposition for 48 hr at room temperature.

Chin et al. have confirmed this extended stability data by demonstrating that paclitaxel solutions in concentrations of 0.3 mg/mL or 1.2 mg/mL mixed in either D5W or NS in polyolefin containers are stable for 48 hr when stored at ambient room temperature (20 to 23°C) and normal fluorescent lighting (24). Likewise, Xu et al. have also confirmed that paclitaxel concentrations of 0.1 mg/mL or 1.0 mg/mL mixed in either D5W or NS are stable for three days at either 2, 22, or 32°C (25). Ongoing studies are attempting to document even longer stability times and are using a broader concentration range.

Paclitaxel solutions may develop haziness upon standing (1,4,6). This haziness has been attributed to the surfactant vehicle as no paclitaxel precipitation or loss in potency is noted (4,6).

Paclitaxel concentrate for injection must be diluted prior to use. Solutions prepared by diluting paclitaxel to concentrations of 0.3 mg/mL to 1.2 mg/mL in common intravenous solutions are stable for at least 27 hr at room temperature. Paclitaxel solutions may develop haziness over time; however, this does not indicate a loss of potency. A small number of fibers (within acceptable levels of the USP Particulate Matter Test for Large Volume Parenteral (LVPs)) have been observed in paclitaxel solutions, which necessitates administration through an in-line filter with a pore size of no greater than 0.22 μm (2,7). However, solutions exhibiting excessive particulate formation should not be used.

VI. PACLITAXEL COMPATIBILITY WITH OTHER MEDICATIONS

Investigators at the M. D. Anderson Cancer Center examined the visual and turbidometric compatibility of paclitaxel with 59 other drugs commonly used in cancer patients (26,27). A 4-mL sample of paclitaxel 1.2 mg/mL in D5W was mixed with a 4-mL sample of each test drug to simulate "Y-site" administration. Table 1 shows the drugs that were determined to be visually and turbidometrically compatible—as evidenced by no precipitation, color change or gas production, and unchanged turbidity over a 4-hr period. The five drugs where visual and/or turbidometric compatibility were uncertain are shown in Table 2. Chlorpromazine, hydroxyzine, methylprednisolone, and mitoxantrone produced a lower turbidity than might be expected. The combination of paclitaxel and amphotericin B resulted in an increase of turbidity and separated into two layers after 24 hr. However, clinicians must be careful in applying these data because visual and/or turbidometric compatibility does not guarantee chemical compatibility.

A study determining the visual and chemical compatibility of paclitaxel combined with doxorubicin has been performed (28). Paclitaxel and doxorubicin were mixed in polyolefin containers at concentrations of 0.14 and 0.04 mg/mL, 0.28 and 0.08 mg/mL, and 0.44 and 0.15 mg/mL, respectively. Paclitaxel was analyzed by HPLC and doxorubicin was analyzed by visible spectrophotometry.

Table 1 Drugs Determined to Be Visually and Turbidometrically Compatible with Paclitaxel 1.2 mg/mL[a]

Drug	Conc. (mg/mL)	Drug	Conc. (mg/mL)
Acyclovir sodium	7	Ganciclovir sodium	20
Amikacin sulfate	5	Gentamicin sulfate	5
Aminophylline	2.5	Haloperidol lactate	0.2
Ampicillin sodium/Sulbactam sodium	20/10[b]	Heparin sodium	100[c]
Bleomycin sulfate	1[c]	Hydrocortisone sodium phosphate	1
Butorphanol tartrate	0.04	Hydrocortisone sodium succinate	1
Calcium chloride	20	Hydromorphone hydrochloride	0.5
Carboplatin	5	Ifosfamide	25
Ceforanide	20	Lorazepam	0.1
Cefotetan disodium	20	Magnesium sulfate	100
Ceftazidime	40	Mannitol	150[d]
Ceftriaxone sodium	20	Meperidine hydrochloride	4
Cimetidine hydrochloride	12	Mesna	10
Cisplatin	1[d]	Methotrexate sodium	15

Drug	Value	Drug	Value
Cyclophosphamide	10	Metoclopramide hydrochloride	5^d
Cytarabine	50^d	Morphine sulfate	1
Dacarbazine	4	Nalbuphine hydrochloride	10^d
Dexamethasone sodium phosphate	1	Ondansetron hydrochloride	0.5
Diphenhydramine hydrochloride	2	Pentostatin	0.4^b
Doxorubicin hydrochloride	2^d	Potassium chloride	0.1^e
Droperidol	0.4	Prochlorperazine edisylate	0.5
Etoposide	0.4	Ranitidine hydrochloride	2
Famotidine	2	Sodium bicarbonate	$1^{d,e}$
Floxuridine	3	Vancomycin hydrochloride	10
Fluconazole	2^d	Vinblastine sulfate	0.12^b
Fluorouracil	16	Vincristine sulfate	0.05
Furosemide	3	Zidovudine	4

[a] Paclitaxel and all test drugs dissolved in 5% Dextrose Injection, USP, unless otherwise noted.
[b] In 0.9% Sodium Chloride Injection, USP.
[c] Units per milliliter.
[d] Undiluted solution.
[e] Milliequivalents per milliliter.
Source: Refs. 26 and 27.

Table 2 Drugs with Uncertain Visual and/or Turbidometric
Compatibility with Paclitaxel 1.2 mg/mL

Drug	Concentration (mg/mL)
Amphotericin B	0.6
Chlorpromazine hydrochloride	2
Hydroxyzine hydrochloride	4
Methylprednisolone sodium succinate	5
Mitoxantrone hydrochloride	0.5

Source: Ref. 27.

Solutions were stored in the dark under refrigeration (4°C) and under ambient
room lighting at room temperature (25°C) for up to 96 hr. With the exception of
doxorubicin, which showed about a 12% loss at 96 hr, all of the combinations were
visually and chemically stable under the conditions of this study.

Using stability-indicating HPLC assays, Burm et al. demonstrated that
paclitaxel 0.3 mg/mL or 1.2 mg/mL was compatible with ondansetron 0.03 mg/
mL and 0.3 mg/mL or ranitidine 0.5 mg/mL and 2.0 mg/mL during a "Y-site"
simulation study (29). The solutions were stored in glass containers at room
temperature (23°C) under normal fluorescent lighting. Solutions were assayed at
zero, one, two and four hours after mixing. These investigators also demonstrated
that all three drugs were compatible (paclitaxel 1.2 mg/mL, ondansetron 0.3 mg/
mL, and ranitidine 2.0 mg/mL) under similar conditions.

In the absence of demonstrated chemical compatibility, health care professionals should be very cautious about mixing paclitaxel with any other drug.

VII. CONCLUSIONS

Health care professionals must be knowledgeable about the unique aspects of the
paclitaxel formulation, which requires special considerations for preparation and
administration. Physicians, nurses, and pharmacists should only use administration equipment that has been specifically demonstrated to be paclitaxel-compatible.
However, professional judgment may have to exercised in situations where specific
compatibility studies are lacking and alternative products are unavailable. Portable infusion pumps may be used to deliver paclitaxel, as paclitaxel-compatible
administration sets for these devices have become available.

Chemical stability studies indicate that paclitaxel diluted to clinically used
concentrations in customary infusion fluids is stable for at least 27 hr at room
temperature, allowing for a 24-hr supply to be prepared in a single container.
Although paclitaxel has been demonstrated to be visually and turbidometrically

compatible with many other drugs during "Y-site" simulation studies, supporting chemical compatibility data for the majority of these combinations is lacking.

REFERENCES

1. Bristol-Myers Squibb Co. Taxol (paclitaxel) for Injection Concentrate package insert. Princeton, NJ: December 1992.
2. Adams JD, Flora KP, Goldspiel BR, et al. Taxol (paclitaxel): A history of pharmaceutical development and current pharmaceutical concerns. Monograph Natl Cancer Instit 1993;15:189–194.
3. Venkataramanan R, Burckart GJ, Ptachcinski RJ, et al. Leaching of diethylhexyl phthalate from polyvinyl chloride bags into intravenous cyclosporine solution. Am J Hosp Pharm 1986;43:2800–2802.
4. Waugh WN, Trissel LA, Stella VJ. Stability, compatibility,and plasticizer extraction of taxol (NSC-125973) injection diluted in infusion solutions and stored in various containers. Am J Hosp Pharm 1991;48:1520–1524.
5. Moorhatch P, Chiou WL. Interactions between drugs and plastic intravenous fluid bags: part II. Leaching of chemicals from bags containing various solvent media. Am J Hosp Pharm 1974;31:149–152.
6. Pearson SD, Trissel LA. Leaching of diethylhexyl phthalate from polyvinyl chloride containers by selected drugs and formulation components. Am J Hosp Pharm 1993; 50:1405–1409.
7. National Cancer Institute Clinical Brochure (revised): Taxol NSC 125973. Bethesda, MD: Division of Cancer Treatment, National Cancer Institute, July 1991.
8. Van Dooren. PVC as pharmaceutical packaging material. Pharm Weekbl [Sci] 1991; 13:109–118.
9. Ganning AE, Brunk U, Dallner G. Phthalate esters and their effect on the liver. Hepatology 1984;4:541–547.
10. Garvey LK, Swenberg JA, Hamm T Jr, Popp JA. Di(2-ethylhexyl)phthalate: Lack of initiating activity in the liver of female F-344 rats. Carcinogenesis 1987;8:285–290.
11. Kamrin MA, Mayor GH. Diethyl phthalate: A perspective. J Clin Pharmacol 1991; 31:484–489.
12. Smith A, Thrussell IR, Johnson GW. The prevention of plasticizer migration into nutritional emulsion mixtures by use of a novel container. Clin Nutr 1989;8:173–177.
13. Flaminio LM, De Angelis L, Ferazza M, et al. Leachability of a new plasticizer tri-(2-ethylhexyl)-trimellitate from haemodialysis tubing. Int J Artif Organs 1988; 11:435–439.
14. Rathinam K, Srivastava SP, Seth PK. Hepatic studies of intraperitoneally administered Tris(2-ethyl hexyl)trimellitate (TOTM) and di-(2-ethyl hexyl)phthalate in rats. J Applied Toxicol 1990;10:39–41.
15. Jaeger RJ, Rubin RJ. Plasticizers from plastic devices extraction, metabolism, and accumulation by biological systems. Science 1970;170:460–462.
16. Jaeger RJ, Rubin RJ. Di-2-ethylhexyl phthalate, a plasticizer contaminant of platelet concentrates. Transfusion 1973;13:107–111.
17. Jaeger RJ, Rubin RJ. Migration of a phthalate ester plasticizer from polyvinyl chloride

blood bags into stored human blood and its localization in human tissues. N Engl J Med 1972;287:1114–1118.

18. Trissel LA, Xu QA, Kwan J, Martinez JF. Compatibility of paclitaxel with various administration and extension sets. Presented at the ASHP Annual Meeting, Reno, Nevada, June, 1994.

19. Goldspiel BR, Kohler DR, Koustenis AG, et al. Paclitaxel administration using portable infusion pumps. J Clin Oncol 1993;11:2287–2288. Letter.

20. Tolcher A, Cowan K, Riley J, et al. Phase I study of paclitaxel (T) and cyclophosphamide (CTX) and G-CSF in metastatic breast cancer. Proc ASCO 1994;13:73 (Abstract).

21. Trissel LA, Davignon JP, Kleinman LM, et al. NCI Investigational Drugs: Pharmaceutical Data. Bethesda, MD: National Cancer Institute, 1987.

22. Data on file. Princeton, NJ: Bristol-Myers Squibb Company.

23. Brown, T, Havlin K, Weiss G, et al. A phase I trial of taxol given by a 6-hour intravenous infusion. J Clin Oncol 1991;9:1261–1267.

24. Chin A, Ramakrishnan RR, Yoshimura NN, et al. Paclitaxel stability and compatibility in polyolefin containers. Ann Pharmacother 1994;28:35–36.

25. Xu QA, Trissel LA, Martinez JF. Stability of paclitaxel in 5% dextrose injection and 0.9% sodium chloride injection at various temperatures. Presented at the ASHP Annual Meeting, Reno, Nevada, June, 1994.

26. Trissel LA, Bready BB. Turbidometric assessment of the compatibility of taxol with selected other drugs during simulated Y-site injection. Am J Hosp Pharm 1992;49: 1716–1719.

27. Trissel LA, Martinez JF. Turbidometric assessment of the compatibility of taxol with 42 other drugs during simulated Y-site injection. Am J Hosp Pharm 1993;50: 300–304.

28. Fogel J, Bokser A, Goldspiel BR, et al. Compatibility of admixtures of doxorubicin hydrochloride and taxol in 5% dextrose injection. Presented at the Eastern States Resident's Conference, Baltimore, MD, April 10, 1992.

29. Burm JP, Jhee SS, Chin A, et al. Stability of paclitaxel with ondansetron hydrochloride or ranitidine hydrochloride during simulated Y-site administration. Am J Hosp Pharm 1994;51:1201–1204.

10

Administration: Nursing Implications

JANET RUTH WALCZAK and SUSAN E. SARTORIUS
Johns Hopkins Oncology Center
Johns Hopkins University School of Medicine
Baltimore, Maryland

I. INTRODUCTION

Paclitaxel is a new drug that offers hope for many cancer patients. While this drug will not cure most patients, it may allow them to live longer and fuller lives because of its significant activity in several cancers. Even though the toxicity profile includes adverse effects that are familiar to oncology nurses, paclitaxel administration requires specific considerations due to some unique aspects of this drug. Nurses and patients alike have to be alert to the entire spectrum of adverse effects and administration issues inherent in this drug. Paclitaxel's activity, unique mechanism of action, method of administration, and toxicities are described in detail in other chapters. The focus of this chapter is on the nursing care of the patient receiving paclitaxel: the administration guidelines and the management of adverse effects.

II. ADMINISTRATION

There are several issues in the administration of paclitaxel. These include premedication, infusion setup, stability, compatibility, and length of infusion.

A. Premedication Regimen

A premedication regimen has been used to prevent the occurrence of a hypersensitivity reaction (HSR). Fatal HSRs were first noted in phase I trials of paclitaxel and clinical development was halted until methods for abrogating the HSR were defined (1). Weiss et al. (2) reported that of 301 patients initially treated, there were 27 (9%) who had definite HSRs and 5 who had possible reactions. All but one of the reactions occurred during the first or second course of therapy and 78% occurred in the first 10 min of the infusion; some occurred despite the use of premedication.

Patients who had a definite HSR experienced symptoms and signs related to histamine release, such as hypotension, dyspnea, bronchospasm, urticaria, angioedema, and diaphoresis. There are two possible causes for the HSR: one is the drug itself and the other is the polyoxyethylated castor oil used in the formulation of the paclitaxel. Because paclitaxel is insoluble, the surfactant polyoxyethylated castor oil produces solubility for the drug. Polyoxyethylated castor oil has been implicated by association, since the types of reactions experienced are similar to those seen with other drugs formulated with polyoxyethylated castor oil, such as cyclosporine, tenoposide and vitamin K (1,2).

Because the exact cause of the HSR was not defined and it was noted that there were fewer reactions when the drug was infused over 24 hr, two approaches were utilized to reduce risk: the infusion time was lengthened from the initial 3 hr to 24 hr and a premedication regimen of dexamethasone, diphenhydramine, and cimetidine or ranitidine—as outlined in Table 1—was defined (2).

The premedication regimen begins 12 hr prior to paclitaxel infusion. Time in the hospital or clinic is reduced by use of oral dexamethasone the night before and the morning of the paclitaxel infusion. Significant small bowel dysfunction may dictate that all the dexamethasone be given parenterally. Diphenhydramine and cimetidine or ranitidine are administered in the hospital or clinic at least 30 min before paclitaxel. If there is a significant delay before the infusion is begun, an additional dose of dexamethasone should be considered. For example, at our institution, if there is a delay of more than 8 hr between the last dose of dexamethasone and the beginning of paclitaxel infusion, an additional 10- to 20-mg dose of dexamethasone is given intravenously (3).

While these interventions have reduced the incidence of HSR, they have not

Table 1 Premedication Regimen

Drug/dose	Route	Time
Dexamethasone 20 mg	PO/IV	12 and 6 hr before paclitaxel
Diphenhydramine 50 mg	IV	30 min before paclitaxel
Cimetidine 300 mg or ranitidine 50 mg	IV	30 min before paclitaxel

Abbreviations: mg, milligrams; PO, orally; IV, intravenously; hr, hours; min, minutes.
Source: Refs. 2, 4, and 7.

totally prevented it. So it is important that both nurse and patient be prepared to act promptly if signs and symptoms of HSR occur. The patient must be instructed to report immediately to the nurse any symptoms of wheezing, shortness of breath, chest pain, or dizziness.

The nurse must closely assess the patient, especially during the first 15 min of the infusion. While cardiac monitoring is not required, it is important to take vital signs frequently, especially in the first hour, when HSR is most likely to occur. Blood pressure, respirations, and pulse are taken prior to initiating the paclitaxel infusion and at 5, 10, 15, 30, 60, and 120 min into the infusion. For the 24-hr infusion, additional checking of vital signs every 4 hr is indicated until the infusion is complete. Emergency medications such as epinephrine, diphenhydramine, albuterol, steroids, and oxygen as well as an electrocardiogram machine and respiratory equipment should be readily available on the nursing unit (4).

If a HSR or suspected HSR occurs, the patient can be effectively treated using the guidelines outlined in Table 2. Clinically significant signs of HSR—such as hypotension, respiratory distress, bronchospasm, or urticaria—require that the infusion be stopped immediately. Less life-threatening events (such a rash or facial flushing) can be treated effectively while the paclitaxel infusion continues (4).

Facial flushing, usually without the sensation of warmth or discomfort, can occur within several hours of initiating the 24-hr paclitaxel infusion and lasts until the end of the infusion. The paclitaxel infusion is not stopped but the patient may require diphenhydramine if the symptoms progress. Usually the flushing slowly dissipates after completion of the infusion. With shorter infusions, patients may experience a mild facial flushing after the completion of the infusion (3,4).

Even if a patient experiences a HSR, paclitaxel can be safely administered using the regimen outlined in Table 3. The medication regimen and titration of the

Table 2 Treatment Guidelines for Hypersensitivity Reactions

Dyspnea, wheezing, hypotension, urticaria:
  Stop the paclitaxel infusion
  Administer epinephrine in 0.35 to 0.5 ml IV boluses (no more than 6 doses)
  Diphenhydramine 50 mg IV push
  If hypotension persists: IV fluids
  If wheezing persists: 0.35 ml of nebulized albuterol
  Steroids may prevent recurrent or ongoing reactions
Rash, facial flushing:
  Continue paclitaxel infusion
  Administer diphenhydramine 50 mg IV/PO every 6 hr as needed for symptomatic relief.

Abbreviations: IV, intravenous; PO, orally; ml, milliliters; mg, milligrams.
Source: Refs. 2 and 4.

Table 3   Regimen for Reinfusion of Paclitaxel After
Hypersensitivity Reaction

Dexamethasone 20 mg IV every 6 hr for 4 doses
Begin other premedications with last dexamethasone dose:
  Diphenhydramine 50 mg IV 30 min before paclitaxel
  Cimetidine 30 mg or ranitidine 50 mg IV 30 min before paclitaxel
Begin paclitaxel infusion at 25% of previous rate for 1 hr
Increase rate gradually over the next 3–6 hr to previous rate

Abbreviations: mg, milligrams; IV, intravenously.
Source: Ref. 4.

paclitaxel infusion rate enables the patient to receive the drug without further
HSR. In fact, subsequent courses are usually tolerated without alteration in the
usual administration regimen (5).

B. Infusion Setup

The paclitaxel solution must be prepared in glass or polyolefin containers and
infused through polyethylene-lined tubing in order to avoid contact with polyvinyl
chloride (PVC). The polyoxyethylated castor oil has been shown to leach the
plasticizer, di(2-ethylhexyl)phthalate (DEHP), in significant concentrations from
exposure to the DEHP.

A 20- to 22-μm in-line microporous filter is used in the infusion setup and
placed at the most proximal position to the patient so that there is no other tubing
between the filter and the intravenous device in the patient. The filter removes
particulate matter that may be in the solution. Once paclitaxel is diluted, the
solution may have a hazy appearance from the particulate matter related to the
polyoxyethylated castor oil. The solution can be safely administered through the
in-line filter without loss of potency (4,6,7). Not all commercially available in-line
filters are non-PVC, so it is important that the filter have at least a short inlet and
outlet tubing to minimize the patient's exposure to the DEHP (7).

C. Dilution, Compatibility, and Length of Infusion

Paclitaxel compatibility studies to date have been limited. However, data have
shown that it can be diluted in 0.9% saline, 5% dextrose, or 5% dextrose in
Ringer's lactate. The final concentration for intravenous infusion should be 0.3 to
1.2 mg/ml. At these concentrations, the paclitaxel solution is stable for up to 27 hr
at room temperature and in room light. Because little is known about paclitaxel's
compatibility with other drugs, no other medications should be infused through
the paclitaxel line (4,6,7).

Currently, the recommended dose of paclitaxel is 135 mg/m^2 administered over 3 to 24 hr. It can be administered every 3 weeks if the patient's absolute neutrophil count (ANC) is $\geq$ 1500 and the platelet count is $\geq$ 100,000. Paclitaxel can be administered either by peripheral or central infusion. All venous access devices— i.e., peripheral intravenous catheters, peripherally inserted central catheters (PICCs), Hickman catheters, Groshong catheters, and implanted ports and the needles used to access them—are safe because they do not contain PVC or are lined with silicone (7).

While paclitaxel has not been shown to be a vesicant, it can cause a cellulitis if it extravasates. Thus care should be taken, as with all infusions, to be certain that the infusion is intravenous (4,7).

III. NURSING MANAGEMENT OF ADVERSE EFFECTS

A. Hematological

Neutropenia is the major toxicity associated with paclitaxel. Although the degree of myelosuppression is related to dose and length of infusion, all patients experience a decline in neutrophil count beginning 6 to 8 days after infusion, and have an ANC nadir of $\leq$ 1000/μL for 5 to 7 days (8). Patients who experience severe neutropenia (ANC $\leq$ 500) for more than 7 days or have febrile neutropenia should have hematopoietic colony stimulating factors initiated 24 hr following subsequent paclitaxel infusions. Anemia and thrombocytopenia are rarely associated with paclitaxel (9). However, patients who have received prior chemotherapy may be predisposed to severe neutropenia and thrombocytopenia. Nursing care should include aplasia precautions, with particular emphasis on reporting fever (Table 4).

B. Neurological

1. Myalgia and Arthralgia

Myalgia and arthralgia may occur at doses of 135 mg/m^2 or higher or with multiple doses of paclitaxel (9,10). On day 3 following the paclitaxel infusion, patients may experience muscle cramping and weakness of the lower extremities. This discomfort can progress to neuromuscular pain involving the upper extremities, hips, and shoulders and may continue for 5 to 7 days. The painful myalgias and arthralgia associated with paclitaxel are unique for each patient, requiring individualized pain management. For most patients, the use of acetaminophen and nonsteroidal anti-inflammatory agents provide adequate analgesias. Narcotic analgesia may be necessary for severe symptoms (4). Patients should report any discomfort to their health care provider so that immediate action can be initiated to reduce or stabilize the symptoms (Table 4). In subsequent paclitaxel cycles, it is helpful to instruct

Table 4   Nursing Management of Adverse Effects Associated with Paclitaxel

Adverse effect	Patient information needs	Nursing interventions

Neutropenia	Take temperature 3 to 4 times a day
	Notify nurse if fever is ≥100.5°F; chills, shakes, new cough appear; there is burning on urination
	Avoid aspirin or aspirin containing products
		Monitor CBC and differential weekly and as needed
		Neutropenia precautions:
		  WBC ≤ 1000
		  ANC ≤ 500
		Instruct in use of granulocyte colony stimulating factors if indicated.

Anemia	Increased weakness, excessive tiredness, shortness of breath, dizziness	Anemia precautions: Hct ≤25% Monitor activity level; assess for symptoms of anemia
Thrombocytopenia	Notify nurse of blood in urine/stool, nose bleeds, bleeding gums, excessive bruising/petechiae Avoid aspirin/aspirin-containing products, use of sharp objects, razors, dental floss; wear shoes; use soft toothbrush	Thrombocytopenia precautions: platelets ≤ 70,000 Examine skin for petechiae/bruising; assess for bleeding
Neurotoxicity	Notify nurse if there is new onset of muscle aches; joint pains; numbness, tingling, burning in fingers or toes; difficulty walking; any new change in regular activities Take warm bath, try gentle massage Begin analgesia in AM of day 3 as necessary; if acetaminophen is used, take temperature prior to each dose if WBC is low Wear soft shoes with good support (may need larger-size shoe for comfort) Use cane if necessary Precaution: do not drive; do not operate heavy equipment; avoid extremes in temperatures; use care when cooking and using toaster	Assess patient weekly for signs of paresthesias, perioral numbness, sensory loss, and motor weakness Assess extent of pain, need for analgesia, extent of change in activity Encourage periods of rest Assess ability to button shirt, write; leg weakness; change in gait Assess extent of numbness/tingling; changes in gait; changes in daily activity; sensory/hearing loss For moderate–severe symptoms, notify physician for possible dose modification

Table 4 Continued

Adverse effect	Patient information needs	Nursing interventions
Mucositis	Notify nurse of mouth dryness/ redness, swelling, pain, sores, ulcerations Mouth care: use mouthwash 3 to 4 times/day with saline-based rinse and soft toothbrush; remember that bland foods are less irritating to mucosa Notify nurse of vaginal/vulvar/ rectal itching, burning, or sores; vaginal discharge Vulvar/perineal care: Cleanse with soap and warm water after urination and prn; cleanse anal area after bowel movement; take sitz baths with warm saline solution as needed Do not use suppositories/ creams without physician consent	Assess weekly for changes in mucous membranes; examine oral mucosa for plaques, ulcerations; assess for vaginal/vulvar/rectal itching, burning, vaginal discharge Assess level of pain and need for topical or systemic analgesia
Nausea and vomiting	Notify nurse of persistent or uncontrolled vomiting Take antiemetics as prescribed Drink fluids—up to 3 liters/ day; eat bland diet	Assess for frequency/pattern of vomiting and need for change in antiemetic regimen Assess for weight loss/ dehydration Encourage bland diet/fluids
Diarrhea	Notify nurse of persistent or uncontrolled diarrhea Take antidiarrheal medication as prescribed Drink fluids; eat bland diet	Assess for frequency, consistency, amount of bowel movements Monitor fluid intake; assess for dehydration, need for antidiarrheal medication
Anorexia	Eat small amounts of food more frequently, at least 4 to 6 times a day Eat foods high in calories, protein; drink fluids; consider liquid dietary supplements	Assess for change in appetite/ taste; dietary and fluid intake Nutrition consult as necessary

Table 4   Continued

Adverse effect	Patient information needs	Nursing interventions
Hypersensitivity reactions	Take dexamethasone 20 mg orally at home as prescribed (12 and 6 hr prior to paclitaxel infusion) While receiving paclitaxel, notify nurse of shortness of breath; difficulty breathing; wheezing; rash/itching; feeling flushed; facial flushing; dizziness; light-headedness	Assess vital signs frequently during first hours of infusion: P, R, and BP at baseline, 5, 10, 15, 30, 45, 60, 90, & 120 min into infusion, then every 4 hr when indicated; ECG, emergency medications, fluids, equipment available on unit; administer medications as prescribed (see Table 2) Administer reinfusion regimen as prescribed after patient stabilizes (see Table 3)
Cardiac symptoms	Notify nurse of palpitations, chest pain, headache, dizziness	Assess patient for baseline cardiac history of antiarrhythmic medication, cardiac conduction problems Assess during infusion for changes in well-being; assess for signs and symptoms of change in heart rate and blood pressure: palpitations, headache, chest pain, dizziness ECG as indicated Continue infusion for asymptomatic bradycardia Stop infusion if patient is symptomatic; notify physician; initiate emergency procedures as indicated Cardiac monitor during infusion if indicated to evaluate heart rate and rhythm

Table 4 Continued

Adverse effect	Patient information needs	Nursing interventions
Alopecia	Hair loss will begin about day 14 and be complete after 1 to 2 courses of therapy; other hair loss will be progressive, including eyebrows, eyelashes, axillary hair, pubic hair after 3 to 5 courses Plan for hair loss by purhcase of wig/hair pieces, hats, scarves; use of jewelry, cosmetics Wear hat in the cold weather; sunblock in the sun	Assess extent of hair loss Encourage cosmetic techniques to enhance appearance Assess psychological reactions to hair loss; provide support; refer to "Look Good, Feel Better" program through the American Cancer Society; refer to psychological counselor as indicated
Skin	Daily bathing with mild soap; mild body lotion may be used for dry skin; avoid lotions with perfumes and other potential irritants Notify nurse of any unusual redness or pain at IV sites Discoloration of veins used for treatment not unusual Wear protective clothing in the sun (hat, long sleeves); hats in the winter; sunscreen in the sun	Assess skin integrity; check IV sites for erythema, edema, pain
Extravasation	Notify nurse of local burning, irritation, redness at site during infusion of paclitaxel Use compresses as directed	Assess site for erythema, pain, edema; stop the infusion; aspirate remaining fluid from intravenous device to minimize volume; apply warm compresses intermittently for 24 hr; instruct patients to apply cold compresses at home 3 to 4 times daily Administer analgesia as indicated

Abbreviations: CBC, complete blood count; WBC, white blood count; ANC, absolute neutrophil count; P, pulse; R, respiration; F, Fahrenheit; mg, milligram; AM, morning; ECG, electrocardiogram; BP, blood pressure.

patients to begin pain management on the morning of day 3 and to continue until the symptoms subside.

2. Peripheral Neuropathy

Peripheral neuropathy has occurred in patients at doses of 135 mg/m^2. It is seen more often in doses $\geq$ 200 mg/m^2 and can be a dose limiting toxicity that necessitates dose modifications (9). Patients who are at risk for developing peripheral neuropathy include those who have preexisting neuropathy from previous chemotherapy, have received multiple doses of paclitaxel, or have coexisting peripheral neuropathies associated with diabetes mellitus or chronic alcoholism (11). All patients should be instructed to report numbness, tingling, and burning of their fingers and toes to their health care provider. A careful assessment—including the extent of paresthesias, perioral numbness, stocking-and-glove sensory loss, and motor weakness—is necessary to determine the extent of changes in performance status and activities of daily living. Narcotic analgesia may aid in reducing symptoms. A new alternative under investigation is the use of amitriptyline for patients with severe and painful neuropathic complaints (9).

C. Gastrointestinal

Gastrointestinal (GI) toxicity is not a major side effect of paclitaxel but can include mucositis, nausea, vomiting, diarrhea, and anorexia (Table 4). Mucositis is a dose-related toxicity, and rarely occurs at doses < 175 mg/m^2. However, patients should be instructed in oral care to prevent dryness of the oral mucosal membrane and to report any symptoms such as burning, edema, ulceration, or erythema to their health care provider. Patients who have a history of painful ulcerations while taking chemotherapy and those receiving higher doses (250 mg/m^2) have experienced ulcerations of the oropharynx, esophagus, and—in severe cases—the intestines (4,12). Interventions for this group of patients would include meticulous mouth care using a saline-based solution, topical anesthetics such as lidocaine elixir, and symptomatic narcotic relief for those experiencing severe pain.

Only 25 to 60% of patients report other GI toxicity; among that group, anorexia is the most common (4,9,12). This usually occurs on day 5 and persists for 7 to 10 days, although it can be present continuously with higher doses. Some patients also experience a change in taste that contributes to their anorexia. During this time, patients should be instructed to eat small, frequent meals including foods high in calories and protein and to drink plenty of fluids.

Although nausea and vomiting are rare and antiemetics are not routinely given, some patients do experience this toxicity. The patients most prone to nausea and vomiting are those who have previously had emetogenic therapy (anticipatory) and patients who have bulky intrabdominal disease. Diarrhea can also occur, but it is usually mild and self-limiting (7).

D. Cardiac

Cardiac toxicities such as sinus bradycardia, atrioventricular conduction blocks, atrial arrhythmias, and ventricular tachycardia have been reported in about 5% of patients receiving paclitaxel (9). At present, the National Cancer Institute guidelines for patients on clinical trials including paclitaxel suggest that patients with risk factors such as atrioventricular or bundle branch block, arrhythmias, history of angina, congestive heart failure, or myocardial infarction in the past 6 months should be excluded from paclitaxel protocols (4).

The most common cardiac side effect is transient asymptomatic bradycardia (50%), with the heart rate decreasing to 40 beats/min. Asymptomatic arrhythmias have not necessitated stopping the paclitaxel infusion (13). Currently, continuous cardiac monitoring is not required except for patients with preexisting conduction abnormalities or those who develop a significant conduction abnormality during the paclitaxel infusion (7). Patients should be instructed on cardiac risk factors and told that they will be observed closely during the chemotherapy infusion and that vital signs will be checked frequently (Table 4).

E. Integumentary

1. Alopecia

Alopecia is often the most distressing adverse reaction that patients experience while receiving paclitaxel. Because hair loss usually occurs at doses of ≥ 135 mg/m^2, patients should be informed that scalp hair loss will begin at about day 14 and is usually complete after one to two courses of therapy (9). The initial hair loss can be very sudden, with most of the scalp hair falling out in a day or two. Total body alopecia will usually occur after three to five cycles of therapy and includes loss of pubic hair, axillary hair, eyebrows, and eyelashes. Hair loss is reversible after the completion of paclitaxel therapy.

2. Venous Toxicity

Patients may have local skin changes related to paclitaxel infiltration. The usual signs and symptoms include erythema, tenderness, and edema at the injection site, along the venous pathway, and in surrounding tissue. While paclitaxel is not classified as a vesicant, an infiltration can result in a cellulitis. With the shorter infusion time, the authors have observed that patients who have paclitaxel administered via a peripheral intravenous site report increased tenderness and mild to moderate erythema at the infusion site. If the paclitaxel extravasates, the patient's arm may remain erythematous for up to 10 days, with tenderness at the site of infiltration. The skin often takes on a brawny (rough) appearance (Fig. 1). However, the symptoms resolve completely for most patients, leaving no long-term effects (4).

The treatment goal for an infiltration of paclitaxel is symptomatic relief, since

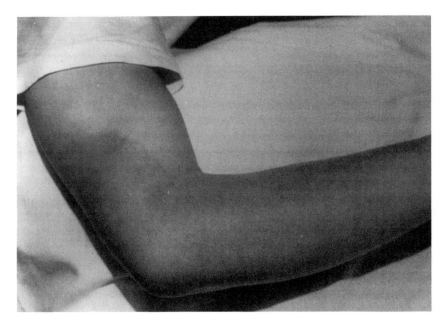

Figure 1 Diffuse erythema and edema on a patient's arm following paclitaxel extravasation.

there is no antidote for the extravasation. When an infiltration occurs, the infusion
is stopped immediately and heat is applied to the site intermittently for 24 hr to
reduce the discomfort and increase vascular reabsorption. Cold compresses can
then be utilized three or four times daily for symptomatic relief until the
extravasation has resolved or the patient is without complaints. For some patients,
acetaminophen or an anti-inflammatory agent may be indicated for managing
residual venous discomfort. Nursing care should reflect careful monitoring of the
IV site and observing for signs and symptoms of erythema, edema, and pain
during the infusion (Table 4) (4).

IV. CONCLUSION

Paclitaxel is a new and exciting antitumor agent that offers hope to many cancer
patients and challenges to oncology nurses. Even though paclitaxel has many
potentially serious adverse effects, patients tolerate the drug well and may
describe an overall improvement in how they feel and in their quality of life while
receiving paclitaxel therapy.

    If paclitaxel is administered via a 24-hr infusion, the patient must be hospitalized for an overnight stay. This not only increases the overall cost of paclitaxel therapy but also adds to the inconvenience and disruption in routine that the patient and family experience. Preliminary data indicate that paclitaxel at doses of 135 and 175 mg/m^2 can be administered over 3 hr (14). As more data indicating the safety and efficacy of the 3-hr infusion become available, patients may be safely treated in the outpatient setting. Because HSR occur in approximately 10% of patients with the longer infusions and premedication regimens (2), home administration of paclitaxel should not be considered until the incidence of HSR can be further reduced or prevented.

Paclitaxel therapy is still evolving. As higher doses and shorter administration times are being investigated, nurses must assess how these changes may affect the toxicities the patient experiences, and how one adverse effect may affect another. Such perhaps is the case with the fatigue that has been reported to occur (7). Fatigue, anorexia, and nadir blood counts all seem to occur concurrently. The degree of fatigue experienced may be compounded by the anorexia and low blood counts as well as the dose of drug received.

As more experience is gained and new data are reported, indications may be redefined and many more patients may be receiving paclitaxel. It is anticipated that there will be new administration guidelines, information about compatibility, and further definition of cardiac risk factors and contraindications for paclitaxel therapy. Also, with the evolution of neurological growth factors, patients may receive more courses of paclitaxel at higher doses without serious neurological effects. Thus, oncology nurses must be alert to the changes, develop new standards of care based on the findings, and teach patients about the indications, regimens, and adverse effects associated with paclitaxel therapy.

REFERENCES

1. Rowinsky EK, Onetto N, Canetta RM, Arbuck SG. Paclitaxel: The first of the taxanes, an important new class of antitumor agents. Semin Oncol 1992;19:646–662.
2. Weiss RB, Donehower RC, Wienik PH, et al. Hypersensitivity reactions from paclitaxel. J Clin Oncol 1990;8:1263–1268.
3. Personal communication: Rowinsky EK, 1993.
4. Lubejko BG, Sartorius SE. Nursing considerations in paclitaxel administration. Semin Oncol 1993;20:26–30.
5. Peereboom DM, Donehower RC, Eisenhauer EA, et al. Successful retreatment with paclitaxel after major hypersensitivity reactions. J Clin Oncol 1993;11:885–890.
6. Waugh WN, Trissel LA, Stella VJ. Stability, compatibility, and plasticizer extraction of paclitaxel (NSC-125973) injection diluted in infusion solutions and stored in various containers. Am J Hosp Pharm 1991;48:1520–1524.
7. Bristol-Meyers Squibb. Paclitaxel Administration Guide. Princeton NJ, 1993.
8. Arbuck SG, Canetta R, Onetto N, Christian M. Current dosage and schedule issues in the development of paclitaxel (Taxol). Semin Oncol 1993;20:31–39.

9. Rowinsky EK, Eisenhauer EA, Chaudry V, et al. Clinical toxicities encountered with paclitaxel (Taxol). Semin Oncol 1993;20:1–13.
10. Rowinsky EK, Gilbert MR, McGuire WP, et al. Sequences of paclitaxel and cisplatin: A phase I and pharmacologic study. J Clin Oncol 1991;9:1692–1703.
11. Chaudry C, Rowinsky EK, Sartorius SE, et al. Peripheral neuropathy from paclitaxel and cisplatin combination chemotherapy: Clinical and electrophysiological studies. Ann Neurol 1994;35:490–497.
12. Rowinsky EK, Burke PJ, Karp JE, et al. Phase I and pharmacodynamic study of paclitaxel in refractory acute leukemias. Cancer Res 1989;49:4640–4647.
13. Rowinsky EK, McGuire WP, Guarnieri T, et al. Cardiac disturbances during the administration of taxol. J Clin Oncol 1991;9:1704–1712.
14. Swenerton K, Eisenhauer E, ten Bokkel-Huirnik W, et al. Paclitaxel in relapsed ovarian cancer: High dose vs low dose and short vs long infusion: A European-Canadian study coordinated by the NCI Canada Clinical Trials Group (abstract 810). Proc Am Soc Clin Oncol 1993;12:256.

11

Ovarian Cancer

WILLIAM P. MCGUIRE
Emory University
Atlanta, Georgia

Paclitaxel, a new and novel antimicrotubule agent, has shown clear activity as a salvage therapy in epithelial ovarian carcinoma. Most important, it is active in tumors that have displayed partial or complete resistance to platinum compounds, a situation in which other salvage therapies have rather unimpressive activity. The role of paclitaxel combined with cisplatin in the initial treatment of advanced disease is currently being explored. Early results in patients with bulky residual disease suggest that this combination is superior to the more commonly used cytoxan and cisplatin (or carboplatin) doublet. Some in the United States have already adopted this combination outside clinical trials as standard therapy for suboptimal disease. Replication of these data may be important depending upon the long-term results from this trial. A trial in less bulky advanced disease is under way but data are too early for any preliminary conclusions.

The major and dose-limiting toxicity of paclitaxel is neutropenia, which makes it an ideal drug to escalate with cytokine support. Cytokines allow escalation of paclitaxel approximately twofold; but at doses $\geq$ 250 mg/m^2, neurotoxicity supervenes, making further escalation difficult or impossible. Further, combining this higher dose of paclitaxel with standard doses of cisplatin is almost certain to lead to cumulative and possibly severe neurotoxicity, since cisplatin alone in doses of 100 mg/m^2 for six courses is frequently associated with modest to severe neurotoxic adverse effects. Although higher doses of paclitaxel are associated with slightly higher response rates, it is not clear that the therapeutic index of more intense doses is better. An ongoing Gynecologic Oncology Group (GOG) trial is addressing the issue of dose intensity of single-agent paclitaxel as first-line salvage therapy. The results of this study will, it is hoped, definitively answer the question of whether more dose-intense paclitaxel has a better therapeutic index.

Also pertinent to this issue, a phase I trial of paclitaxel and carboplatin is nearing completion and may allow escalation of the paclitaxel dose (with cytokine support) while preserving dose intensity of the platinum coordination complex without causing severe neurotoxicity. It is a well-tolerated regimen, with major antitumor activity, and needs confirmation in a phase III study of its relative activity in treating advanced ovarian cancer.

Another major issue that remains to be resolved with paclitaxel is the proper schedule of administration. A single clinical trial demonstrated that paclitaxel given as a 3-hr infusion was just as safe as the 24-hr infusion in terms of incidence of allergic reactions, and that the shorter infusion was significantly less toxic to neutrophils. Unfortunately, the study design did not allow a statistically valid statement regarding equivalent efficacy of this shorter infusion. A single small trial in breast cancer suggests that more prolonged infusions may be associated with improved efficacy. Further research with paclitaxel-based therapy in ovarian cancer must be performed, especially in those patients with potentially curative presentations.

Likewise, paclitaxel is being combined with several other drugs which have single-agent activity in ovarian cancer; ifosfamide, etoposide, topotecan, and hexamethylmelamine. One or more of these doublets may proceed into phase III testing within the decade, depending on their therapeutic index in phase II studies.

It has become clear that when paclitaxel is combined with other agents, a strong sequence dependency may exist. This would make phase I studies more difficult, since the sequence of drug administration may have to be incorporated into the study design. This is even more complicated, since some studies have shown that the sequence with the better antitumor efficacy may also be the sequence with the more serious adverse effects.

The role of paclitaxel-based therapy as an adjuvant in completely resected and early-stage disease is untested. Likewise, the value of intraperitoneal paclitaxel is unknown. It is clear that it is possible to administer paclitaxel safely by this route, that evidence exists for antitumor efficacy, and that a very favorable pharmacological advantage exists (peritoneal:plasma ratio of 1000).

Clinical trials conducted over the next several years will more clearly place paclitaxel in its proper role in the treatment of ovarian cancer. Enough data already exist, however, to state that paclitaxel is the most important drug to enter the therapeutic armamentarium in epithelial ovarian neoplasms since cisplatin appeared in 1975.

I. INTRODUCTION

The past two decades of research have reasonably established that cisplatin-based combination therapy is more effective than single-agent alkylating agents (1) or combinations of drugs which do not incorporate cisplatin into the regimen (2–4) in the treatment of advanced ovarian cancer. Thus, cisplatin-based therapy has become the standard against which other therapies are compared. This improved efficacy may apply only to response rates and disease-free survival (DFS), since no large impact on survival has been noted. The lack of survival advantage for platinum-based therapy may be more apparent than real, however, due to the frequent use of platinum as salvage therapy in patients failing nonplatinum regimens. Approximately 30% to 50% of patients with disease refractory to standard alkylating agents will respond to cisplatin, often for long periods, with probable prolongation of survival (5). Regarding the controversy surrounding the impact of platinum-based therapy on outcome in advanced ovarian cancer, a recent retrospective study from The Netherlands found that patients with ovarian cancer diagnosed between 1981 and 1985 had better survival than a similar group of patients diagnosed between 1975 and 1980. The two major reasons which explained this difference was the more routine use of both aggressive surgical cytoreduction and cisplatin-based therapy (6). The relative roles of each could not be determined. Additionally, Surveillance Epidemiology and End Results (SEER) data suggest that survival in advanced ovarian cancer has increased modestly in the past decade concomitant with the common use of platinum-based primary therapy (7).

When alkylating agents or nonplatinum combinations were utilized in advanced ovarian cancer in the 1970s, the anticipated response rate was, on average, 40% (10% to 20% complete pathological response) with median survivals of 12 to 15 months. Frequently such studies did not subdivide patients by postoperative tumor bulk, making it somewhat difficult to compare results with more contemporary ones using platinum compounds where postoperative disease bulk was more uniformly reported. Nevertheless, in the era of primary therapy with cisplatin-based combinations, the response rates have generally risen to 70% to 80% (20% to 50% complete pathological response), with the greatest activity noted in patients who were optimally cytoreduced.

To date there has not been a definitive prospective study comparing cisplatin as a single agent with a cisplatin-containing combination in advanced ovarian cancer. Some investigators argue that single-agent cisplatin is just as effective as platinum-based combinations, is less toxic, and is less likely to lead to secondary tumors. Nevertheless, a recent metaanalysis of more than 8000 cases of advanced ovarian cancer (> 6500 deaths) suggested very strongly that platinum-containing combinations were statistically superior to single-agent cisplatin (8). Nevertheless, following the decade of platinum-based therapy, a major problem remained: the emergence of resistant cell lines and progressive ovarian cancer in the majority of patients presenting with advanced disease. Salvage therapies in the 1980s were generally poor, since nearly all patients had received cisplatin, and cisplatin-refractory ovarian cancer characteristically responded poorly to second- and third-line therapy.

The emergence of paclitaxel as a valid salvage therapy in refractory ovarian carcinoma sparked intense interest as well as some misconceptions among both medical and lay individuals. The drug is nearly as active against cisplatin-resistant ovarian cancer as cisplatin-sensitive ovarian cancers. Early data on paclitaxel combined with cisplatin suggest that it is well tolerated and more active than the standard regimen of cytoxan and cisplatin in bulky-disease patients in terms of response rate and improved progression-free survival. Overall survival data are still immature. The true role of this drug in the overall treatment of ovarian cancer remains to be defined. Although hope, anticipation, and current press releases assume that incorporation of an active new drug into primary treatment strategies will advance the therapeutic envelope for ovarian cancer, history tells us that no such assumption should be made. Only well-performed clinical trials that use paclitaxel as part of primary therapy will ultimately determine whether paclitaxel, like cisplatin, improves response rates, progression-free survival, and other outcome measures in the disease. More important, however, will be the long-term effect of this agent. Only if the question "Does paclitaxel definitively improve the chance for cure in the patient with ovarian cancer?" is answered with a resounding yes should one accept this new drug as a mandatory part of treatment. We must also look at paclitaxel and paclitaxel-based combinations in terms of therapeutic index to determine if this drug adds anything to quality of life or duration of life aside from cure.

This chapter will review what we know about paclitaxel as an agent for treating ovarian cancer, what studies are currently under way, and what studies still have to be performed to properly assess the role of this new agent in a treatable but still too often fatal disease.

II. PACLITAXEL IN OVARIAN CANCER

During the initial phase I trials of paclitaxel, several responses were reported in patients with ovarian cancer. Based upon this activity, especially in heavily pretreated patients, ovarian cancer was targeted for the first group of phase II trials. Unlike other investigational drugs at this stage of development, most signal tumors—e.g., lung cancer, breast cancer, and colon cancer—were not included in early phase II trials due to a severe limitation in drug supplies.

A. Initial Phase II Studies

Phase II trials were initiated in ovarian, gastric, and renal carcinoma and melanoma based on hints of activity in phase I trials. The most exciting initial clinical activity was in ovarian cancer based on a trial performed at Johns Hopkins (9). Subsequent trials confirmed this activity, noted, importantly, in patients with cisplatin-refractory disease as well as those with drug-sensitive relapse. A summary of those results is shown in Table 1. In the Hopkins study there was 1 pathologic complete response and 11 clinical partial responses in 40 evaluable patients (response rate of 30%). Response durations ranged from 1 to 17 months (median, 6 months). Additionally, there were 7 patients with less than partial responses who had resolution of symptoms and tumor reductions not meeting the 50% criterion. These "responses" were frequently of long duration (median, 7 months). All patients in this study had been very heavily treated prior to paclitaxel (mean prior chemotherapy regimens, 2.7), necessitating significant dose reductions (average dose 110–135 mg/m^2), yet responses were observed in peritoneal, nodal, pulmonary, and hepatic sites. Perhaps most impressive was the observation of responses in patients who were refractory to platinum therapy (24% in the Hopkins study; 27% overall in four studies). Though the amount of prior therapy differed in these four trials and the dose of paclitaxel varied, all these studies used a 24-hr schedule of paclitaxel infusion and a standard antiallergy premedication scheme consisting of dexamethasone, diphenylhydramine, and an H_2 antagonist.

The toxicity in this heavily treated patient group was primarily neutropenia, grade III or IV, occurring in > 80% of patients even at doses of 110 to 135 mg/m^2. Nevertheless, this toxicity was brief, was rarely associated with fever, and was

Table 1 Single-Agent Studies of Paclitaxel in Ovarian Cancer

Institution	# pts	CR	PR	MR	Response rate		
					CDDP-senst	CDDP-resist[a]	Overall
Johns Hopkins	40	1[b]	11	7	6/15 (40%)	6/25 (24%)	30%
GOG	41	5	10	NA	7/14 (50%)	8/27 (30%)	37%
Einstein	30	1[b]	5	NA	3/NA	3/NA	20%
NCI[c]	44	6	15	5	NA	NA	48%
Total	155	13	41	12	13/29 (45%)	14/52 (27%)	35%

Abbreviations: CR, complete response; PR, partial response; MR, minor response; NA, not available.

[a]Platinum-resistant: Defined as progression while on or within 6 months after completion of a platinum-based regimen.

[b]Pathologically verified complete response.

[c]Study performed with paclitaxel + G-CSF.

never cumulative, so that the schedule of every 3 weeks could always be maintained. Neurotoxicity was expected to be common since paclitaxel is a known neurotoxin, all patients had significant prior cisplatin therapy, and many of the patients had residual neuropathy at the initiation of paclitaxel therapy. Fortunately, no clear development or progression of peripheral neuropathy was observed in the study even in patients receiving > 12 courses of therapy.

Similar degrees of activity were seen in two other phase II studies evaluating paclitaxel in less heavily treated patients (one prior regimen in the GOG study (10) and unstated in the study from Einstein (11)). Even in these studies, dose reductions from the starting dose of 170 mg/m^2 in the GOG study and 250 mg/m^2 in the study from Einstein were required. Neutropenia predominated in the GOG study and was dose-limiting, while both neutropenia and neuropathy were observed in the study from Einstein and both accounted for dose reductions. Median survivals in the Hopkins, GOG, and Einstein trials were 8.2, 15.9, and 6.5 months, respectively. The overall median survival was 11.1 months (17.3 months for those not resistant to platinum and 9.2 months for resistant patients). The longer median survival in the GOG study was probably due to the patient population, which was limited to those with a single prior treatment regimen, and 33% of patients had platinum-sensitive disease.

B. Paclitaxel with Cytokines

Since neutropenia is dose-limiting in most studies of paclitaxel at doses < 200 mg/m^2 and thrombocytopenia is uncommon, exploration of escalating doses of paclitaxel with granulocyte colony stimulating factor (G-CSF) were initiated to determine if there was a dose-response relationship. It should be reiterated, however, that in the study from Hopkins, with significant variations in dose from 110 to 250 mg/m^2, no evidence was seen of such a relationship. In fact, the only pathological complete response was in a patient receiving 110 mg/m^2 on each course because of very heavy prior therapy and recurrent febrile neutropenia while on paclitaxel.

Investigators at the National Cancer Institute (NCI) initially performed a phase I study escalating paclitaxel from 135 mg/m^2 to 300 mg/m^2 in conjunction with G-CSF starting the day after paclitaxel and continuing until recovery of the neutrophil count (12). Five of 14 patients had objective responses, and a safe dose was determined to be 250 mg/m^2 of paclitaxel with 5 μg/kg G-CSF. Dose-limiting toxicity was peripheral neuropathy. The same investigators (13) then performed a phase II trial using a dose of 250 mg/m^2 with flexible dosing of G-CSF (sometimes requiring G-CSF doses as high as 20 μg/kg). Neutropenia was not severe with this schedule and dose-limiting peripheral neuropathy predicted by the phase I study precluded further dose escalations. There were 47 patients treated, with 21/44 (48%) of evaluable patients showing a partial response or better (6 complete clinical responses and 15 partial clinical responses). Thus, paclitaxel dose intensification, at least in this study, is associated with an enhanced rate of response over that seen in other phase II studies using lower doses in a similar population of patients. Of note, however, is the apparent lack of any improvement in progression-free survival (median 6.2 months) or survival (median 11.5 month) as compared with end-result data from those phase II studies cited above using lower doses of paclitaxel, progression-free survival (median 7.2 months) or survival (11.1 months). The additional expense of higher doses of paclitaxel and the extraordinary expense of flexible dose G-CSF in the face of no apparent survival advantage requires a randomized study before dose escalation of paclitaxel with cytokine support can be recommended in the salvage treatment of ovarian cancer. It must be remembered that all patients in the salvage setting are destined to die from ovarian cancer; one must, then, question the validity of a more expensive therapy that does not, at a minimum, prolong survival. An ongoing GOG study addresses in a randomized fashion this very question. It is discussed further in a subsequent section.

C. Broad-Based Application of Paclitaxel as Salvage Therapy and Licensing

The four phase II studies described above of paclitaxel used as salvage therapy in ovarian cancer were the basis of the application to the Food and Drug Administration leading to its licensing for that indication in January 1993. Prior to that approval, there was a clamor from patients with recurrent ovarian cancer who wanted access to paclitaxel.

The NCI made the drug available through a protocol that provided paclitaxel, 135 mg/m^2, as a 24-hr infusion with standard premedications through the NCI-designated comprehensive cancer centers to patients with ovarian cancer who had failed at least three prior regimens. Results from that "trial" demonstrate further both the safety and efficacy of the drug (14) in refractory ovarian cancer on a large scale. This trial accepted patients with heavy prior therapy, any performance status except 4, and mildly abnormal renal and hepatic function; in short, a rather poor group of patients in terms of chance for response to cytotoxic therapy. Nevertheless, 22% of patients had documented responses (4% complete and 18% partial) and the median survival was 9.0 months, not dissimilar to that seen in the studies mentioned previously. Many of the patients had dose reductions below the starting dose of 135 mg/m^2, again bringing into question whether a significant dose-response relationship exists in the salvage setting and suggesting again that little survival advantage is gained with higher doses of therapy in this setting. The toxicity of the therapy in this trial was, as anticipated, primarily granulocytopenia, with 78% experiencing grade III or IV effects. The incidence of fever (33%) was somewhat higher than seen in other studies and probably reflects the overall poor performance status of many entered on this trial. Cardiac, neurological, and mucosal toxicities were rare and clinically unimportant. Treatment-related death occurred in 1.6% of patients, an acceptable number in view of the poor risk of the population. This trial lent support to paclitaxel having both safety and efficacy in advanced and heavily pretreated ovarian cancer in a large, multi-institutional trial and further suggested that results from single-institution studies did not have inflated response rates due to patient selection and its associated bias.

D. Dose and Schedule Considerations

As data emerged that paclitaxel was active as salvage therapy in ovarian cancer and would likely be marketed for that indication, Bristol-Myers Squibb sponsored a trial to test the effects of both dose and schedule of administration as salvage therapy in ovarian cancer. In that trial (15), which had a bifactorial design, 407 patients with one or two prior regimens were randomized to one of two doses of paclitaxel (135 mg/m^2 or 175 mg/m^2) and to one of two schedules (3-hr or 24-hr) after a standard regimen to prevent allergic reactions. The concern about the acute safety of the short infusion schedule was clearly answered by the trial, since the incidence of severe hypersensitivity reactions was only 1.3% and there was no effect of dose or schedule on their occurrence. Additionally, the incidence of grade IV granulocytopenia was, surprisingly, found to be significantly less in the 3-hr infusion schedules (18%) as compared to the 24-hr schedules (71%); $p = 0.0001$. All episodes of febrile neutropenia occurred in the 24-hr schedules. Other toxicities appeared to be more common in the higher-dose arms and were not clearly schedule-dependent: an arthralgia/myalgia syndrome ($p = 0.01$) and peripheral neuropathy ($p = 0.008$).

In all, 382 patients were evaluable for response and 66 (17%) responded. Even after adjustment for imbalance in the four treatment groups based upon known prognostic factors, no significant effect of either dose or schedule could be identified for clinical response. The small differences in dose intensity (30%) in the two arms in this study make it unlikely that any relationship will be seen between dose and response.

It is certainly plausible that the significantly greater adverse effect of more prolonged infusions of paclitaxel on the granulocytic precursors could also be operational at the level of antitumor effects or, conversely, that shorter infusions may be less effective. Lending support to this hypothesis are data in several cell culture systems of human ovarian, lung, breast, colon, and pancreatic cancers that suggest total exposure time to paclitaxel is significantly more important than drug concentration. The IC$_{50}$ ranged from 2.5 to 7.5 nM and concentrations above 50 nM had no further effect. Very high doses of paclitaxel actually had a salutary effect on cell survival. Prolonging exposure time from 24 to 72 hr increased cytotoxicity from 5- to 200-fold (16).

The factorial design used in this study does not allow one to look at each individual cell within the four assignments. Although there is a statistically significant prolongation of progression-free survival ($p = 0.02$) for the 175-mg/m^2 group, this represents only a 5-week delay in time to progression with the higher dose therapy. The recommendation, then, that paclitaxel should be used at 175 mg/m^2 as a 3-hr infusion is not statistically possible from this trial. Additionally, overall survival and median survival are similar in both dose and both schedule groups.

It must be emphasized that in a group of patients with recurrent and cisplatin-refractory disease who are destined to die from ovarian cancer and for whom this therapy is purely palliative, the 3-hr regimen in an ambulatory care setting is very attractive, should be the initial method of treatment in the salvage setting, and has been so approved by the Food and Drug Administration. Extrapolation of these results to the setting of primary therapy, however, is to be discouraged at this time. The data, discussed below, of primary therapy with paclitaxel and cisplatin are still maturing. Nevertheless, these data strongly suggest that this new doublet is superior to the "standard" of cytoxan and cisplatin and that use of a possibly inferior schedule could abrogate outcome in a patient population where long-term survival is the goal. Additionally, data from other tumors, e.g., breast cancer, suggest that patients who fail salvage therapy with paclitaxel with short infusion schedules may respond with continuous infusion approaches (Norton L., personal communication, February 1994).

E. Paclitaxel in Combination with Cisplatin in Ovarian Cancer (Phase I/II)

After demonstration of activity of paclitaxel as a single agent in ovarian cancer, the next logical step was combination of paclitaxel with cisplatin, the other very active agent in this tumor. This combination seemed particularly attractive, since both drugs were active and, with the possible exception of peripheral neuropathy, had no overlapping toxicities. The Johns Hopkins group carried out a phase I study of the drug combination using alternating sequences of the two drugs, and cohorts were treated with escalating doses of one or the other drug (17). Paclitaxel was administered as a 24-hr infusion and cisplatin was administered at 1 mg/min. Patients were treated with both sequences of drug, i.e., paclitaxel as a 24-hr infusion followed immediately by cisplatin or cisplatin followed by paclitaxel.

Prospective neurometric evaluations were carried out on all patients, with the fortunate finding that mild to modest neurotoxicity occurred in only 27% of patients and most of these patient had preexisting neuropathy secondary to alcoholism. The neurotoxicity was often detected by neurometric evaluation and was usually not clinically evident. Several episodes (5) of asymptomatic ventricular irritability were observed in patients on this trial, leading the NCI to restrict patient entry to subsequent trials of paclitaxel for any type of preexisting cardiac disease. With further evaluation in several larger single-agent trials of paclitaxel and a single large trial of the paclitaxel/cisplatin doublet (18), it has become clear that the electrical abnormalities apparently induced by paclitaxel or its excipient, polyoxyethylated castor oil, are rarely associated with functional cardiac disease. It is the opinion of this author that patients who are clinically candidates for therapy with paclitaxel should not be excluded on the basis of preexisting cardiac disease.

Neutropenia was dose-limiting in this study, with both depth and length of granulocyte nadirs being less severe with the schedule in which paclitaxel preceded cisplatin administration. Additionally, the paclitaxel $\rightarrow$ cisplatin sequence was more active than the cisplatin $\rightarrow$ paclitaxel sequence in vitro in L1210 cells (19). The recommended phase II/III dose at the completion of this trial was cisplatin and paclitaxel at doses of 75 mg/m^2 and 135 mg/m^2, respectively. During the course of this phase I trial, 6 patients with suboptimally debulked stage III or stage IV ovarian cancer were treated with the two-drug combination as initial therapy. Five of the patients responded (1 pathological complete response (pCR), 1 clinical complete response (cCR)/pathological partial response (pPR), and 3 clinical partial responses (cPRs)).

F. Intraperitoneal Paclitaxel (Phase I)

Paclitaxel may be uniquely suited for intraperitoneal administration, since it should be poorly cleared from the peritoneal cavity (bulky molecule); it is probably primarily metabolized in the liver, making it a potential first-pass drug; and it is rapidly cleared from plasma (α half life = 5.5 hr). Cell culture data suggest that antimicrotubule effects are both concentration- and time-dependent (20) such that intraperitoneal therapy with high concentration and long dwell times may be clinical beneficial. With doses of 25 to 200 mg/m^2 of paclitaxel given intraperitoneally every 3 to 4 weeks, abdominal pain was found to be dose-limiting at doses > 175 mg/m^2 (21). Exposure of the peritoneal cavity to paclitaxel was approximately 1000-fold greater than the systemic compartment, yet concentrations in the systemic compartment exceeded those shown to produce cytotoxicity in experimental tumor systems. Clinically relevant concentrations of paclitaxel persisted in the peritoneal cavity for up to 168 hr following administration. Systemic toxicity was not severe at doses < 175 mg/m^2, although some leukopenia was noted at the higher doses. Evidence of antitumor activity was seen even in a population that was heavily pretreated and had bulky intraperitoneal disease.

Based upon encouraging results from this study, a second phase I trial using a weekly schedule was initiated. The rationale and goal of this study was to expose the peritoneal cavity continuously to clinically cytotoxic concentrations of paclitaxel. This study has just been closed to patient entry (22), with doses ranging from 20 to 75 mg/m^2 weekly for 16 weeks. Abdominal pain was dose-limiting at 75 mg/m^2. The recommended phase II dose is 60 mg/m^2, and pharmacokinetics at this dose level reveal intraperitoneal concentrations in the range of 100 μM (3 logs higher than required to exert cytotoxicity in experimental systems). Delayed pharmacokinetic studies reveal that with weekly administration, the peritoneal cavity is continuously exposed to relevant concentrations of paclitaxel. Serum levels at the 60-mg/m^2 dose were also in excess of 0.1 μM. Clinical activity was seen at the recommended phase II starting dose. Based upon these two phase I studies, a phase II study in patients with small-volume residual ovarian cancer has been initiated by the GOG but data are too preliminary. Currently, the role of intraperitoneal therapy in the treatment of ovarian cancer is unknown. If paclitaxel is active, as it may well be based on early data, a phase III trial will be necessary to evaluate its role in the treatment of low-volume primary disease. The only parameter that may adversely affect its efficacy in local/regional disease is the size of the molecule and the requirement that most drug delivery via this route is by passive diffusion, which may be conformationally hampered.

G. Paclitaxel/Cisplatin Combination in Primary Treatment (Phase III)

Based upon a recommended II/III starting dose of cisplatin and paclitaxel, the GOG initiated a phase III randomized trial in patients with suboptimally debulked stage III and stage IV ovarian cancer comparing cisplatin and paclitaxel (75 mg/m^2 and 135 mg/m^2) with their standard regimen, cisplatin and cytoxan (75 mg/m^2 and 750 mg/m^2). The study was closed to patient entry in March 1992 after accrual of 410 patients. The patients in this study were well balanced with regard to known prognostic factors including stage, performance status, age, cell type, measurable disease, and histological grade.

The results of that study remain immature (23) with respect to survival, but definite and reportable trends are emerging. Using the Kruskal-Wallis Rank Test to assess differences in severity of toxicity, the cisplatin/paclitaxel regimen was significantly more toxic in terms of leukopenia ($p = 0.01$), febrile neutropenia ($p = 0.01$), alopecia ($p = 0.001$), and allergic reactions ($p = 0.01$) than the cisplatin/cytoxan regimen. Documented septic events were distributed equally between the two regimens (3%). Additionally, all cardiac events more severe than grade 1 were noted in the cisplatin and paclitaxel arm but were primarily asymptomatic. The only fatal event, an acute myocardial infarction, was confirmed at autopsy to be associated with severe coronary artery disease and was not temporally related to paclitaxel infusion. Importantly, this increase in toxicity was not reflected in differential discontinuation of treatment for adverse effects; these occurred in 14/202 (7%) in the cisplatin/cytoxan regimen and 11/186 (6%) in the cisplatin/paclitaxel regimen. Thus, although more toxic statistically, the cisplatin/

paclitaxel regimen could be given on schedule in most patients. The cisplatin/ paclitaxel regimen was administered in over 100 institutions safely and without inordinate clinical toxicity; thus, one can assume that this regimen is easily transferable to the community hospital setting. In fact, the overall dose of cisplatin administered was the same in both arms, and the overall dose intensity was better in the cisplatin/paclitaxel regimen due to more frequent treatment delays with the cisplatin/cytoxan regimen.

Clinical response was determined in 219 patients with measurable disease; surgical response was assessed in patients with clinical complete responses or those patients entered on study who had nonmeasurable disease and no evidence of interval progression. Tables 2 and 3 portray the outcomes of these patients. There is a significant improvement in clinical response ($p = 0.02$) favoring the cisplatin/ paclitaxel regimen. Of those patients undergoing reassessment laparotomy, the differences in negative second look were similar; however, there was a greater incidence of macroscopically negative but microscopically positive patients in the cisplatin/paclitaxel arm. These latter patients have characteristically behaved intermediate between those with a negative reassessment laparotomy and those with macroscopically persistent disease (24). Whether this group with low-volume persistent disease—which was significantly more common ($p = 0.005$) in the cisplatin/paclitaxel arm—will influence survival awaits further maturity of data.

Figure 1 depicts progression-free survival (PFI) in this trial. Median PFI, a single-point analysis, is not reported; relative risk is reported, which evaluates the entire curve rather than a single point. The cisplatin/paclitaxel regimen reduces the risk of recurrence by 32% over that achieved with cisplatin/cytoxan. Survival data are expected to be mature enough for reporting by the end of 1994.

Table 2   Clinical Response in Randomized Trial Comparing Cisplatin/Cytoxan and Cisplatin/Paclitaxel

	Treatment		
Clinical response[a]	DDP/CTX	DDP/TAX	Total
Complete response	37 (33%)	52 (54%)	89 (43%)
Partial response	34 (31%)	22 (23%)	56 (27%)
None	40 (36%)	22 (23%)	62 (30%)
Not evaluated	6 (5%)	6 (5%)	12 (5%)
Total	117	102	219

[a]There is a statistically significant difference ($p = 0.02$) in clinical response rate.

Table 3 Surgical Response in Randomized Trial Comparing
Cisplatin/Cytoxan and Cisplatin/Paclitaxel

	Treatment		
Surgical response[a]	DDP/CTX	DDP/TAX	Total
Negative	34 (19%)	40 (25%)	74 (22%)
Microscopically positive	10 (6%)	26 (16%)	35 (11%)
Macroscopically positive	63 (36%)	56 (35%)	119 (35%)
Clinical progression	69 (39%)	38 (24%)	107 (32%)
Not done	26 (13%)	26 (14%)	52 (13%)
Total	202	186	388

[a]There is no significant difference in surgical complete response.

H. Other Paclitaxel-Based Combinations

Paclitaxel is being combined with other drugs that have known activity in ovarian
cancer (ifosfamide, carboplatin, etoposide) and an agent with unknown activity in
ovarian cancer (topotecan). These phase I studies are each being conducted in a
population of advanced ovarian cancer patients as either initial therapy (carboplatin) or first-line salvage therapy (ifosfamide, etoposide, and topotecan).

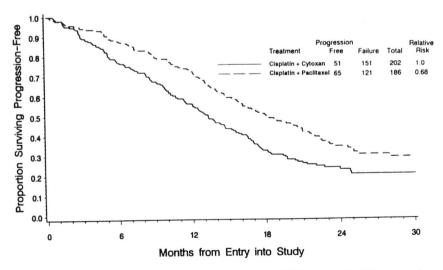

Figure 1 Progression-free survival by treatment in GOG Protocol #111 comparing
cisplatin/cytoxan and cisplatin/paclitaxel in patients with suboptimally debulked stage III
and stage IV ovarian cancer.

1. Paclitaxel and Carboplatin

Paclitaxel has been combined with carboplatin in a study that uses the Calvert formula (25) for the dosing of the carboplatin while using a fixed dose of paclitaxel. The study is still accruing (26) patients but early results allow the following statements to be made: (1) A paclitaxel dose of 135 mg/m^2 given as a 24-hr infusion followed by carboplatin given to an area under the curve (AUC) of 7.5 is well tolerated and can be given for 6 cycles every 22 days with minimal treatment delays; neutropenia rather than thrombocytopenia is dose-limiting. (2) A paclitaxel dose of 175 mg/m^2 given as a 3-hr infusion followed by carboplatin given to an AUC of 7.5 is well tolerated and can be given for 6 cycles every 22 days with minimal treatment delays; neutropenia is prominent but not dose-limiting and further escalation of carboplatin continues with G-CSF as needed. (3) The clinical response rate with this regimen is very high (> 80%). As the carboplatin dose is further escalated with G-CSF, thrombocytopenia is anticipated to become dose-limiting. When grade 3 thrombocytopenia is noted, recombinant human inter-leukin-6 (rhuIL-6) will be added to the regimen to determine if further carboplatin dose escalation is feasible.

2. Paclitaxel and Ifosfamide

Paclitaxel has been combined with ifosfamide in a phase I trial conducted by the GOG in patients with ovarian cancer who have failed first-line therapy not containing either drug. The paclitaxel dose is fixed at 135 mg/m^2 administered as a 24-hr infusion followed by escalating doses of ifosfamide given as a bolus for 4 consecutive days (days 2–5). It appears that the maximal tolerated dose of ifosfamide is 1200 mg/m^2, with neutropenia being the dose-limiting toxicity (Markman, M., personal communication, February 1994). Since there are data that paclitaxel and other drugs display significant sequence dependence, the reverse sequence is being explored in additional patients, i.e. ifosfamide on days 1 to 4 followed by paclitaxel. It is not obvious that this doublet will ever be evaluated in a phase III trial in refractory ovarian cancer; however, completion of the phase I trial is deemed important, since this doublet may be of interest in primary or salvage treatment of other malignancies.

3. Paclitaxel and Etoposide

Paclitaxel has been combined with etoposide in a phase I trial in the GOG in patients with ovarian cancer who have failed first-line therapy not containing either drug. This study was designed to assess the effects of sequence on toxicity but has not been accomplished due to significant toxicity at early levels (Roth B. J., personal communication, February 1994). Paclitaxel at 135 mg/m^2 administered over 24 hr followed by etoposide at 50 mg/m^2 daily for 3 days was excessively toxic to the neutrophils and sequence dependency could not be evaluated. Current plans are to administer the paclitaxel at 135 mg/m^2 as a 3-hr infusion with

50 mg/m^2 of etoposide given daily for 3 days. This is based upon a significant decrease in hematological toxicity with the shorter paclitaxel infusions and a desire to complete this phase I study for possible use in other malignancies. It is unlikely that this doublet will be randomly compared to other therapy in a phase III trial in ovarian cancer.

4. Paclitaxel and Topotecan

Paclitaxel has been combined with topotecan, an analog of the topoisomerase I inhibitor camptothecin, in a phase I trial in the GOG patients with ovarian cancer who have failed first-line therapy not containing either drug. Topotecan has some activity as a single agent in cisplatin-refractory ovarian cancer (27). This study was designed to assess the effect of sequencing on toxicity, but this has not been possible due to the significant toxicity at low doses (Rowinsky E. K., personal communication, February 1994). The major toxicity has been neutropenia and thrombocytopenia and there have been three treatment-related deaths. The probable maximally tolerated dose is paclitaxel 135 mg/m^2 as a 24-hr infusion and topotecan 1.25 mg/m^2 daily for 5 days.

5. Paclitaxel with Cisplatin and Cytoxan

Patients with newly diagnosed stage III and IV ovarian cancer have been treated with the triple regimen of cisplatin, cytoxan, and paclitaxel in doses of 100 mg/m^2, 750 mg/m^2, and 250 mg/m^2, respectively (28). In all patients, G-CSF is used. Patients have been treated with up to 12 cycles of therapy without apparent neurotoxicity. Dose-limiting toxicity was allergic reactions (cycles 5–9) felt to be due to cisplatin (6/12), such that cisplatin was discontinued after 6 cycles. Dose-limiting toxicity after this adjustment has not been reported. The response rate is high; 75%. Accrual continues. Longer follow-up to assess possible late neurotoxicity is important in this trial, since significant neurotoxicity would be predicted with 6 cycles of cisplatin at doses of 100 mg/m^2. Phase III testing of this combination against the cisplatin/paclitaxel combination may be in order in the future.

III. ONGOING NATIONAL STUDIES

A. Exploration of Cisplatin/Paclitaxel in Optimal Disease

The GOG, having seen improved outcomes with cisplatin/paclitaxel in suboptimal disease, is now evaluating the same regimen in optimal disease. This is the disease in which the incorporation of platinum coordination complexes appears to have had its major impact in terms of improving survival, and the hope is that the cisplatin/paclitaxel regimen will further improve outcome in this patient population. The schema of the study is depicted in Figure 2. The initial study design compared the same two regimens previously compared in suboptimal disease with a third arm

216   McGuire

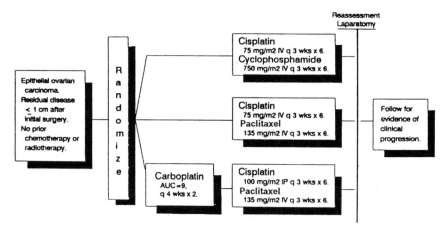

Figure 2 Schema for GOG Protocol #114 comparing cisplatin/cytoxan with cisplatin/ paclitaxel with high-dose carboplatin followed by intravenous paclitaxel and intraperitoneal cisplatin.

that initially treated with two courses of moderately high-dose carboplatin followed by intraperitoneal cisplatin and intravenous paclitaxel for 6 courses. After the initial end results data from the study in suboptimal disease showed superiority of the cisplatin/paclitaxel regimen, the cisplatin/cytoxan arm was dropped. Additional accrual and longer follow-up will be necessary to determine the impact of paclitaxel-based therapy on optimally debulked ovarian cancer.

B. Exploring the Components of Cisplatin/Paclitaxel in Suboptimal Disease

Figure 3 shows the current trial being performed by the GOG in suboptimal ovarian cancer. Fully 15 years after cisplatin was incorporated into the primary therapy of ovarian cancer, there has not been a definitive trial to assess whether or not one could accomplish the same goals with single-agent platinum coordination complex as opposed to combinations based on platinum. A large metaanalysis suggests that combination therapy is superior (29). In this trial the components of the cisplatin/paclitaxel combination are evaluated in a three-arm study in which patients receive the cisplatin/paclitaxel combination or each component as a single agent in higher dose. Patients failing or relapsing after monotherapy will generally be crossed over to the other monotherapy. This will allow one to compare response rates with combination therapy versus monotherapy as well as look at survival as a function of receiving combination therapy or sequential single agents. Additionally, this trial may allow identification of pretreatment characteristics that

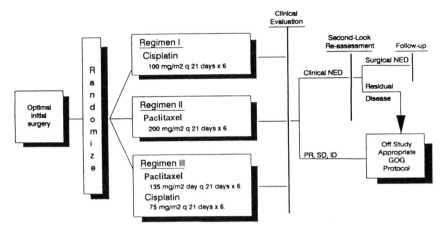

Figure 3 Schema for GOG Protocol #132 comparing cisplatin/paclitaxel and its component parts in suboptimally debulked stage III and stage IV ovarian cancer.

define patients unlikely to respond to single-agent paclitaxel, since this is the first trial to test paclitaxel as monotherapy in previously untreated ovarian cancer. The trial is anticipated to close in less than a year.

C. Exploration of Dose-Response Relationships

As previously noted, there are hints of a dose-response relationship with paclitaxel in ovarian cancer without a clear survival advantage. The study shown in Figure 4 is a trial designed to assess this question more definitively in a randomized study. Patients failing first-line therapy not containing paclitaxel are randomized to one of three doses of paclitaxel monotherapy as salvage. Unfortunately, after this study was designed and opened, accrual fell dramatically due to the commercial availability of paclitaxel and the frequent incorporation of paclitaxel into primary therapy. Candidates for salvage therapy without prior paclitaxel exposure were more difficult to recruit. Thus, the low-dose arm, 135 mg/m², was discontinued and only the two higher-dose arms are continuing accrual. Even with this change, accrual remains slow. This is the only trial in ovarian cancer that may answer the issue of dose as it relates to outcome. Since patients on the two lower-dose arms are to have dose reductions rather than G-CSF administration to maintain dose intensity, these two lower-dose arms may be collapsed into one comparing low- or moderate-dose therapy without the expense of cytokines and high-dose therapy with cytokines. Since higher-dose therapy is more expensive and potentially more toxic, a significant improvement in survival would be mandatory before high-dose

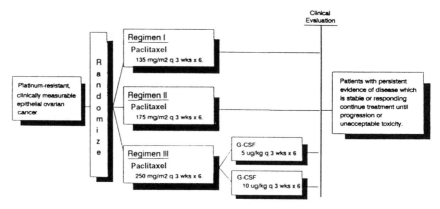

Figure 4 Schema for GOG Protocol #34 evaluating dose intensity of paclitaxel in patients with platinum-refractory ovarian cancer.

therapy could be recommended in the salvage setting. Perhaps more pertinent is the need for a high-dose and low-dose comparison as part of initial therapy where long-term disease control or cure are still possible.

IV. FUTURE DEVELOPMENTS OF PACLITAXEL IN OVARIAN CANCER

It has now been a full decade since paclitaxel was initially placed into clinical trials. Something is known regarding the value of paclitaxel in ovarian cancer; much is yet to be clarified. In the area of ovarian cancer, issues that still have to be addressed include the following:

1. Determine the role of intraperitoneal paclitaxel in low-volume persistent disease that was responsive to intravenous paclitaxel.
2. Determine the role of intraperitoneal and/or intravenous paclitaxel as part of adjuvant therapy in low-stage/high-risk ovarian cancer.
3. Explore in a randomized fashion the value of high-dose paclitaxel and low-dose paclitaxel (monotherapy or in combination) in patients without prior cytotoxic therapy.
4. Explore in a randomized fashion the effect of schedule (short versus long infusions) of paclitaxel administration on outcome in primary therapy.
5. Explore the value of prolonged continuous infusion of paclitaxel on response in patients refractory to shorter infusion schedules.
6. Explore in a randomized fashion the relative therapeutic index of cisplatin/ paclitaxel and other paclitaxel-based regimens.

7. Possibly replicate the cisplatin/paclitaxel and cisplatin/cytoxan study in suboptimal disease outside the United States.
8. Explore the role of paclitaxel as consolidation therapy in patients who were incomplete responses initially.

V. DOCETAXEL

The other major taxane under clinical investigation is docetaxel, a compound prepared by esterification of 10-deacetyl baccatin III which is extracted from the needle of the western European yew, *Taxus baccata*. This compound has had extensive phase I testing, which demonstrated both neutropenia and mucositis to be dose-limiting. During these phase I trials, which were heavily subscribed to by patients with ovarian cancer, unequivocal clinical activity was noted. Phase II studies have verified activity ranging from 32% to 40% in patients with cisplatin-sensitive and refractory states. Hypersensitivity reactions may be less common with this compound, which is not formulated in polyoxyethylated castor oil. An unfortunate adverse effect seen with repetitive doses of docetaxel is a fluid-retention syndrome with pleural and pericardial effusion. This syndrome is very slow to resolve and has slowed clinical development of this agent. Interested readers are referred to a recent comprehensive review (30).

REFERENCES

1. Williams CJ, Mead GM, Macbeth FR, et al. Cisplatin combination chemotherapy versus chlorambucil in advanced ovarian carcinoma: Mature results of a randomized trial. J Clin Oncol 1985;3:1455–1462.
2. Neijt JP, ten Bokkel Huinink WW, van der Burg ME, et al. Randomised trial comparing two combination chemotherapy regimens (HEXA-CAF vs CHAP-5) in advanced ovarian cancer. Lancet 1984;2:594–600.
3. Omura G, Blessing JA, Ehrlich CE, et al. A randomized trial of cyclophosphamide and doxorubicin with or without cisplatin in advanced ovarian carcinoma: A Gynecologic Oncology Group Study. Cancer 1986;57:1725–1730.
4. Omura GA, Brady MF, Homesley HD, et al. Long-term follow-up and prognostic factor analysis in advanced ovarian carcinoma: the Gynecologic Oncology Group experience. J Clin Oncol 1991;9:1138–1150.
5. Wiltshaw E, Subramarian S, Alexopoulos C, Barker GH. Cancer of the ovary: A summary of experience with cis-dichlorodiammineplatinum (II) at the Royal Marsden Hospital. Cancer Treat Rep 1979;63:1545–1548.
6. Balvert-Locht HR, Coebergh JW, Hop WC, et al. Improved prognosis of ovarian cancer in The Netherlands during the period 1975–1985: A registry-based study. Gynecol Oncol 1991;42:3–8.
7. Ozols RF. The case for combination chemotherapy in the treatment of advanced ovarian cancer. J Clin Oncol 1985;3:1445–1447.

8. Williams CJ. Systematic overview of randomised trials in advanced ovarian carcinoma: Results and implications for future trials. Proc Intl Gynecol Cancer Soc 1991;3:49.

9. McGuire WP, Rowinsky EK, Rosenshein NB, et al. Taxol: A unique antineoplastic agent with significant activity in advanced ovarian epithelial neoplasms. Ann Intern Med 1989;111:273–279.

10. Thigpen JT, Blessing JA, Ball H, et al. Phase II trial of paclitaxel in patients with progressive ovarian carcinoma after platinum-based chemotherapy: a Gynecologic Oncology Group study. J Clin Oncol 1994;12(9):1748–1753.

11. Einzig AI, Wiernik PH, Sasloff J, et al. Phase II study and long-term follow-up of patients treated with taxol for advanced ovarian adenocarcinoma. J Clin Oncol 1992; 10(11):1748–1753.

12. Sarosy G, Kohn E, Stone DA, et al. Phase I study of taxol and granulocyte colony-stimulating factor in patients and refractory ovarian cancer. J Clin Oncol 1992;10: 1165–1170.

13. Kohn EC, Sarosy G, Bicher A, et al. Dose-intense taxol: High response rate in patients with platinum-resistant recurrent ovarian cancer. J Natl Cancer Inst 1994; 86:18–24.

14. Trimble EL, Adams JD, Vena D, et al. Paclitaxel for platinum-refractory ovarian cancer: Results from the first 1,000 patients registered to National Cancer Institute treatment referral center 9103. J Clin Oncol 1993;11:2405–2410.

15. ten Bokkel Huinink WW, Eisenhauer E, Swenerton K. Preliminary evaluation of a multicenter, randomized comparative study of TAXOL (paclitaxel) dose and infusion length in platinum-treated ovarian cancer. Canadian-European Taxol Cooperative Trial Group. Cancer Treat Rev 1993:19(Suppl C):79–86.

16. Liebman JE, Cook JA, Lipschultz C, et al. Cytotoxic studies of paclitaxel in human tumour cell lines. Br J Cancer 1993;68:1104–1109.

17. Rowinsky EK, Gilbert MR, McGuire WP, et al. Sequences of taxol and cisplatin: A phase I and pharmacologic study. J Clin Oncol 1991;9:1692–1703.

18. Rowinsky EK, McGuire WP, Guarnieri T, et al. Cardiac disturbances during the administration of taxol. J Clin Oncol 1991;9:1704–1712.

19. Rowinsky EK, Citardi MJ, Noe DA, Donehower RC. Sequence-dependent cytotoxic effects due to combinations of cisplatin and the antimicrotubule agents taxol and vincristine. J Cancer Res Clin Oncol 1993;119(12):727–733.

20. Chang A, Keng P, Sobel S, Gu CZ. Interaction of radiation (XRT) and taxol. Proc Am Assoc Cancer Res 1993;34:A2168.

21. Markman M, Rowinsky E, Hakes T, et al. Phase I trial of intraperitoneal taxol: A Gynecologic Oncology Group study. J Clin Oncol 1992;10:1485–1491.

22. Francis P, Rowinsky E, Hakes T. Phase I trial of weekly intraperitoneal (IP) taxol in patients with residual ovarian carcinoma: A GOG study. Proc Am Soc Clin Oncol 1993;12:A813.

23. McGuire WP, Hoskins WJ, Brady MF, et al. A phase III trial comparing cisplatin/cytoxan and cisplatin/taxol in advanced ovarian cancer. Proc Am Soc Clin Oncol 1993;12:A808.

24. Omura GA, Brady MF, Homesley HD, et al. Long-term follow-up and prognostic

factor analysis in advanced ovarian carcinoma: The Gynecologic Oncology Group experience. J Clin Oncol 1991;9:1138–1150.

25. Calvert AH, Newell DR, Gumbrell LA, et al. Carboplatin dosage: Prospective evaluation of a simple formula based on renal function. J Clin Oncol 1989;7:1748–1756.

26. Ozols RF, Kilpatrick D, O'Dwyer P, et al. Phase I and pharmacokinetic study of taxol and carboplatin in previously untreated patients wit advanced epithelial ovarian cancer: A pilot study of the Gynecologic Oncology Group. Proc Am Soc Clin Oncol 1993;12:A824.

27. Rowinsky EK, Grochow LB, Hendricks CB, et al. Phase I and pharmacologic study of topotecan: A novel topoisomerase I inhibitor. J Clin Oncol 1992;10:647–656.

28. Kohn E, Reed E, Link C, et al. A pilot study of taxol, cisplatin, cyclophosphamide, and G-CSF in newly diagnosed stage III/IV ovarian cancer patients. Proc Am Soc Clin Oncol 1993;12:A814.

29. Williams CJ. Systematic overview of randomised trials in advanced ovarian carcinoma: Results and implications for future trials. Proc Intl Gynecol Cancer Soc 1991;3:49.

30. Pazdur R, Kudelka AP, Kavanagh JJ, et al. The taxoids: Paclitaxel and docetaxel. Cancer Treat Rev 1993;19:351–386.

12

Breast Carcinoma

FRANKIE ANN HOLMES and VICENTE VALERO
University of Texas M. D. Anderson Cancer Center
Houston, Texas

I. INTRODUCTION

Although paclitaxel was first discovered in 1963, factors reviewed by Rowinsky et al. (1)—namely, limited supply, difficulties with clinical formulation, hypersensitivity reactions, and its success in platinum-resistant ovarian cancer—limited its availability for phase II trials in other solid tumors. In 1986, the National Cancer Institute (NCI) solicited letters of intent for phase II trials of paclitaxel in breast carcinoma. Although a trial proposed by the University of Texas M. D. Anderson Cancer Center was approved in 1986, drug unavailability precluded opening that trial until January 1990. Persistent limitations in supplies of the drug curtailed the usual number of studies that would have been performed at multiple centers to evaluate this drug. Until Food and Drug Administration approval of paclitaxel for ovarian cancer in December 1992 and increased drug availability from more efficient methods of drug recovery, additional studies were planned only as the results of current studies became available. The increase in drug availability since 1992 has finally led to the proliferation of studies necessary to optimally define the activity and role of paclitaxel.

In this chapter we address the published studies chronologically (Table 1), consider the issue of anthracycline resistance, and preview studies in progress to define issues of schedule, dose, drug combinations, resistance, combination with

Table 1 Overview of Published Trials of Paclitaxel in Breast Cancer

Study type	Other comments; dose (schedule)[a]	Author-institute	Result
Phase II, limited prior rx	250 (24), no G-CSF	Holmes et al., MDACC	56% responses
	250 (24), G-CSF	Reichman et al., MSKCC	62% responses
	175 v 135 (3), no G-CSF	Nabholtz, Spielman, Bristol-Myers Squibb Taxol Study Group	29% v 22% responses
Phase I with Dox; initial chemo for metastases	Sequence Tax (24) with Dox by 48-hr infusion	Holmes et al., MDACC	MTD depends on sequence
	Simultaneous Tax + Dox (72)	O'Shaugnessey et al., NCI	MTD: Tax/Dox = 180/60 160/75
	Dox by rapid injection; Tax (24); alternate sequence	Sledge et al., Indiana U	sequence-dependent toxicity
Phase II, initial chemo for metastases	Alternate Tax and Dox q 3 wk	Sledge et al., Indiana U	10 pts; 2 CR, 5 PR;
Phase II, extensive prior rx	G-CSF; $\geq$ 2 prior; Tax 200	Seidman et al., MSKCC	2 prior: 36% $\geq$ 3 prior: 21%
	No G-CSF; $\geq$ 3 prior: Tax 150 (24); 2 prior: Tax 175 (24)	Holmes et al., MDACC	3 prior: 18% 2 prior: 20%
	No G-CSF; $\geq$ 2 prior; Tax 135 (24)	NCI, TRC 9202	22% responses
	G-CSF; 2 prior; Tax 140 (96); doxorubicin resistance	Wilson et al., NCI	48% responses

[a]All doses are given in mg/m^2; schedule, in parentheses, is shown in hours.
Abbreviations: rx, regimens; Tax, paclitaxel; Dox, doxorubicin; G-CSF, granulocyte colony stimulating factor; MTD, maximum tolerated dose; CR, complete response; PR, partial response; MDACC, M. D. Anderson Cancer Center; MSKCC, Memorial Sloan-Kettering Cancer Center; U, university.

radiotherapy, and use in adjuvant therapy (Table 2). Docetaxel, the other active taxoid in clinical trials, is also discussed.

II. PHASE II TRIALS IN PATIENTS WHO HAD LIMITED PRIOR CHEMOTHERAPY

A. M. D. Anderson Cancer Center

1. Design

The M. D. Anderson trial (2) was designed to evaluate paclitaxel at a starting dose of 250 mg/m^2 given by 24-hr infusion every 21 days. For patients considered at high risk of myelosuppression—as defined by a history of irradiation to 30% or more of marrow-bearing bones, prior treatment with mitomycin, or poor hematological tolerance of previous chemotherapy manifested by the need for dose reductions because of neutropenia and fever—the starting dose was 200 mg/m^2. Granulocyte colony stimulating factor (G-CSF) was not used. Therapy was to be continued for at least six cycles past maximum response or stable disease. Escalated doses for patients who experienced minimal toxic effects were 275 mg/m^2 and 300 mg/m^2. Reduced dose levels for patients who experienced unacceptable toxic effects were 200, 180, 160, and 130 mg/m^2. Grade 3 toxic effects (3) or a granulocyte count less than 250/mm^3 necessitated reduction of dose by one level; grade 4 toxic effects, by two levels. All patients were treated and observed in an ambulatory treatment center.

Eligible patients were allowed to have had only one prior chemotherapy treatment, either as an adjuvant or for metastatic disease. Bidimensionally measurable or evaluable disease was required. There was no restriction on the length of the disease-free interval or the number of prior hormonal therapies.

2. Results: Patient Characteristics

Twenty-five patients were entered over a 6-month period (January through July 1990). Their characteristics are shown in Table 3. The group was almost equally divided between those whose prior therapy had been administered as an adjuvant to surgery and those whose prior therapy was for metastatic disease. The median disease-free interval—that is, the time from initial diagnosis of primary breast cancer until the time of diagnosis of metastatic breast cancer—was 18 months. The median time from diagnosis of the first metastasis until treatment with paclitaxel was 10 months (range, 1–126 months). This means that half of the patients had received 10 or more months of therapy for metastatic disease before starting paclitaxel. Almost one-third (8 of 25) had over 2 years of therapy. All but two patients had received doxorubicin, and six were considered resistant to doxorubicin. Doxorubicin resistance was defined as development of progressive disease within 6 months of completion of a doxorubicin-based adjuvant regimen or

Table 2 Ongoing Trials of Paclitaxel in Breast Cancer

Study type	Question	Dose (schedule)[a]	Institute
Phase II, infusion duration	3 vs 24 hr	Tax 175	Bristol-Myers Squibb 071
	3 hr: initial & salvage rx, no G-CSF	Tax 250 (initial) Tax 175 (salvage)	MSKCC, Hudis
	3 vs 96 hr	Tax 200 (3) vs Tax 140 (96)	MDACC, MSKCC
	14 day	Tax 2.5/day	NCI Medicine Branch, O'Shaughnessy
Phase II, retreatment interval	14 days	Tax 90 (3) + CDDP 60	Vancouver, Gelmon
	14 days	Tax 250 (24) × 3; part of sequential regimen for high-risk adjuvant	MSKCC, Norton
Phase II, dose	3 hr: with/without G-CSF	Tax 250 + G-CSF v 175	U. Wisconsin, Schiller
Phase III, initial rx comparisons	single agent vs combination	Tax 150 (24) + Dox 50 vs Tax 175 (24) vs Dox 60	ECOG
	Single-agent activity	Tax 200 (3) vs CMFP	Bristol-Myers Squibb 075
		Tax 200 (3) vs Dox 75	EORTC
Phase III, refractory disease	Compare Tax to vinblastine	Tax 175 (3 hr) vs vinblastine 5.5 mg/m² weekly	NCI TRC 93-01 (BMS 132)
	Compare Tax to Mitomycin	Tax 175 (3) q 3 wk vs mitomycin 12 q 6 wk	Bristol-Myers Squibb 047
Phase I, combinations	Cyclophosphamide	Tax 160 (72) + CTX 900 × 3	NCI Medicine Branch, O'Shaughnessy
		Tax 135 (24) + CTX 750 also study sequence	Hopkins
		Tax 175 (3) + CTX 600 also study sequence	Bellinzona
Phase II, combination	CDDP	Tax 135 (24) + CDDP 75	Brown U
		Tax 250 (24) + CDDP 75	New York U
		Tax 90 (3) + CDDP 60 given every 2 weeks	Vancouver, Gelmon
	Dox (bolus)	Tax 175, 225 (3) with Dox 60; also study sequence	INT Milan, Munzone
		Tax 135 (3) + Dox 60	J Hopkins
		Tax 75 (24) d8, 21 + Dox given every 2 weeks	Wayne State U
		Tax 135 (3) + Dox 40	Finsen (Copenhagen)
	Dox (bolus)	Tax 175 (3) + Dox 60 also study sequence	INT-Milan

Phase I, sequential	Dox (bolus)	Dox 20 wk 1 & 3 Tax 75 (3) wk 2 & 4 every 6 wk; ↑ Dox and Tax alternately w/ each level	Wayne State U, LoRusso
	Edatrexate (10-EDAM)[b]	Tax 135 (3), ↑ edetrexate from 40; then fix edatrexate and ↑ Tax given every 2 weeks	MSKCC, Rigas
	Vinorelbine (Navelbine)	Tax 175 (3) ↑ vinorelbine from 36 administer simultaneously	MDACC, Ibrahim
	Estramustine[b]	estramustine 600 PO qd ↑ Tax (96) from 80	Fox Chase, Hudes
Phase II, modulate multidrug resistance	R-verapamil Quinidine Cyclosporine		NCI, O'Shaugnessey U. Arizona, Miller Stanford, Sikic Columbia, Schiff
Phase I, radiation sensitizer	Radiation for locally advanced breast cancer		
Phase I, hepatic insufficiency	Dose modification needed for 24- and 3-hr infusion	Tax 50 (24) if bili > 3.0 Tax 75 (24) if bili 1.6–3.0 Tax 100 (24) if ↑ AST only Too early for 3-hr data	CALGB, Venook
Phase II, adjuvant therapy	Evaluate full-dose single-agent Tax in sequential regimen for patients with ≥ 10 positive nodes	Sequential Dox 90 × 3, Tax 250 × 3, CTX 3000 × 3; each repeated q 2 wk and each G-CSF	MSKCC, Hudis
	?	still planning	NSABP, B. Fisher

[a]All doses are given in mg/m^2; schedule, in parentheses, is shown in hours. Retreatment interval is 21 days unless otherwise specified.
[b]These are open phase I trials, not limited to breast cancer.

Abbreviations: Tax, paclitaxel; vs, versus; CALGB, Cancer and Leukemia Group B; MDACC, M. D. Anderson Cancer Center; MSKCC, Memorial Sloan-Kettering Cancer Center; CDDP, cisplatin; G-CSF, Granulocyte colony stimulating factor; NCI TRC, National Cancer Institute—USA Treatment Referral Center; q, every; Dox, doxorubicin; ECOG, Eastern Cooperative Oncology Group; rx, regimen; CMFP, cyclophosphamide, methotrexate, 5-fluorouracil, prednisone; EORTC, European Organization for the Research and Treatment of Cancer; CTX, cyclophosphamide; INT-Milan, Instituto Nacional Tumori at Milan; NSABP, National Surgical Adjuvant Breast Project; bili, bilirubin.

Table 3 Patient Characteristics in Phase II Trials of Paclitaxel by 24-hr Infusion in Patients Who Had Received Limited Prior Chemotherapy

	M. D. Anderson	Memorial Sloan-Kettering
Number of evaluable patients	25	26[b]
Median age, yr (range)	51 (34–70)	52 (30–67)
Median disease-free interval, mo (range)[a]	18 (0–94)	20 (12–47)
Median no. sites (range)	2 (1–10)	2 (1–≥3)
Dominant disease site		
Soft tissue	6	5
Bone	4	4
Viscera	15	19
Patients w/ prior adjuvant/metastatic hormones	2/9	5/2
No. with both adjuvant and metastatic hormones	4	4
No. pts w/ prior adjuvant/metastatic chemotherapy	14/11	16/0
No. pts with prior doxorubicin	23	8
No. pts doxorubicin resistant	6	0

[a]In the Memorial Sloan-Kettering study, this is the time from *completion* of adjuvant therapy until treatment with paclitaxel. The disease-free interval in the M. D. Anderson study is the time from diagnosis of primary breast cancer until diagnosis of metastatic disease. Thus, these two numbers are not strictly comparable.
[b]Total patients 28, but 2 were not evaluable for response. This explains the total number listed by dominant disease site.

progressive metastatic disease while receiving a doxorubicin-based regimen, either after an initial response (secondary resistance) or without any intervening response at all (primary resistance).

3. Results: Responses

As Table 4 shows, 297 courses were administered, with a median of 13 courses per patient (range, 2–21 courses). Three patients had complete responses (CR) and 11 patients had partial responses (PR). The objective remission rate was 56% [95% confidence interval (CI), 35%–76%]. In only two patients, progressive disease (PD) continued unimpeded. The median time to documentation of a PR was 3.5 months (range, 1–7 months). However, the median time to first objective demonstration of improvement in patients who later demonstrated an objective response was 6 weeks (range, 3–22 weeks). The median duration of response was 9 months (range, 3–19 months); the median survival duration was 20 months (range, 5–27 months). Two of the patients with CR had soft tissue disease, and one had lung disease. The durations of CR were 5.3 and 18.7 months for the patients with soft tissue disease and 14.7 months for the patient with lung metastases. Of eight

Table 4 Response Rates in Patients Who Had Received Limited Prior
Therapy by Study (Paclitaxel by 24-hr Infusion)

	M. D. Anderson (25 patients)	Memorial Sloan-Kettering (26 patients)
Total number of courses	297	178
Median number of courses/patient (range)	13 (2–21)	6 (1–19)
Responses:		
CR, %	12	12
PR, %	44	50
Minor, %	32	15
No change, %	4	0
Progression, %	8	23
% CR + PR	56	62
95% Confidence Interval	35–76	41–80
Responses by prior therapy: adjuvant vs metastatic		
No. patients who had prior adjuvant vs metastatic therapy	14 vs 11	16 vs 0[a]
CR	14% vs 9%	19% vs 0%
PR	43% vs 46%	44% vs 60%
Minor/no change	43% vs 27%	12% vs 20%
Progression	0% vs 18%	25% vs 20%
Response rates by age: <50 vs ≥50 yr		
No. <50 vs ≥50 yr	12 vs 13	14 vs 12
Complete and partial	50% vs 62%	79% vs 42%[b]
Progressive disease	17% vs 0%	?

[a]Ten patients had had no prior chemotherapy; responses are shown for them.
[b]Two-sided $p = 0.105$ by Fischer's exact method.
Abbreviations: CR, complete response; PR, partial response.

patients who had minor responses (MR), the median duration of response was 2.6
months (range, 0.7–14.4 months); however, three patients had MR lasting 7.6,
9.9, and 14.4 months. Of all 25 patients, 8 had responses lasting greater than 12
months (range, 12.6–18.7 months). At the time of this writing (November 1993),
one patient, who had a PR in soft tissue disease, is alive. When responses were
analyzed by age, we found that 6 of 12 patients less than 50 years old and 8 of 11
patients 50 years or older had objective responses. Of interest, however, was that
the only two patients who showed no response to paclitaxel were younger than 50
years.

Responses were seen in all sites of disease. Each patient's disease was classified by the dominant site of metastasis—i.e., the site with the poorest prognosis. The dominant sites, in order of decreasing risk, are viscera, bone, and soft tissue. Of 15 patients with viscera-dominant disease, one had a CR and four had PR. Of six patients with soft tissue–dominant disease, two had CR, three had PR, and one had a MR. Of four patients with bone-dominant disease, two had PR and one had a MR. Because the criteria for complete remission in bone requires complete remineralization of lytic lesions, complete remissions are uncommon in bone metastases.

Responses were analyzed by prior chemotherapy. Of 14 patients, 8 (57%) treated with prior adjuvant chemotherapy had objective responses (2 CR, 6 PR), and 6 of 11 patients (54%) who had prior chemotherapy for metastatic disease had objective responses (1 CR, 5 PR). The one patient whose disease was unchanged and the two patients who had continued progression of disease were in the group previously treated for metastatic disease. Of these latter two, one had responded to the initial chemotherapy, the other had not.

Responses were also assessed by history of therapy with vinca alkaloids. Only patients who had received prior adjuvant therapy had received vincas: vincristine (three patients), vinblastine (one patient), or both (four patients). Of these eight patients, one had a CR, four had PR, and three had MR to paclitaxel. Doxorubicin sensitivity is discussed later in this chapter.

Of 13 patients who had received prior hormonal therapy, 8 had PR and 5 had MR to paclitaxel. Only three patients from each of these two groups had responded to the hormonal therapy.

The median paclitaxel dose in all patients was 200 mg/m^2, but doses ranged from 130 mg/m^2 to 250 mg/m^2. As the study was initially designed, dose reduction was required if the granulocyte count was less than 250/mm^3. However, after it became apparent that patients were not experiencing any untoward effects from a brief period of neutropenia, doses were not reduced for neutropenia alone. Analysis of courses 1 through 3 showed that 25 patients received courses 1 and 2 and 23 patients received course 3, totaling 73 treatments. Of these 73 treatments, doses were reduced in 26 for the following reasons: 7 patients were considered at high risk of myelosuppression and started at 200 mg/m^2; 11 patients had granulocyte counts less than 250/mm^3; 5 had neutropenia with fever or infection; 2 had febrile neutropenia with neuropathy; and 1 had disabling myalgias/neuropathy. Thus, nearly half of the dose reductions were empirical for clinically uncomplicated neutropenia.

4. Hematological Toxicity

Figure 1 shows the median lowest recorded granulocyte counts and platelet counts by course number. Ranges are not included for the granulocyte count but for all courses the range included 0 cells/mm^3. As doses were reduced for granulocytopenia or other problems, the median lowest recorded granulocyte counts rose. The median duration of granulocyte counts less than 500/mm^3 was 7 days (range, 2–15

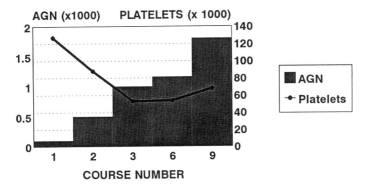

AGN = absolute granulocyte nadir

Figure 1   Hematologic toxic effects in selected courses in M. D. Anderson Cancer Center phase II trial of paclitaxel by 24-hour infusion in patients who had received limited prior therapy.

days); the median day of the lowest recorded granulocyte counts was day 12 (range, 11–14 days). In contrast, however, the platelet count was unaffected by the treatment. Only three patients received transfusion of red cells for anemia.

5. Nonhematological Toxicity

Table 5 shows nonhematological toxic effects by percentage of patients and percentage of courses affected. This allows representation of both the worst toxic effects experienced by the patients and the long-term toxic effects over the entire course of their treatments, which continued for a median of about 7 months. In general, therapy was well tolerated. Forty-four percent of patients had neutropenic fever or infection; after appropriate dosage adjustment, however, only 6% of courses were affected. This tells us that while a substantial minority of patients did experience neutropenic fever or infection as complications of their therapy, over the entire course of their treatment the complications were limited. Grade 3 stomatitis was not seen, but grade 3 myalgia was noted in four patients. This was clearly related to the dose level and resolved with reduction of the dose. Nausea and vomiting were mild and occurred in a minority of patients.

6. Other Toxic Effects

Alopecia was seen in all patients. Hypersensitivity reactions were not seen, although most patients did develop erythroderma of the face and sometimes of the anterior neck and chest in sun-exposed areas, within 24 hr after premedication with dexamethasone; this is a well-known cutaneous reaction to high doses of corticosteroids. Cardiac events were noted in only four patients, and none required any therapy. Two patients experienced sinus bradycardia; one patient had sinus

Table 5   Nonhematologic Toxic Effects in Phase II Trials of Paclitaxel by 24-Hr Infusion in Patients Who Had Received Limited Prior Therapy by Percentage of Patients and Percentage of Courses

Toxic effect	M. D. Anderson		Memorial Sloan-Kettering	
	% of patients $(n = 25)$	% of courses $(n = 232)$[a]	% of patients $(n = 28)$[b]	% of courses $(n = 178)$
Neutropenia (neutrophil count <500/mm³)	100	86	57 (data for course 1 only)	Data for course 1 only
Infection during neutropenia[c]	8	0.9	7	1
Febrile neutropenia	44	4.7	21	4
Stomatitis				
Grade 2	32	6	0	0
Grade 3	0	0	4% grade 4[d]	0
Myalgias				
Grade 2	68	48	36	?
Grade 3	16	3	0	0
Neuropathy				
Grade 2	52	n/a	7	n/a
Grade 3	8		0	
Diarrhea				
Grade 2	60	14	0	0
Grade 3	4	0.4	0	0

[a]232 courses were reported initially (Ref. 2).
[b]28 patients were evaluable for toxicity; 26 patients were evaluable for response.
[c]Neutropenia, <1000 granulocytes/mm³.
[d]One patient with hepatic insufficiency.
Abbreviations: n/a, not applicable.

pause. The fourth had mitral valve prolapse with a history of atypical chest pain and experienced another episode of pain associated with ventricular ectopy 3 days after completion of her second course. It is unclear whether this was related to paclitaxel.

B. Confirmatory Trial: Memorial Sloan-Kettering Cancer Center

1. Design

After the results of the M. D. Anderson study were critically reviewed by the NCI, a confirmatory trial was instituted by Memorial Sloan-Kettering (4) using the same dose, 250 mg/m^2, repeated every 21 days. Dose levels were identical to those of the M. D. Anderson study, but G-CSF 5 µg/kg was given from days 3 through 10 or until the absolute neutrophil count recovered to 2000/mm^3 or greater for 3 consecutive days. Because the supplies of paclitaxel were limited, the treatment was to be continued only for 2 cycles after best response or a maximum of 10 cycles for stable disease. The eligibility criteria were similar: patients who had received one prior chemotherapy treatment were eligible, but in this trial only previous adjuvant therapy was allowed. Prior chemotherapy for metastatic disease was cause for exclusion. There were two other exclusion criteria: only patients who had been disease-free for at least 1 year after completion of all adjuvant therapy were eligible, and patients must not have received more than two hormonal therapies, one each as adjuvant therapy and for metastatic disease. The intent was to avoid patients with long tumor histories who might have developed resistance to therapeutic drugs.

2. Results: Patient Characteristics

Table 3 shows the characteristics of the 26 evaluable patients. Two other patients were treated but were considered inevaluable for response. One of these required interruption of paclitaxel treatment for urgent irradiation; the second was found to have received two prior hormone regimens for metastatic disease. However, four patients who were considered evaluable had received two prior hormonal therapies, one each as adjuvant therapy and for metastatic disease.

The characteristics of the patients in this trial are similar to those of the patients on the M. D. Anderson trial. The disease-free interval was not measured, but rather the time after completion of adjuvant therapy. This suggests that for the 17 patients who received adjuvant chemotherapy and the 9 patients who received adjuvant hormone therapy, the disease-free interval exceeded 20 months. Forty percent of patients had not received any prior chemotherapy. Of the 17 patients who had received prior adjuvant chemotherapy, 8 had received a doxorubicin-based regimen. No patient was resistant to doxorubicin as defined above. Two patients had received adjuvant vincristine. The dominant disease site was viscera.

3. Results: Responses

As Table 4 shows, 178 courses were given, with a median of 6 (range, 1–19) courses per patient. The overall response rate was remarkably similar to that of the M. D. Anderson study. Three patients had CR and 13 patients had PR, for an objective remission rate of 62% (95% CI, 48%–80%). Four patients had MR, and six (23%) had outright disease progression. All three of the CR were in soft tissues of the lymph nodes and skin except in one patient, who also had a pleural effusion. Striking to the investigators was the histologically documented CR in one patient who was experiencing recurrence in a previously irradiated chest wall. Responses were seen in all sites of disease.

At 5 weeks (range, 1–14 weeks), the median time to first objective response was much shorter than that in the M. D. Anderson study. However, one of the patients who ultimately had a CR in previously irradiated chest wall continued to improve until pathological CR could be documented at 57 weeks.

The study design made it impossible to assess the duration of response. Patients who responded were removed from the study after two courses; many received other therapy to maintain or consolidate their responses.

Analysis of responses by prior therapies showed that approximately 60% of patients had objective responses (CR and PR) regardless of whether they had received adjuvant chemotherapy. One of the two patients who had received vincristine as part of adjuvant chemotherapy had a PR. Similarly, 60% of patients who had received prior hormonal therapy, either as an adjuvant or for metastatic disease, had objective responses.

Analysis of responses by age showed a trend for younger patients (those under 50 years old) to have a greater number of objective responses (79% versus 42%, two sided $p = 0.105$ by Fischer's exact method). The median age of the responding patients, 45.5 years (range, 30–67 years), was lower than that of nonresponders, 55 years (range, 37–64 years).

4. Hematological Toxic Effects

Neutropenia was the chief toxic effect and the reason for all dose reductions except one, in a patient who had nausea and emesis. A majority of patients required at least one dose reduction; the median dose per course was 200 mg/m^2 (range, 160–300 mg/m^2). Granulocyte colony stimulating factor (G-CSF) was not included in the original study design, but because the initial two patients experienced such profound and durable myelosuppression, with granulocyte count nadirs of 0.1 and 0.2 cells/mm^3 lasting for 7 and 8 days, G-CSF was added to the treatment plan for the remaining 26 patients. All patients recovered to granulocyte counts of at least 1500 granulocytes/mm^3 by day 21.

The incidence of infectious complications is shown in Table 5. Although 21% of patients had febrile neutropenia, this represented only 4% of all courses. The effect of G-CSF is well shown by analysis of the granulocyte count nadirs during cycle 1. Of 28 patients evaluable for toxic effects, 16 (57%) had absolute neutrophil counts below 500/mm^3. This contrasts sharply with nadirs of 300/mm^3 or less observed in 22 of 25 patients (8 patients had nadirs of 0/mm^3) in the M. D. Anderson study, in which 7 patients started at a dose of 200 mg/m^2. In the 57% of patients who had grade 4 neutropenia, the median time to recovery to a granulocyte count of over 500 granulocytes/mm^3 was 3.5 days, compared with 7 days in the M. D. Anderson study. Clinically important thrombocytopenia and grade 4 mucositis occurred in one patient with extensive liver metastases who had a nearly 10-fold elevation of the aspartate aminotransferase (AST) level and mild hyperbilirubinemia. This patient had fulminant disease, and her hepatic insufficiency undoubtedly contributed to the pancytopenia and stomatitis she experienced.

5. *Other Toxic Effects*

Other toxic effects were mild; they are shown in Table 5. Myalgias and arthralgias (paroxystic pain) were mild but were exacerbated by treatment with G-CSF. All patients had total alopecia. There were no hypersensitivity reactions and no cardiac toxic effects.

6. *Pharmacokinetic Studies*

Plasma paclitaxel levels were examined twice during the last 2 hr of cycle of 1. In nine patients, the intrapatient variation was greater than 50%. Four of these patients had neutropenia with fever in cycle 1. Only 2 of the remaining 18 patients had neutropenic fever. Rowinsky reported that a minimum clinically effective paclitaxel level (1) is 0.1 μmol/L. The median of the mean paclitaxel levels was 1.04 μmol/L. Subset analysis was performed to evaluate the effect of mean paclitaxel levels on the incidence of neutropenic fever or response, but no significant correlation with either the incidence of neutropenic fever or response was found. Data from Jamis-Dow et al. in 48 patients with ovarian cancer treated at a dose of 250 mg/m^2 over 24 hr did not show any significant correlation between plasma concentrations of paclitaxel and toxic effects or responses. The reasons for this were (a) 92% of patients had grade 3 or 4 hematological toxic effects, (b) only 8% of patients had grade 3 or 4 nonhematological toxic effects, and (c) there was a low degree of interpatient variation in plasma concentration of paclitaxel (5).

C. Comments on These Studies

These two published studies clearly establish the activity of paclitaxel in metastatic breast cancer. Paclitaxel produced responses in 50% to 60% of these patients, and only 8% to 23% of patients had de novo disease progression. Only the M. D. Anderson study design addressed the question of durability of response, but that study showed median response durations of 9 months, similar to the duration of response to standard first-line chemotherapy for metastatic disease. Additional studies will be needed to confirm this.

The two studies did not define an optimal dose and schedule. Using the same 24-hr infusion schedule and identical doses and dose-reduction criteria as the M. D. Anderson study, Memorial Sloan-Kettering found that the addition of G-CSF reduced the incidence of grade 4 neutropenia from nearly 100% to 57% and halved the duration of granulocyte counts less than 500 cells/mm^3 (from 7 to 3.5 days) (2,5). However, doses were reduced for nadir counts below 250/mm^3, so the full impact of G-CSF was not apparent. Because both trials showed no clinical consequences of these episodes of severe neutropenia, a separate Memorial Sloan-Kettering trial was designed to allow administration of full doses of paclitaxel without regard to the depth or duration of neutropenia (6). The schedule of administration was identical to that of their initial trial: paclitaxel 250 mg/m^2 by 24-hr infusion with G-CSF on days 3 to 10. The target population was similar except that this study included only patients who had received one prior chemotherapy regimen for metastatic disease whether or not adjuvant chemotherapy had been received. More than half of the patients had also received prior adjuvant chemotherapy. Of 25 patients, 11 (44%) had objective responses (95% CI, 24%–65%), of which 2 (8%) were CR and 9 (36%) were PR. This response rate was similar to those of the previous trials. However, despite the use of G-CSF, one-third of patients still required dose reduction to 175 to 200 mg/m² by cycle 4, primarily for neutropenia with fever. A few patients had doses reduced for neuropathy, fatigue, and myalgias.

Two small differences were noted in these studies: the median time to response and the age differential of responding patients. The median times to response were 14 weeks in the M. D. Anderson study and 5 weeks in the Memorial Sloan-Kettering study. As noted above, however, even in the M. D. Anderson study, most patients who responded had objective evidence of improvement by 6 weeks. Patients with bone and liver lesions had clinical evidence of improvement by course 2. However, criteria for an objective response were not met for an additional two to six courses.

The second difference was the analysis of response by age (Table 4). In the Memorial Sloan-Kettering study, responses were more common in patients younger than 50 years, whereas the reverse was seen in the M. D. Anderson study, although the absolute difference in response rates between age groups was less. Even in the Memorial Sloan-Kettering study, however, this difference was not significant ($p = 0.105$ by Fischer's exact method). Given the heterogeneity of breast cancer, the obvious explanation for both these differences is the small sample sizes.

D. Bristol-Myers Squibb (European-Canadian) Taxol Study Group

1. Design

Preliminary data have been presented in abstract form of an ongoing randomized phase II trial comparing two doses of paclitaxel, 135 mg/m² and 175 mg/m², given by 3-hr infusion in patients who had undergone only limited prior chemotherapy (7). Patients were stratified by time to disease progression or relapse after completion of adjuvant chemotherapy: less than or equal to 6 months versus greater than 6 months. Standard premedication was given. Eligibility criteria included the usual requirements for a phase II trial. The only restriction was that patients may have received only one prior chemotherapy regimen for metastatic disease. Patients may or may not have received adjuvant therapy; thus, some patients may have received as many as two prior regimens.

2. Patient Characteristics

A total of 471 patients have been randomized from 14 countries, including many European nations, Canada, and Israel. Preliminary reports on the initial 117 patients have been updated to include 245 patients (52% of the total); selected data are shown in Table 6 (8). Fifty-nine percent of patients had relapsed 6 months or less after completion of adjuvant chemotherapy. Nearly one-third of patients on each arm had had two prior chemotherapy regimens (i.e., both as adjuvant therapy and for metastatic disease), and approximately 70% of patients had received anthracyclines. Of these patients, 50% to 60% had received the anthracyclines for metastatic disease and about 10% for both adjuvant therapy and metastatic disease. Seventy percent of patients had visceral disease involving a median of two to four sites.

3. Results

Interim analysis was performed on the 245 patients who were evaluable for response after a median of five (range, 1–10) courses for the entire group and after

Table 6 Patient Characteristics by Arm in Bristol-Myers Squibb (European-Canadian) Taxol Study Group Randomized Trial Comparing Paclitaxel 135 mg/m^2 to 175 mg/m^2 by 3-Hr Infusion

	135 mg/m^2 ($n = 122$)	175 mg/m^2 ($n = 123$)
Relapse after adjuvant chemotherapy		
≤ 6 mo, %	59	59
> 6 mo, %	41	41
ECOG performance status 0–1, %	84	85
Median age, yr (range)	50 (25–75)	48 (25–70)
Prior chemotherapy, %		
Adjuvant	31	32
Metastatic	38	37
Adjuvant + metastatic	30	32
Prior anthracycline, %	69	72
Adjuvant only	31	38
Metastatic only	58	48
Adjuvant + metastatic	11	13
Dominant site, %		
Soft tissue	15	24
Bone (± soft tissue)	8	7
Viscera (± bone ± soft tissue)	76	70
Number of disease sites, %		
1	9	13
2–4	64	62
≥5	26	25

Abbreviations: ECOG, Eastern Cooperative Oncology Group.

a median of five (range, 1–10) courses and six (range, 1–9) courses, respectively, for the 135 mg/m^2 and 175 mg/m^2 arms. The overall response rate was 26%, with 3% CR and 23% PR. Of the 245 patients, 105 (43%) were still on treatment and had stable disease. Responses were analyzed by prior therapy. For patients who had undergone prior adjuvant, metastatic, or adjuvant and metastatic therapy, response rates were 32%, 20%, and 26%, respectively. Analysis of results by anthracycline sensitivity is discussed later in this chapter.

Responses are analyzed by treatment arm in Table 7. Of 117 patients in each arm who were evaluable for response, the objective response rates were 22% in the lower-dose group and 29% in the higher-dose group (one-sided $p = 0.295$). Subset analysis by prior therapy suggested that patients who had received only prior adjuvant therapy had the highest rates of response, 29% (lower dose) and 35% (higher dose); but patients who had received both adjuvant and metastatic chemotherapy fared only slightly worse, with objective response rates of 22% (lower dose) and 29% (higher dose). The median times to progression were 3.1 and 4.2 months, respectively, for the lower- and higher-dose arms ($p =$ not significant).

4. Toxic Effects

This outpatient regimen was well tolerated. Selected toxic effects are shown by treatment arm in Table 8. World Health Organization (WHO) grade 3 or 4 neutropenia was more frequent in the 175 mg/m^2 arm than in the 135 mg/m^2 arm: 66%

Table 7 Results by Arm in Bristol-Myers Squibb (European-Canadian) Taxol Study Group Randomized Trial Comparing Paclitaxel 135 mg/m^2 to 175 mg/m^2 by 3-Hr Infusion

	135 mg/m^2 ($n = 117$)	175 mg/m^2 ($n = 117$)
Complete response, %	1 ⎱ 22%[a]	6 ⎱ 29%[a]
Partial response, %	21 ⎰	23 ⎰
Stable disease, %	45	45
Progressive disease, %	32	25
Adjuvant	31	32
Metastatic	38	37
Adjuvant + metastatic	30	32
Response by prior chemotherapy, %		
Adjuvant only	29	35
Metastatic only	16	24
Adjuvant + metastatic	22	29
Median time to progress, mo	3.1	4.2
95% confidence interval (CI)	2.6–4.3	3.2–4.6

[a]$p = 0.295$ for the difference in objective response rates between arms.
Overall response (95% CI) for each arm: 22% (17%–28%); 29% (23%–35%).

Table 8 Toxic Effects by Arm in Bristol-Myers Squibb (European-Canadian) Taxol Study Group Randomized Trial Comparing Paclitaxel 135 mg/m² to 175 mg/m² by 3-Hr Infusion

Toxic effect, worst WHO grade,[a] by % patients	135 mg/m², % patients (n = 117)	175 mg/m², % patients (n = 117)[b]
Neutropenia[c]		
Grade 3	30	39
Grade 4	21	27
Fever	21	18
Infection	10	18
Severe infection	1	0
Peripheral neuropathy		
Grade 3	44	63
Grade 4	3	6
Mucositis		
Grade 3	11	23
Grade 4	1	3
Arthralgia/myalgia		
Any	56	51
Severe	10	13
Hypersensitivity reactions		
Any	29	37
Severe	0	0

[a]WHO, World Health Organization.
[b]Denominator varies from 116 to 119.
[c]Grades 3–4, 135 vs 175 mg/m²: $p = 0.03$.

and 51%, respectively. Fever or infectious complications were found in 31% of the lower-dose group and 36% of the higher-dose group and were mild except in one patient on the lower-dose arm who developed pneumonia. Grade 3 thrombocytopenia or anemia occurred in fewer than 5% of patients on either arm.

There were no adverse cardiac events or significant hypersensitivity reactions, although nearly 30% to 40% of patients on each arm experienced mild symptoms such as flushing, rash, or alterations in blood pressure. The occurrence of grade 3 or 4 peripheral neuropathy and mucositis was related to dose, although, at least in this early analysis, the occurrence of myalgia/arthralgia syndrome was unrelated to dose.

5. Conclusions

Results from the full study of 471 patients were analyzed in November 1993 (8). With the larger number of patients and longer follow-up, it appears that the higher dose is superior in terms of response rates, especially in patients who are resistant to anthracyclines (see below). Response durations are similar in both arms. The response rates are lower than would have been predicted from the results of earlier phase II studies, but nearly one-third of the patients had had two prior regimens, and even the highest dose level is still somewhat low in comparison to the doses used in the previous two studies. Grade 4 neutropenia occurred in only 21% of the lower-dose arm and 27% of the higher-dose arm, whereas it occurred in 100% in the M. D. Anderson study and 57% in the Memorial Sloan-Kettering study, which used higher doses of G-CSF. Toxic events were more common in the higher-dose arm but were, in general, mild, suggesting that even higher doses could be used safely. This study was the basis for the Oncology Drug Advisory Committee's recommendation to the Food and Drug Administration that paclitaxel be approved for the palliative therapy of patients with metastatic breast cancer whose tumors progressed after or during therapy with anthracyclines.

III. COMBINATION STUDIES WITH DOXORUBICIN

Once the activity of paclitaxel was confirmed, the next step was to combine it with other agents. The obvious choice for the initial empirical combination was doxorubicin, because it is clearly the most active agent in breast cancer. Because of the high levels of activity of both drugs, and to better define the efficacy of this combination, only patients without prior chemotherapy for metastatic disease were eligible. Again, scarce drug supplies limited the number of studies until recently. Only three U.S. phase I combination trials had been reported, all in abstract form, as of October 1993 (9–16). A second generation of combination studies, with doxorubicin or cisplatin were initiated in the USA, Canada, and Europe and were reported or discussed at the Seventh European Conference on Clinical Oncology and Cancer Nursing (ECCO-7) in November 1993 (17–19) (also see Table 2). These are discussed after the doxorubicin studies.

A. Phase I Trials with Doxorubicin by Continuous Infusion

In 1990, the NCI (11–13) and M. D. Anderson (9,10) designed parallel studies of paclitaxel and doxorubicin, administered by different schedules, as the initial chemotherapy for metastatic disease. However, each study reached markedly different maximum tolerated doses (MTD), so both studies were expanded to evaluate pharmacokinetics and schedule-dependent interactions.

1. M. D. Anderson Trial

a. Design. The treatment plan was as follows: paclitaxel over 24 hr followed immediately by a fixed dose of (60 mg/m^2) doxorubicin over 48 hr (Tables 1 and 9). On days 5 through 19, G-CSF 5 µg/kg was administered subcutaneously.

Table 9 Design and Patient Characteristics in Phase II Combination Trials of Paclitaxel with Doxorubicin in Patients Who Had Received Limited Prior Chemotherapy

Schedule	M. D. Anderson		NCI-USA	Indiana U
	sequential Tax → Dox	sequential Dox → Tax	simultaneous Tax + Dox	alternate sequence between and within patients
Paclitaxel duration, hr	24	24	72	24
Doxorubicin duration, hr	48	48	72	Rapid IV[a]
G-CSF, µg/kg	5	5	10	5
Number of patients treated	10	21	18	12
Median age, yr	48	47	?	?
Range	36–62	32–66		
Median disease-free interval, mo	18	18 26	?	?
Range	0–72	0–96		
Number who had received				
prior adjuvant chemotherapy	6	15	4	
prior adjuvant doxorubicin	3	5	0	
Dominant disease site	Viscera	Viscera	Viscera	
Median number of sites	2	2	2	?
Range	1–9	1–6	?	?

[a] A 4-hr interval was inserted between completion of one drug and administration of the next drug, irrespective of the sequence.
Abbreviations: Dox, doxorubicin; Tax, paclitaxel; IV, intravenous; G-CSF, granulocyte colony stimulating factor.

Paclitaxel doses would be escalated from a starting dose of 125 to 150, 180, and 210 mg/m^2. Standard premedication, administered to all patients, was oral dexamethasone 20 mg given 14 and 7 hours before paclitaxel and intravenous cimetidine 300 mg with diphenhydramine 50 mg given 1 hr before paclitaxel.

Patients were eligible if they had not received prior chemotherapy for metastatic disease and were sensitive to doxorubicin. Patients considered sensitive to doxorubicin were those who had received no prior doxorubicin or had relapsed more than 6 months after receiving an adjuvant chemotherapy regimen that contained doxorubicin. The total prior dose of doxorubicin was limited to 300 mg/m^2 if given by rapid infusion or 400 mg/m^2 if given by 48-hr or longer infusion. Patients must also have had adequate cardiac function demonstrated by gated cardiac scan. The patients must have met standard criteria for measurable or evaluable disease, adequate performance status, and good organ function and have signed an informed consent. Dose-limiting toxicity was defined as the occurrence of grade 3 toxic effects (excluding hematological effects and alopecia) in any two patients at a given dose level or grade 4 toxic effects in any one patient at a given dose level. Because the profound myelosuppression seen in the phase II trial performed at M. D. Anderson without G-CSF had no serious clinical consequences, dose-limiting hematological toxicity was defined as infection or fever during granulocytopenia (granulocyte count $\leq$ 500/mm^3), a granulocyte count of less than 250 granulocytes/mm^3 for 5 days or more, failure to recover to a count of 1500 granulocytes/mm^3 by day 22, or a platelet count of less than 20,000/mm^3.

b. *Results (Table 10).* Only 10 patients were required to determine the MTD. The median age was 48 years (range, 36–62 years), and the median disease-free interval was 18 months (range, 0–72 months). In eight patients, the dominant site of disease was the viscera; the median number of disease sites was two (range, 1–9). Six patients had received prior adjuvant chemotherapy, and in three it was a doxorubicin-based regimen. Dose-limiting stomatitis or neutropenia with fever was seen in three of six patients treated at the starting dose, so lower doses were tested: paclitaxel/doxorubicin (mg/m^2) 125/48, 125/40, 100/40, and 90/36. Paclitaxel 125 mg/m^2 and doxorubicin 48 mg/m^2 was the MTD for the first course. In subsequent courses, however, cumulative thrombocytopenia (Fig. 2) required further dose reductions. Despite the use of G-CSF, 60% of patients (6% of courses) had neutropenia with fever. The other significant toxic effect was stomatitis of grade 2 or greater in all patients (60% of courses). One patient had a CR in liver and soft-tissue disease; seven patients had PR (95% CI, 44%–98%). The median duration of response was 6.5 months (range, 3–13 months). All patients relapsed, and four patients had died when this report was prepared. The poor prognosis of this group is underscored by the observation that 3 of these 10 patients developed leptomeningeal metastases; in 2 of them, it was the first site of failure while they were receiving paclitaxel and doxorubicin. The median duration of survival is 16.5 months (range, 8–22+ months).

Table 10 Preliminary Results of Phase I Trials of Paclitaxel with Doxorubicin

Trial	M. D. Anderson: Tax → Dox	M. D. Anderson: Dox → Tax	NCI: Tax + Dox	Indiana University: Tax ↔ Dox
No. patients	10	21	18	6
No. courses	102	239	?	?
Dose-limiting toxic effect	Mucositis, neutropenic fever	Neutropenic fever	Mucositis-diarrhea, abdominal pain (typhlitis)	Sequence-dependent[a] mucositis
Other chronic toxic effect	Thrombocytopenia	Thrombocytopenia	Thrombocytopenia	?
Maximum tolerated dose, mg/m²				
Tax	125	150	160 & 180	150
Dox	48	60	75 & 60	50
No. CR (%)	1 (10)	1 (5)	1 (6)	?
No. PR (%)	7 (70)	10 (57)	10 (56)	?
No. minor response/no change (%)	2 (20)	11 (43)	7 (38)	?
No. progressing (%)	0	0	0	?
95% Confidence interval for % CR + PR	44%–98%	34%–78%	36%–83%	?

[a]Tax → Dox: grade 3–4 mucositis in three patients; Dox → Tax: none.
Abbreviations: Tax, paclitaxel; Dox, doxorubicin; CR, complete response; PR, partial response.

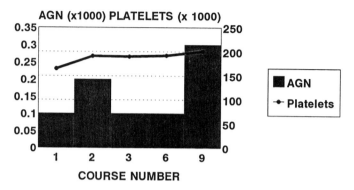

AGN = absolute granulocyte nadir

Figure 2 Hematologic toxic effects in selected courses is M. D. Anderson Cancer Center phase I trial of paclitaxel preceding doxorubicin as initial chemotherapy for metastatic breast cancer.

c. *Reverse Schedule.* Meanwhile, preliminary data from the NCI study, which administers both drugs by 72-hr continuous infusion, showed a much higher MTD and a different pattern of toxic effects (see below). We inferred a schedule-dependent interaction and instituted a reverse schedule, using the new starting dose of doxorubicin 48 mg/m^2 and paclitaxel 125 mg/m^2 (Table 1). Twenty-one patients were treated. The median age was 47 (range, 32–66 years). The median disease-free interval was 18 months (range, 0–96 months). All patients had visceral disease, and the median number of sites was two (range, 1–6 sites). Fifteen patients had had prior adjuvant chemotherapy, and in five it was doxorubicin-based. The dose-limiting toxic effect for the first course was neutropenic fever, and the MTD was paclitaxel 150 mg/m^2, doxorubicin 60 mg/m^2. In subsequent courses, dose-limiting mucositis and cumulative thrombocytopenia also occurred. One patient had a CR and 11 had PR, for an objective response rate of 57% (95% CI, 34%–78%) (Table 9). The median duration of response is greater than 6.5 months (range, 3–12 months), and the median survival is greater than 11 months (range, 6–17+ months). A total of 3 patients died, and 11 patients continued on the study as of October 1993.

d. *Pharmacokinetic Studies.* Because the MTDs for each schedule were so different, we hypothesized that pretreatment with paclitaxel alters doxorubicin pharmacokinetics and tested this hypothesis in a small trial (14). Five patients were treated with the lower MTD, paclitaxel 125 mg/m^2 and doxorubicin 48 mg/m^2. For course 1, three patients received paclitaxel followed by doxorubicin and two received doxorubicin followed by paclitaxel. Doses of drugs were held constant, but the sequence of administration was reversed in the second course. Preliminary pharmacokinetic data confirmed the clinical observation and our hypothesis. In seven of eight patients, doxorubicin plasma levels at the end of the infusion were 72% higher in the group receiving paclitaxel before doxorubicin compared to the reverse sequence. Doxorubicin clearance was decreased by an average of 30% in the group receiving paclitaxel before doxorubicin compared to the reverse sequence. It appears that immediate sequencing of paclitaxel before doxorubicin impairs doxorubicin disposition by unknown mechanisms.

2. NCI Trial

a. Design (Tables 1 and 9). The starting dose was paclitaxel 160 mg/m^2 and doxorubicin 45 mg/m^2; then planned dose escalation was to increase doxorubicin to a maximum of 75 mg/m^2, and then to increase paclitaxel in increments of 20 mg/m^2. Both drugs were given simultaneously by 72-hr infusion. Granulocyte colony stimulating factor was given at a higher dose, 10 μg/kg. Dose-limiting toxicity was defined as any grade 3 or 4 nonhematological toxic effect excluding nausea or vomiting that could be controlled with medication. Dose-limiting hematological toxicity was defined as a granulocyte count less than 500/mm^3 for more than 5 days, a platelet count less than 20,000/mm^3, or any toxic effect that prohibited retreatment at full doses by day 22. Eligibility criteria were similar to those of earlier trials except that patients who had received any prior doxorubicin were excluded.

b. Results (Table 10). A total of 18 patients were treated to determine the MTD of paclitaxel in combination with doxorubicin 60 mg/m^2 (11–13); 12 other patients were treated to determine the MTD of paclitaxel in combination with doxorubicin 75 mg/m^2. Finally, another 12 patients were treated to evaluate the pharmacokinetics of this combination, for a total of 42 patients.

Of the original 18 patients required for determination of the MTD, 4 had received prior adjuvant chemotherapy and had a median of two sites of disease; 10 patients had liver metastases. At doses of paclitaxel 180 mg/m^2 and doxorubicin 75 mg/m^2, dose-limiting toxicity, grade 3 diarrhea, and abdominal pain with radiographic changes supportive of a diagnosis of typhlitis occurred (22,23). The MTD was paclitaxel 180 mg/m^2 with doxorubicin 60 mg/m^2. Subsequently, the dose of paclitaxel was decreased to 160 mg/m^2 and that of doxorubicin was escalated. The MTD for this combination was paclitaxel 160 mg/m^2, doxorubicin 75 mg/m^2.

Anemia and thrombocytopenia were common and cumulative, and platelet transfusion was required in a small fraction of the patients. In over half of all cycles, patients required hospitalization for neutropenic fever (47%) or documented infection (8%). In the first 18 patients, all evaluable, the objective responses were CR 6% and 10 PR (56%), for an overall rate of 62% (95% CI, 36%–83%). When the entire cohort of 42 patients was evaluated, 39 patients were evaluable, and the response data were slightly better: 72% objective responses

(95% CI, 55%–85%), of which 10% were CR. The median duration of response was 7 months (13).

c. *Pharmacokinetic Studies.* The pharmacology of paclitaxel was evaluated in four groups of patients (15). The intent was to determine whether there was any difference in paclitaxel or doxorubicin pharmacokinetics when they were given together versus when they were given separately. In group 1, paclitaxel and doxorubicin were administered at the MTD for course 1 and doxorubicin alone for course 2. In group 2, courses 1 and 2 were as for group 1, but reversed; i.e., doxorubicin was given alone for course 1, etc. In group 3, paclitaxel and doxorubicin were given at the MTD for course 1; paclitaxel was given alone at the same dose as in the combination for course 2. In group 4, courses 1 and 2 were as for group 3, but reversed; i.e., paclitaxel was given alone for course 1. No difference in the steady-state plasma concentrations of paclitaxel or doxorubicin were seen whether the drugs were given alone over 72 hr or in combination (15). The concentrations of doxorubicinol, a metabolite that is less cytotoxic than the parent drug, were increased 1.5-fold. However, the absolute concentration was very low (0.016–0.025 μM) and not considered clinically important.

B. Phase I Study with Doxorubicin by Rapid Injection

After release of preliminary reports of the studies described above and recognizing that doxorubicin administered by continuous infusion causes a higher incidence of mucositis and that most physicians administer it as a rapid intravenous infusion (i.e., a bolus, or "IV push"), Sledge et al. (16–18) performed two pilot trials evaluating this combination as a prelude to an Intergroup phase III study designed to compare the efficacy of the combination with that of each of its components.

1. *Phase II Study of Alternating Paclitaxel and Doxorubicin*

The first trial investigated a sequential combination of paclitaxel and doxorubicin (17). Paclitaxel 200 mg/m² alternated with doxorubicin 75 mg/m² every 3 weeks. Eligible patients may have received only one prior chemotherapy regimen.

Preliminary results were presented at the 1993 annual meeting of the American Society for Clinical Oncology (ASCO) (Table 10). Of the initial 10 patients with measurable disease, 2 had CR and 5 had PR. The incidence of febrile neutropenia was identical with both drugs, 17%. As expected, however, the incidence of thrombocytopenia was greater when doxorubicin was given.

2. *Phase I Trial of Paclitaxel and Doxorubicin*

The second trial (18) evaluated the simultaneous combination of paclitaxel with doxorubicin (given by bolus) as initial chemotherapy for metastases (Tables 1 and 10). To further define any schedule-dependent toxicity, the sequence of administration of each drug was alternated not only between patients but also within patients, changing with each cycle. The two schedules comprised doxorubicin given first by bolus, followed 4 hr later by paclitaxel by 24-hr infusion, and the reverse. The 4-hr interval between completion of one drug and the start of the next drug was used in both sequences. Two dose levels were evaluated: paclitaxel 150 mg/m^2 with doxorubicin 50 mg/m^2 and paclitaxel 175 mg/m^2 with doxorubicin 60 mg/m^2. On days 3 through 12, G-CSF 5 μg/kg was given subcutaneously.

Results. Only 12 patients were needed to determine the MTD, 6 at each level. As expected, the frequency of toxic effects was higher in the group that received the higher doses. Neutropenic fever or infection occurred in 18% of the lower-dose group and 30% of the higher-dose group. Four courses were complicated by grade 3/4 mucositis in three patients who were treated at the higher dose level, but only when they received the sequence in which paclitaxel preceded doxorubicin; no patients receiving the reverse sequence had mucositis. Response data were not reported.

3. *Phase III Trial Comparing Paclitaxel Alone, Doxorubicin Alone, and the Combination of Paclitaxel and Doxorubicin*

The two trials already described provided the framework for a multicenter study comparing each of the single agents to the combination (16). This Intergroup trial, in which the Eastern Cooperative Oncology Group (ECOG), the North Central Cancer Treatment Group (NCCTG), and the Southwest Oncology Group (SWOG) will participate, will test paclitaxel alone (175 mg/m^2 by 3-hr infusion), doxorubicin 60 mg/m^2 alone, and the combination of paclitaxel 150 mg/m^2 and doxorubicin 50 mg/m^2 with G-CSF 5 μg/kg/day. Besides testing the relative efficacy and toxicity of these regimens, the crossover efficacy will also be evaluated. Secondary study objectives include determining the effects of these regimens on quality of life and the relationship of steady-state paclitaxel levels to responses. Accrual is targeted for 730 patients, of whom 660 (90%) are expected to be eligible for analysis.

IV. PHASE II TRIALS IN PATIENTS WHO HAVE HAD EXTENSIVE PRIOR THERAPY

As more paclitaxel has become available, it has been possible to test it in patients with advanced stage IV disease. Only preliminary data are available from these studies, some of which are still in progress. An important component of these trials of palliative therapy is the assessment of quality of life (24), an issue that has been difficult to evaluate quantitatively in a standardized manner. The complexity of the analysis of these data will require a separate report delivered after response data have been fully analyzed.

A. Memorial Sloan-Kettering Cancer Center—24-Hr Infusion

This trial essentially repeated Memorial Sloan-Kettering's initial phase II trial but was targeted to patients who had undergone two or more prior chemotherapy regimens (6,25). Paclitaxel 200 mg/m^2 was given by 24-hr infusion with G-CSF. Fifty-one patients were quickly enrolled. The tumors of 22 (51%) of these patients had primary resistance to doxorubicin or mitoxantrone, and those of 27 (53%) had secondary resistance; i.e., the tumors had a transient response before progressing. In two patients, stable disease was the best response to either drug. A total of 22 patients (43%) had received two prior regimens and 29 patients (57%) had received three or more. Fourteen percent of patients had received high-dose chemotherapy regimens that required transplant of autologous bone marrow or transfer of peripheral blood stem cells, with growth factor support. Two-thirds had received palliative irradiation.

Results

Only preliminary results (Table 11) have been reported (6,25), but the study has been completed and the final report is forthcoming. Partial responses were observed in 14 patients (27%; 95% CI, 16%–42%). The median duration of response was 7 months. Responses were analyzed by number of prior regimens. Responses were seen in 36% (95% CI, 16%–56%) and 21% (95% CI, 8%–40%), respectively, of the 22 patients who had received two prior regimens and the 29 who had received three or more regimens.

As expected, myelosuppression was the dose-limiting toxic effect, but thrombocytopenia (<50,000 platelets/mm^3) occurred in 10 patients (19%). At the time of the initial report, no patients had had their doses escalated, whereas doses had to be reduced in 47% of patients, generally for hematological toxic effects. However, four patients had other toxic effects: profound weakness (one patient), severe myalgia and arthralgia (one patient), or severe stomatitis (two patients).

Table 11 Preliminary Results of Paclitaxel by 24-Hr Infusion in Four Studies in Patients Who Had Received Extensive Prior Therapy

	Memorial Sloan-Kettering		M. D. Anderson	
No. prior chemotherapy regimens	2	≥3	2	≥3
Range	—	(3–6)	—	(3–7)
Dose, mg/m^2	200	200	175	150
G-CSF	Yes	Yes	No	No
Number of evaluable patients	22	29	35	33
Response rates, % (95% CI)				
CR	0	0	0	0
PR	36 (16–56)	21 (8–40)	20 (8–39)	18 (7–35)

Abbreviations: G-CSF, Granulocyte-colony stimulating factor; CI, confidence interval; CR, complete response; PR, partial response.

B. M. D. Anderson Cancer Center—24-Hr Infusion

1. Patients Who Had Received Three or More Prior Regimens

a. Design and Patient Characteristics. Because the dose-response data for paclitaxel were still unknown but the cost of colony stimulating factors was high, a trial was designed to evaluate paclitaxel administered by 24-hr infusion without G-CSF (10,26). The target population was patients who had received three or more prior regimens, inclusive of adjuvant therapy. The starting doses were 150 mg/m^2 for patients at standard risk of complicated myelosuppression and 135 mg/m^2 for patients at high risk. We defined complicated myelosuppression as the occurrence of fever or infection during neutropenia. We defined patients as being at high risk for complicated myelosuppression if (1) they had undergone irradiation of up to 25% of the marrow-bearing bones, (2) they had had prior chemotherapy with mitomycin-C or high-dose regimens requiring rescue by autologous stem cells, or (3) they had evidence of poor hematological tolerance to prior chemotherapy manifested by dose reductions or delays. If infectious complications occurred, dose reduction, not addition of G-CSF, would be used for subsequent courses. Recognizing the palliative nature of this therapy, we included a formal assessment of quality of life (27). Patient characteristics are shown in Table 11 and compared with those of the patients in the Memorial Sloan-Kettering trial. The patients in this trial were slightly older and had a median of four prior chemotherapy regimens (range, 3–7 regimens).

b. Results. Analysis of 35 patients with a median of 4 courses per patient, showed 6 PR (18%; 95% CI, 7%–35%) (Table 11). Neutropenia and fever or infection occurred in 21% of all cycles. The median duration of response was greater than 5.5 months (range, 2–7 months).

2. Patients Who Had Received Two Prior Regimens

To better define the role of G-CSF and dose in patients who had received only two prior regimens, a second arm was added to the study for patients in this category. The starting doses were 175 mg/m^2 for patients at standard risk of myelosuppression and 150 mg/m^2 for those at high risk. Of 35 patients, PR was seen in 20% (95% CI, 8–39%) (Table 11).

C. National Cancer Institute, Medicine Branch—96-Hr Infusion

1. Design and Rationale

As noted above, Fojo and other researchers at NCI showed that administration of drugs susceptible to P-glycoprotein–mediated multidrug resistance by a slow, long-duration infusion retarded expression of P-glycoprotein (28,29). Wilson et al. exploited this concept in a phase I trial of paclitaxel by 96-hr infusion in patients with breast cancer or lymphoma (30,31). The MTD was 140 mg/m^2, and the limiting toxic effect was mucositis. A subsequent phase II trial for patients with breast cancer or lymphoma tested this dose with the addition of G-CSF. Neither of these trials used the standard prophylactic medications for prevention of hypersensitivity reactions. The rationale for this omission was that the concentration of the apparent cause of this reaction, the diluent polyoxyethylated castor oil, would be much less than one-fourth of that administered by the standard 24-hr schedule. Moreover, from a practical standpoint, the 4-day duration of the infusion made it illogical to premedicate patients only on day 1.

Another important objective of this study was to evaluate P-glycoprotein expression in patients whose disease could be biopsied.

2. Eligibility

Only patients who had received two prior chemotherapy regimens were eligible. Additionally, they must have received doxorubicin and developed progressive disease while receiving it.

3. Results

Preliminary results were presented at the 1993 Annual Meeting of ASCO (30), but mature data were published in late 1994 in the *Journal of Clinical Oncology* (31). Of 33 evaluable patients with a median age of 49 and a median Zubrod performance status of 1, 16 (48%) had PR (95% CI, 31%–66%). Only 21% of patients had outright progression of disease. The preliminary results of the biopsy studies to evaluate multidrug resistance were unrevealing; P-glycoprotein expression was uniformly low in all specimens.

D. National Cancer Institute Protocol TRC-9202—24-Hr Infusion

Before approval and wider availability of paclitaxel, the NCI developed a Treatment Referral Center (TRC) program for compassionate use. The starting doses were 175 mg/m^2 for patients at standard risk of myelosuppression and 135 mg/m^2 for high-risk patients, both by 24-hr infusion without G-CSF. High-risk patients were those who had received prior irradiation to more than 30% of the bone marrow or a cumulative mitomycin-C dose of at least 20 mg/m^2. Eligibility criteria were standard and targeted patients who had received two or more prior regimens for metastatic disease. However, patients with both measurable and evaluable disease were eligible. The duration of therapy was three courses after best response or a maximum of eight cycles if patients had stable disease.

1. Results

a. Patient Characteristics. The results of this study were presented at December 1993 hearings of the Oncology Drug Advisory Committee to the Food and Drug Administration and were presented at the combined European Organization for the Research and Treatment of Cancer (EORTC)/NCI-USA meetings in March 1994 (32). From November 1992 through February 1993, 44 centers registered 267 patients. Because 11 patients were never treated, and data are missing for 9 patients, 247 were evaluable for toxic effects. Of these 247 patients, 164 were evaluable for response. A total of 83 patients were excluded from response analysis because they did not have measurable disease (80 patients) or were not eligible (3 patients). Most responses and charts had not yet been audited by NCI at the time of this report (December 1993). The median age was 51 years (range, 23–85 years); the median ECOG performance status was 1 (range, 0–2). Sixty-nine percent of the patients had measurable disease. Sixty percent had had three or more prior chemotherapy regimens, and 88% were considered not to be candidates for doxorubicin therapy. However, fewer than half of these patients were resistant to doxorubicin as already defined. In the majority of patients, additional therapy with doxorubicin was not possible because they had received their cumulative maximum dose (39%) or other medical contraindications existed (24%). A total of 1137 courses were given to the 247 patients evaluable for toxicity. The median number of courses was four (range, 1–13).

   b. *Responses and Toxic Effects.* Preliminary results as of November 1993 showed a 22% overall response rate (95% CI, 16%–29%), of which 2% were CR. The median duration of response was 5 months (range, 2–10+ months). Nearly one-third of patients started at the lower dose; 37% had dose reductions; 24% had dose delays longer than 1 week; and 42% received G-CSF. Grade 4 neutropenia occurred in 70% of patients, but infections were documented in only 7%. However, 46% of patients experienced febrile neutropenia, and 34% of these episodes occurred in course 1, which did not include the use of G-CSF. Other non-hematological toxic effects were generally mild and occurred in fewer than half of all patients. Analysis of response by prior doxorubicin status is discussed below.

V. DOXORUBICIN RESISTANCE AND PACLITAXEL

Since both paclitaxel and doxorubicin are susceptible to P-glycoprotein–mediated multidrug resistance, an important question that arose early in paclitaxel trials was the issue of cross-resistance. The definition of doxorubicin resistance in metastatic disease is clear: development of progressive disease during treatment with a doxorubicin-based regimen. However, for patients who received adjuvant doxorubicin or doxorubicin for metastatic disease and discontinued it for reasons other than progressive disease (generally after reaching a specified cumulative total dose), the definition is less clear. Development of metastatic disease within 6, 12, and 12 months, respectively, after completing adjuvant chemotherapy were the definitions used by M. D. Anderson, Memorial Sloan-Kettering, and the Istituto Nazionale Tumor (INT—Milan) in Italy (2,4,19,33). In a later update (19), however, INT-Milan further categorized anthracycline resistance as primary or secondary. Primary resistance was defined as absence of response to doxorubicin or recurrence within 6 months after any response that was not a CR. Secondary resistance was defined as recurrence or progression more than 6 months after completion of anthracycline-based chemotherapy. Vermorken et al. (35) defined resistance as disease progression while receiving a chemotherapy regimen containing doxorubicin or epirubicin within 4 to 12 weeks before starting paclitaxel. At the NCI, the definition of Wilson et al. was no response or failure to achieve a CR after a complete course of doxorubicin- or mitoxantrone-based therapy (31). Only very limited information is available from a trial by Uziely et al. (36) in patients with resistance to doxorubicin and tumor accessible to biopsy. With these definitions in mind, the results of subset analysis by study of patients with doxorubicin resistance whose disease was treated with paclitaxel are shown in Table 12. What is striking is that the response rates in anthracycline-resistant patients, with the exceptions of the very small number of patients in the initial M. D. Anderson trial and those reported in the preliminary results of the INT-Milan trial, are identical to those of the overall study from which they are derived. The only described mechanisms of paclitaxel resistance are P-glycoprotein–mediated resistance and alterations in tubulin binding. Because doxorubicin does not function as a microtubule binding agent, the only common pathway for doxorubicin and paclitaxel resistance is through P-glycoprotein. The apparent lack of cross-resistance evinced by these studies suggests that many cases of doxorubicin resistance are not mediated by P-glycoprotein. Indeed, many mechanisms of resistance to doxorubicin have been described, most importantly qualitative and quantitative alterations in topoisomerase II. Although only limited information is currently available from the study by Uziely et al., in which patients who were resistant to doxorubicin had biopsies for P-glycoprotein before and after paclitaxel therapy, this will be an important study (36).

A. Bristol-Myers Squibb Taxol Study Group

Updated results from this study have been included in Table 12. They show that anthracycline sensitivity had no clear effect on response in the 175 mg/m^2 arm, but patients who received 135 mg/m^2 and were anthracycline-resistant had a lower response rate (7,8). However, the numbers of patients in these subsets are too small for definitive conclusions.

B. INT-Milan Study

This is a phase II study focused on patients who relapsed within 12 months after completion of anthracycline-based adjuvant chemotherapy or who progressed while receiving anthracycline therapy for metastatic disease. The first patients were treated at 175 mg/m^2 by 3-hr infusion (33). When no dose-limiting toxic effects were seen, 13 additional patients were treated at 225 mg/m^2 (34). All the patients who had adjuvant anthracyclines received it as neoadjuvant therapy, so assessment of response to anthracycline therapy was possible in all patients.

Table 12 Paclitaxel and Anthracycline Resistance in Available Clinical Trials[a]

Trial (ref)	Total no. patients	CR + PR, %	No. resistant to anthracycline	CR + PR, %
M. D. Anderson, one prior rx (2)	25	56	6	33
Memorial Sloan-Kettering, two prior rx (4)	72	28	37	30
NCI-≥ two prior, 96-hr infusion (30,31)	17	53	17	53
European Canadian, 3 hr (7,8)				
175 mg/m²	235	29	38	27
135 mg/m²	236	22	30	15
NCI-TRC 9202 (32)	164[b]	22	145	23
INT-Milan, 3 hr 175, 225 mg/m² (19,33)	28	36	28	Primary 27[c] Secondary 47 see[d]
U Southern California, 135 mg/m² 24 hr, biopsy for Pgp[d] (36)	36	>17	32	

[a]Definitions of resistance varied. The NCI definition was no response to doxorubicin or mitoxantrone or failure to achieve a CR to a complete course of therapy. M. D. Anderson and the European-Canadian study included the NCI definition and progression within 6 months after completion of an adjuvant regimen for patients with newly diagnosed metastatic disease. Memorial Sloan-Kettering was least stringent and considered progression within 12 months after adjuvant therapy in addition to the NCI criterion.

[b]Of 247 treated patients, 164 were evaluable for response.

[c]Primary resistance: absence of response to doxorubicin or recurrence within 6 months from a noncomplete response; secondary resistance: recurrence or progression more than 6 months after completing anthracycline-based chemotherapy.

[d]Pgd, P-glycoprotein as a mediator of multidrug resistance. Insufficient data from abstract. However, responses were seen only in patients with weak or absent immunostaining for Pgp. See text.

Abbreviations: CR, complete response; PR, partial response; rx, regimen.

Of the 28 patients reported in the update (34), 16 had had neoadjuvant therapy and 12 had had palliative therapy. All patients had measurable disease. The overall response rate was 36% (95% CI, 19%–56%), with 4 CR, 6 PR, and 10 stable disease. Response rate was reported not to be dose-related. The median duration of response was 5 months (range, 1–11.5 months), and five patients were continuing therapy. World Health Organization grade 4 neutropenia was seen in only 3% and 7% of cycles at 175 mg/m^2 and 225 mg/m^2, respectively. As noted in Table 12, the response rate in patients with primary anthracycline resistance was only 60% of that in patients with secondary anthracycline resistance (27% versus 47%).

C. European Cancer Center Trial (Amsterdam)

Preliminary data were reported by Vermorken et al. on 17 patients who would fit Gianni's classification of primary anthracycline resistance described above (35). Paclitaxel 250 mg/m^2 by 3-hr infusion with escalation to 300 mg/m^2 and G-CSF support was given every 3 weeks. Only 3 PR (18%) were seen, disease was unchanged in six patients, five had progressive disease, and three died soon after therapy. The interpretation of the final reports of these two trials will certainly be influenced by the considerations of schedule addressed below.

VI. UNANSWERED QUESTIONS: TRIALS IN PROGRESS

A search for clinical trials of paclitaxel in patients with breast cancer or open trials for patients with solid tumors in the Physicians Data Query (PDQ) database of NCI-sponsored protocols yielded 34 ongoing studies in January 1994. Each well-designed trial generates as many questions as it answers. Many of these trials have secondary end points. This brief review will focus on the major questions to be answered. A partial listing of these studies is found in Table 2.

A. Optimal Schedule: Infusion Duration and Retreatment Interval

1. Infusion Duration

Two randomized studies are addressing different aspects of this issue.

   a. Bristol-Myers Squibb 071: 3- Versus 24-Hr Infusion. Data from trials in ovarian cancer have shown that the 3-hr infusion schedule is safe, well tolerated, and as effective as the 24-hr infusion schedule at doses of 135 mg/m^2 and 175 mg/m^2, but the spectrum of toxic effects was different (37). Neutropenia was much less frequent, 17% and 74%, respectively, with equal doses given over 3- and 24-hr. The occurrence of neuropathy was related only to the total dose. Whether this schedule is as effective in breast cancer is still unproved. Although clinical trials have proceeded on that assumption, editorial comment by Chabner (38) on the data presented at the Oncology Drug Advisory Committee to the FDA and by Arbuck (39) on the higher dose 3-hr infusion schedule (see B.1, below) have refocused attention on this question. Recent preclinical data in a number of cell lines show that, above a plateau concentration, cytotoxicity was more dependent on duration of exposure than on dose (40,41).

Bristol-Myers Squibb has completed accrual on a study that compares the 3- and 24-hr schedules in breast cancer. Over 500 patients have been accrued to this study, which uses paclitaxel at a dose of 175 mg/m^2 as second-line therapy. This sample size should provide a clear answer to the schedule question. A similar trial that was to have been performed by the Cancer and Leukemia Group B (CALGB) was never activated, presumably because of the data from the ovarian cancer studies.

b. *Memorial Sloan-Kettering: 3-Hr Infusion.* Memorial Sloan-Kettering is testing the 3-hr infusion schedule of paclitaxel without G-CSF as initial and salvage therapy for metastatic breast cancer (NCI protocol T92-0166). The dose for patients who have received no prior chemotherapy for metastatic breast cancer ("initial therapy group") is 250 mg/m^2. The dose for patients who have received two or more prior regimens is 175 mg/m^2. Doses will be reduced to 150 mg/m^2 and 125 mg/m^2 if necessary. Granulocyte colony stimulating factor will be added if patients develop febrile neutropenia after reduction of the dose to 125 mg/m^2. Quality of life will be assessed. Results for both the initial and salvage groups will be reported at the 1994 Annual Meeting of ASCO (42).

c. *M. D. Anderson/Memorial Sloan-Kettering: 3- Versus 96-Hour Infusion.* Another study, a phase II trial comparing the 3- and the 96-hr schedules, will be performed by M. D. Anderson and Memorial Sloan-Kettering and their affiliates. The target population will be patients who have received two or more prior regimens. All patients must have received anthracyclines or anthracenediones, and every effort will be made to document evidence of progressive disease during administration of doxorubicin or mitoxantrone. The intent is to determine whether the superior response rates reported by Wilson et al. (30,31) are as clearly schedule-dependent as suggested by the data and warrant the extra effort required by a 4-day infusion of a drug that has only a 27-hr stability. Starting doses will be 250 mg/m^2 and 140 mg/m^2, respectively, for the 3- and 96-hr infusion groups. Granulocyte colony stimulating factor will not be used unless patients develop fever during neutropenia, but it will be added in lieu of dose reduction for the initial episode. Dose escalation will be permitted. Tumors that can be biopsied will be evaluated for P-glycoprotein and microtubule bundling in consenting patients.

d. *Memorial Sloan-Kettering: 96-Hr Infusion.* Independently of the above trial, the NCI will sponsor a trial of 96-hr infusion of paclitaxel in patients whose disease has progressed on 3- or 24-hr infusion schedules. Patients whose disease has progressed while receiving docetaxel will also be treated on this trial.

e. *National Cancer Institute, Medicine Branch: 14-Day Infusion.* A phase I trial is under way. The initial infusion duration will be escalated from 8 to

12 to 14 days, after which the doses will be escalated. The target starting dose for the 14-day infusion is 2.5 mg/m²/day.

2. Retreatment Interval

In patients who received little prior therapy or are receiving G-CSF, granulocyte recovery is generally adequate for retreatment by day 14. In the early phase I trials in leukemia, which used a much higher dose, retreatment at intervals of less than 21 days resulted in severe cumulative mucositis. Two studies currently in progress are examining the 14-day retreatment interval.

a. *Vancouver: Paclitaxel with Cisplatin.* Gelmon is testing low doses of paclitaxel (90 mg/m²) by 3-hr infusion with cisplatin 60 mg/m² repeated every 14 days in patients with metastatic breast cancer in first relapse (20). Preliminary results were reported in a symposium format at the Seventh European Cancer and Clinical Oncology and Nursing (ECCO-7) meetings in November 1993. There were 16 evaluable patients, and objective responses were seen in 94% of them. Neutropenia was the dose-limiting toxic effect, and neurotoxic effects were minimal. Most patients receive treatment as outpatients.

b. *Memorial Sloan-Kettering: High-Risk Adjuvant Trial.* This trial evaluates paclitaxel in the postoperative adjuvant setting as a single agent at high doses for patients with 10 or more involved lymph nodes (43). The rationale for this regimen is twofold. First, Buzzoni et al. reported superior results in a study of adjuvant single-agent doxorubicin in sequence with cyclophosphamide, methotrexate, and 5-fluorouracil (44). Second, the Day-Norton reanalysis of the Goldie-Coldman hypothesis suggests that a series of high doses of multiple single agents may be more effective in treating resistant cells and in preventing the development of resistance than the simultaneous use of them at lower doses (45,46). The treatment schedule comprises three courses of each single agent repeated every 14 days in the order paclitaxel 250 mg/m², doxorubicin 90 mg/m², and cyclophosphamide 3 g/m². Granulocyte colony stimulating factor is given on days 3 through 10 of each cycle. Oral communications with Dr. Larry Norton about patient tolerance indicate that some patients develop noncardiogenic peripheral edema and dermatitis by the end of the paclitaxel courses. This is similar to the reported toxic effects of docetaxel (see below). However, with a maximum of only three cycles, the problem is self-limiting. Updated data will be presented at the 1994 ASCO meeting.

B. Optimal Dose

As noted above, the optimal dose is still unknown. The ovarian cancer studies, which used the 3-hr infusion schedule, suggest that dose may be important. This is a loaded question for health care planners, because the question of dose always brings up the need for hematopoietic support with G-CSF, which adds substantially to the cost of an expensive drug. However, the economics of the issue depend on the science of the question. The European-Canadian Paclitaxel Breast Study Group results (7,8), presented earlier, suggest an emerging advantage for the higher dose. A recently published study has addressed the question of optimal dose.

Wisconsin: Phase I Paclitaxel (3-Hr Infusion) With and Without G-CSF

The University of Wisconsin performed a phase I trial for patients with advanced cancer for whom no standard therapy was available. The study had two parallel arms, one in which patients received no G-CSF and one in which they received G-CSF 5 μg/kg beginning day 2 through 14 or until the absolute granulocyte count was above 10,000/mm^3 after the nadir. Final results were published in February 1994 (47). The MTD for the arms with and without G-CSF, respectively, were 250 mg/m^2 and 210 mg/m^2. As was expected, the dose-limiting toxic effect for the group that received G-CSF was peripheral neuropathy and that for the group that received no G-CSF was neutropenia. The neuropathy was related to dose and was cumulative. One patient treated at the 300 mg/m^2 dose became wheelchair-bound and unable to use her hands. She had previously received 600 mg/m^2 of cisplatin 6 months earlier. The mean absolute neutrophil counts with and without G-CSF were 4,500/mm^3 and 840/mm^3, respectively, and the durations of neutropenia (neutrophil counts less than 500/mm^3) were 0 and 2.5 days, respectively. Grade 3 myalgias and arthralgias were dose-dependent, were seen in 24% of courses, and were ameliorated by narcotics and corticosteroids. One of the 35 patients (2.8%) experienced a grade 3 anaphylactoid reaction.

C. Comparisons of Single-Agent Paclitaxel and Single-Agent Doxorubicin or Combinations

Although the initial phase I trials described above of paclitaxel with doxorubicin performed by the NCI and M. D. Anderson were not designed to evaluate responses, their preliminary results do not suggest that this dose and schedule combination are synergistic. Preclinical data recently published by Hahn et al. suggest there is less than additive in vitro cytotoxicity when paclitaxel is combined with doxorubicin (48). Earlier studies by Rose in a murine system showed similar results (49). However, a number of clinical trials are ongoing, and the preliminary results of at least one suggest that there is potential for synergy between the two agents (34).

ECOG: Paclitaxel Versus Doxorubicin Versus Paclitaxel Plus Doxorubicin

This is a randomized trial comparing paclitaxel 175 mg/m^2 by 24-hr infusion with doxorubicin 60 mg/m^2 by bolus injection and with the combination of paclitaxel 150 mg/m^2 by 24-hr infusion with doxorubicin 50 mg/m^2 by rapid injection with

G-CSF. This is an important study, because it addresses the issues raised by the phase I trials at M. D. Anderson and NCI (10,12).

Other trials with similar intents will evaluate patients who have received no prior chemotherapy for metastatic disease and compare paclitaxel with doxorubicin and with the standard regimen of cyclophosphamide, methotrexate, 5-fluorouracil, and prednisone (CMFP). In patients with refractory disease, two phase III trials will compare paclitaxel to salvage regimens that use vinblastine or mitomycin.

D. Combination Trials

A host of trials evaluating combinations of paclitaxel with cyclophosphamide, cisplatin, doxorubicin, edatrexate, vinorelbine, and other agents are underway. The high response rates in the study by Gelmon of cisplatin were described earlier (20). Reports of a similar combination but different schedule being tested at New York University did not confirm this level of activity (21). The INT-Milan trial results will also address the issue of schedule-dependent mucositis in doxorubicin and paclitaxel therapy. Preliminary reports suggest that the combination of paclitaxel by 3-hr infusion preceding doxorubicin given as a bolus injection does not produce the sequence-dependent mucositis and pharmacodynamic alterations reported by Holmes et al. (9,10) and Sledge et al. (18) for the 24-hr paclitaxel infusion.

Two other trials with microtubule-active agents are ongoing. One, at M. D. Anderson, combines vinorelbine and paclitaxel. Preliminary preclinical data in breast cancer cell lines suggest that the two agents are synergistic when administered simultaneously (50). This synergy was lost when the drugs were given sequentially. If vinorelbine precedes paclitaxel, the effects are additive, but if the sequence is reversed, there is antagonism. This study just opened for patient accrual at the time of this writing.

The second study, a phase I evaluation at the Fox Chase Cancer Center of fixed doses of estramustine with escalating doses of paclitaxel by 96-hr infusion, is nearing the MTD. Estramustine binds to microtubule-associated proteins (MAPs) to produce disruption of microtubules (51), whereas paclitaxel binds to tubulin. Although estramustine itself is only a weak antineoplastic agent, its action on the microtubules may enhance the activity of paclitaxel.

E. Resistance

Because P-glycoprotein-mediated multidrug resistance is a proven mechanism of resistance to paclitaxel (1), a number of trials are in progress to document its occurrence or evaluate methods to prevent or reverse it. R-verapamil, quinidine, and cyclosporine are among the agents under evaluation.

Preliminary results from a trial correlating the presence of P-glycoprotein in baseline biopsies of advanced breast tumors with response to paclitaxel were reported at the American Society of Clinical Oncology by Uziely et al. (Table 12) (36). She treated 36 patients with metastatic breast cancer and tumor accessible to biopsy with paclitaxel 135 mg/m^2 over 24 hours. Of these 36, 32 were classified as resistant to doxorubicin, as defined by progressive disease during treatment; 35 had pretreatment biopsies for P-glycoprotein which were double stained using monoclonal antibodies C219 and JSB1. Of 34 evaluable patients, 2 had CR, 4 had PR, and 2 were improved. Responses were seen only in patients with weak or absent immunostaining for P-glycoprotein. No responses occurred in patients with moderate or high expression. The final report should correlate baseline P-glyco-protein levels with prior therapy with anthracyclines and vinca alkaloids and subsequent response to paclitaxel. An interesting follow up question in this study will be whether or not any of the 8 responding patients developed P-glycoprotein expression upon failure to paclitaxel. The final data from this study are eagerly awaited.

A related issue is the definition of the contribution of the diluent, polyoxyethyl-ated castor oil, to the activity of paclitaxel by its ability to reverse P-glycoprotein–mediated multidrug resistance (52). The concentration of polyoxyethylated castor oil required to solubilize paclitaxel is higher than with any of the other drugs with which it is used, approximately 16 ml for a dose of 200 mg/m^2 (53). Recent studies suggest that paclitaxel doses of 135 mg/m^2 and 175 mg/m^2 given by 3-hr infusion produce sufficiently high plasma levels of polyoxyethylated castor oil to function as an inhibitor of P-glycoprotein (54). This issue will be important, especially if taxoids with more aqueous solubility are synthesized to be formulated without polyoxyethylated castor oil (55).

With wider experience, additional mechanisms of resistance to paclitaxel will undoubtedly be described. Glutathione depletion by L-buthionine sulfoximine has recently been shown to produce resistance to paclitaxel in the MCF-7 breast cancer cell line (56).

F. Radiation Sensitization

As discussed earlier in this volume by Schiff, paclitaxel's mechanism of action causes accumulation of cells in the mitotic phase of the cell cycle, the phase most sensitive to radiation. Preclinical data confirm that this sensitization is enhanced even at paclitaxel doses that are not cytotoxic (57). Currently, Schiff et al. are evaluating the combination of paclitaxel with irradiation in patients with inoper-able locally advanced breast cancer. Patient accrual to date has been slow because of safety concerns, but since no unexpected toxic effects have been seen in the initial patient, rapid completion of the study is anticipated.

G. Safety in Hepatic Insufficiency

Both the Memorial Sloan-Kettering and NCI Medicine Branch trials showed that patients who had hepatic insufficiency experienced more severe toxic effects than patients without hepatic insufficiency: pancytopenia and mucositis and their consequences (4,30,31). Wilson et al. noted that this occurred in his 96-hr infusion study when the AST was elevated as little as twofold (30,31). Pharmacokinetic studies, detailed earlier by Rowinsky et al., showed that clearance of paclitaxel was slower in patients with hepatic insufficiency.

Currently, there are no firm guidelines for administration of paclitaxel to patients with hepatic insufficiency (1). However, this is an important issue for oncologists treating breast cancer. A phase I trial to evaluate this is in progress in the CALGB. Preliminary data were presented at the NCI in September 1993 and will be updated at the 1994 ASCO meeting (58). Patients were grouped in three cohorts based on an empiric assessment of the extent of liver dysfunction. Group 1 had elevation of transaminases alone; group 2 had elevation of bilirubin to levels of 1.6 to 3.0 mg/dL; group 3 had bilirubin levels greater than 3.0 mg/dL. Starting doses were 200 mg/m², 150 mg/m², and 100 mg/m² by 24-hr infusion, respectively, for the three groups. Group 3 patients were not treated, however, until preliminary results were obtained from groups 1 and 2. Significant toxic effects occurred at the starting doses for groups 1 and 2, including severe mucositis and pancytopenia. Thus, a "reverse phase I" study of dose reduction was conducted. The recommended dose for patients with bilirubin levels exceeding 3.0 mg/dl is 50 mg/m² by 24-hr infusion. The doses for groups 1 and 2 are still being explored; 75 mg/m² is currently under evaluation for group 2 and 100 mg/m² for group 1. Preliminary pharmacokinetic data showed that, since paclitaxel clearance is nonlinear with the 24-hr infusion, other mechanisms must be responsible for the serious toxic effects observed. Evaluation of the 3-hr infusion schedule is ongoing (January 1994), with a starting dose of 50 mg/m².

H. Adjuvant Therapy

Both the National Surgical Adjuvant Breast Project (NSABP) and Memorial Sloan-Kettering (as described earlier) (43) will be evaluating paclitaxel in the adjuvant setting. To familiarize NSABP investigators with paclitaxel, a pilot trial in patients being treated for metastatic disease will precede the adjuvant trial. It is hoped that paclitaxel will have a major impact on the curative potential of adjuvant and neoadjuvant therapies.

VII. DOCETAXEL

A. Background

Docetaxel, the first clinically useful taxoid, is a semisynthetic taxane prepared from a noncytotoxic precursor, 10-deacetyl bacattin III, which is extracted from the needles of the European yew, *Taxus baccata* (59,60). The docetaxel molecule differs from paclitaxel at two sites: position 10 on the baccatin ring and position 3 on the side chain. The mechanism of action and the effects on the cell cycle are similar to those of paclitaxel: they promote assembly of unusually stable micro-tubules and block cells in the M phase. However, docetaxel accomplishes this differently from paclitaxel in three important aspects. First, it is 2.5 times as potent, as measured by an in vitro tubulin assay. Second, the microtubules formed by docetaxel contain the normal complement of 13 protofilaments, while micro-tubules formed under the influence of paclitaxel contain only 12 protofilaments. Third, docetaxel affects certain classes of microtubules, especially those that are Tau-dependent, differently from paclitaxel.

In vitro cytotoxicity assays in murine and human tumor cell lines and in vivo preclinical antitumor activity in murine and human xenografts show that docetaxel has greater cytotoxicity than paclitaxel. Docetaxel is synergistic with cyclo-phosphamide, 5-fluorouracil, etoposide, vincristine, and edatrexate but not with cisplatin or doxorubicin. Incomplete cross-resistance between the two taxoids was observed in vitro in human cell lines. Docetaxel is inactive against the P388 cell line that is resistant to doxorubicin, but it is active in other cell lines expressing the multidrug-resistance phenotype. Like paclitaxel, docetaxel is a radiation sensi-tizer (61). In preclinical toxicology studies, the toxic effects of a repeated-dose schedule were more severe than those of a single-dose schedule and were dose-dependent.

B. Phase I Trials

Six human phase I trials using different schedules were conducted internationally in 238 patients in 1990 (62). The MTD was determined using a short 1-hr/1-day infusion. The dose-limiting toxic effect was grade 4 neutropenia, which was independent of schedule, noncumulative, dose-dependent, of brief duration (less than 7 days), and rarely associated with infection. There was no significant anemia or thrombocytopenia. Gastrointestinal mucositis was schedule-dependent and was more frequent and severe when longer or repeated infusions were given (6-hr, 24-hr, or 5-day schedules). Other toxic effects and the frequency of their occurrence were total alopecia, in more than half of all patients; mild nausea, vomiting and diarrhea, in less than 30%; reversible paresthesias, in less than 20%; and anaphy-lactoidlike reactions, in 20% of all patients but severe in only 4%. Myalgias occurred as a minor side effect. Two unexpected toxic effects occurred: dermatitis and a fluid-retention syndrome. The dermatitis was seen only in patients who received the short infusion. The fluid-retention syndrome occurred only after multiple doses. Significant clinical activity was documented, with 17 objective responses, 8 of which were in breast cancer (60). The recommended dose for the phase II trials was 100 mg/m^2 over 1 hour every 21 days.

C. Phase II Trials

Six major phase II studies of docetaxel have been conducted in metastatic breast cancer in Europe and North America: three in untreated patients, one in patients who had undergone prior therapy, and two in anthracycline-resistant patients. A summary of the preliminary results is shown in Table 13.

1. EORTC—Clinical Screening Group

There were 32 evaluable patients of 35 treated at a dose of 100 mg/m^2 in the first study conducted by the EORTC-Clinical Screening Group (CSG) (62,63). Thirty-seven percent of these patients had received adjuvant chemotherapy and in 91% of these it was anthracycline-based. Objective responses were seen in 18 patients (72%), 16% of which were CR. The response rates were similar in patients who received prior adjuvant chemotherapy and those who did not. The mean duration of response is estimated to be 34 weeks.

A second study using a dose of 75 mg/m^2 produced an objective response rate of 55%; however, the extent of prior therapy was not mentioned.

2. National Cancer Institute of Canada

The National Cancer Institute of Canada (NCIC) studied 51 patients, 49 of whom were evaluable for toxicity and 45 for response (64,65). The initial 34 patients received 100 mg/m^2; the remaining group, 75 mg/m^2. The response rate in the initial group was 69%, with 3 (9%) CR and 20 PR. The preliminary response rate in the second cohort of patients was 58%.

3. Memorial Sloan-Kettering

Memorial Sloan-Kettering treated 35 patients with metastatic breast cancer who had received no prior chemotherapy for stage IV disease; 29 were evaluable for

Table 13 Phase II Studies of Docetaxel in Metastatic Breast Cancer

Institution (ref)	Prior therapy	No. of patients	CR + PR, %	No. CR (%)	No. PR (%)
EORTC-CSG (62, 63)	No	32	72	5 (16)	18 (56)
NCI-Canada (64, 65)	No	34	69	3 (9)	20 (60)
Memorial Sloan-Kettering (66)	No	29	76	2 (7)	20 (69)
EORTC-ECTG (67)	Yes	32	50	2 (6)	14 (44)
M. D. Anderson (68)	Anthracycline (refractory)	33	55	0 (0)	18 (55)
UT–San Antonio (69)	Anthracycline (refractory)	26	60	3 (11)	11 (43)

Abbreviations: CR, complete response; PR, partial response; EORTC-CSG, European Organization for the Research and Treatment of Cancer—Clinical Study Group; NCI-Canada, National Cancer Institute—Canada; EORTC-ECTG, Early Clinical Trials Group; UT, University of Texas.

objective responses (66). Sixty percent had received adjuvant chemotherapy. Objective responses were seen in 22 patients (76%), of which two (7%) were CR.

4. EORTC-ECTG

The EORTC-Early Clinical Trials Group (ECTG) trial was targeted to patients who had received one prior chemotherapy regimen for metastatic disease regardless of whether they had received prior adjuvant chemotherapy (67). Of the 39 patients treated, 32 patients were evaluable for response; 16 (50%) objective responses were seen, with a 6% rate of CR.

5. Anthracycline-Resistant Breast Cancer

Two studies have been performed in patients with anthracycline-resistant breast cancer. The criteria for anthracycline resistance were stringent. Primary anthracycline resistance in patients with metastatic breast cancer was defined as initial failure to respond to anthracyclines. Secondary anthracycline resistance was defined as progression of disease after an initial response while receiving treatment with anthracyclines. Patients who developed progressive disease while receiving anthracyclines as adjuvant therapy were considered to have primary resistance.

a. M. D. Anderson. Of 35 treated patients, 33 were evaluable for response (68). The median number of prior chemotherapy regimens was 1.5 (range, 1–3); the median number of metastatic sites was 3 (range, 1–6). Objective responses were seen in 18 patients (55%), with a median time to progression in responding patients of 7.5 months.

b. San Antonio. A similar study was performed at the University of Texas Health Science Center in San Antonio (69). Objective responses were seen in 54% (11 PR and 3 CR) of 26 patients.

In summary, docetaxel is extremely active as a single agent, with response rates of 55% to 76% in untreated patients and 50% to 55% in pretreated patients, including those who are resistant to anthracycline. Objective responses were seen in 70% of the untreated patients with liver metastases and in 50% of the refractory patients with liver metastases. These data are still preliminary, so duration of response and overall survival data are not yet available for most studies.

D. Toxic Effects

1. Hematological Toxicity

Anemia and thrombocytopenia have been mild: fewer than 20% of the courses have been associated with effects of grade 2 or greater. Grade 3 or 4 neutropenia has been seen in all patients in all studies. In untreated patients, grade 4 neutropenia occurred in 80% to 90% of courses (62–66) and in pretreated patients, 100% (68,69). The median nadir granulocyte count was approximately $300/mm^3$. The median nadir day of neutropenia was day 8 (range, 6–15). The median duration of grade 4 neutropenia was approximately 7–8 days. Although the EORTC-CSG reported no episodes of neutropenic fever or infection in 168 courses, these effects were seen in 12% of 191 courses at M. D. Anderson.

2. Nonhematological Toxic Effects

Hypersensitivity reactions identical to those described for paclitaxel were noted in approximately 20% of the patients who received docetaxel and 10% of the courses, but with significant variation between studies (Table 14) (70). Because of the frequency and severity of this complication, premedication with a regimen of antihistamines and corticosteroids, similar to that used prior to paclitaxel, was started. This treatment has nearly abolished this complication (Table 14): the incidence decreased from 50% to 5% of the patients in our institution (71) as well as the NCIC (65) and EORTC trials (72).

The incidence and severity of alopecia and gastrointestinal toxic effects were similar to those for paclitaxel. Peripheral neuropathy occurred but was uncommon, mild, and, as with paclitaxel, mainly sensory. Moderate to severe fatigue/

Table 14 Incidence of Hypersensitivity Reactions and Skin Toxicity to Docetaxel Before and After Use of Routine Premedication Regimen

Institution (ref)	Before premedication No. patients	Reaction	After premedication No. patients	Reaction
Hypersensitivity reaction				
NCI-Canada (65)	21		25	
Any reaction		67%		36%
Significant reaction		57%		0%
Amsterdam (67)	24	17%	—	—
M. D. Anderson—All studies (71)	81	50%	87	5%
EORTC-ECTG (72)	334	26%	50	7%
Skin toxic reaction[a]				
NCI-Canada (65)	21	86%	25	44%
M. D. Anderson—breast (68)	81	53%	87	14%

[a]The NCI-Canada premedication regimen was identical to the standard premedication regimen for paclitaxel, namely, dexamethasone 20 mg orally 12 and 6 hr before docetaxel with standard H_1 and H_2 blockers. The M. D. Anderson regimen used dexamethasone 8 mg twice daily for 5 days starting 24 hr before treatment. The longer duration of the M. D. Anderson regimen was associated with a lesser incidence of skin toxic effects.
Abbreviations: HSR, hypersensitivity reactions; NCI-Canada, National Cancer Institute-Canada; EORTC-ECTG, European Organization for the Research and Treatment of Cancer, Early Clinical Trials Group.

asthenia was seen in 30% to 60% of courses and myalgia in 20% to 40% of courses.

Skin toxic effects were documented in 25% to 60% of the patients and in 20% to 35% of the courses before premedication with antihistamines and corticosteroids was implemented. Skin biopsies showed nonspecific perivascular lymphocytic infiltration (68). Six dermatological syndromes were seen: (1) focal, scattered maculopapular eruptions with desquamation, usually localized to the extremities; (2) alterations in the fingernails and toenails, including thinning, subungual erythema, ridging of the nails plates, proximal or distal shedding, and subungual hemorrhage; (3) the hand-foot syndrome (acral erythema, palmar-plantar erythema); (4) photodermatitis; (5) reactive dermatitis; and (6) folliculitis. In some patients the lesions appeared in areas of prior injury or areas of pressure. A 5-day treatment regimen of corticosteroids beginning on the day before treatment somewhat decreased the incidence and severity of these cutaneous reactions. In the M. D. Anderson trial, the incidence of skin toxic effects greater than grade 2 decreased from 21% to 11% of courses, and the incidence of the hand-foot syndrome decreased from 21% to 2% after routine implementation of the premedication regimen (68). In contrast, the use of a short course of corticosteroids, as used in the EORTC-ECTG, was not effective (70).

The fluid-retention syndrome initially presented as a progressive increase in weight. Later, patients developed peripheral edema, mainly in the lower extremities. With continued administration of docetaxel, this progressed to pleural or pericardial effusions, ascites, and anasarca. However, all these effects were seen only in patients receiving a cumulative dose of more than 400 mg/m^2. No renal, cardiac, liver, pulmonary, or endocrine dysfunctions have been documented in these patients. The possibility of a capillary leak syndrome has been considered, but some of the clinical manifestations of the docetaxel fluid-retention syndrome are different from those previously described with the capillary leak syndrome. For example, pulmonary edema is not part of the fluid-retention syndrome.

Two strategies to circumvent this toxicity have been used in a small number of patients. First, the NCI-Canada and the EORTC used a lower dose of docetaxel, 75 mg/m^2, but this had no apparent benefit. Second, the NCIC, the EORTC, and M. D. Anderson used premedication with steroids. The NCIC used a short course of premedication similar to the one used with paclitaxel, but this did not change the severity or frequency of the syndrome. However, long-term administration of steroids appears to delay the onset and the severity of this syndrome. In the M. D. Anderson (68) and EORTC trials (70), administration of steroids for 5 or more days appeared to decrease the incidence of the syndrome or at least delay its appearance from the time the patient had received a cumulative total dose of 400 mg/m^2 until the time that the cumulative dose reached 800 mg/m^2. Several ongoing pilot studies, as well as a major randomized trial of different premedication regimens, will address this problem (72).

VIII. CONCLUSION: FUTURE DIRECTIONS

Intensive laboratory and clinical research is ongoing in the development of the taxoids. For docetaxel, major efforts are under way to understand the pathophysiology of the skin toxicity and fluid-retention syndrome and to develop effective preventive and therapeutic measures to circumvent these toxic effects. Preclinical and clinical studies to develop synergistic combinations of both paclitaxel and docetaxel with other active agents are ongoing.

In addition to the studies listed in Table 1 for paclitaxel, phase I and II studies are in progress to evaluate combinations of docetaxel with anthracyclines, cyclophosphamide, and vinorelbine. Other agents that affect different aspects of microtubule function are under development and may offer possibilities of synergism when used in combination with paclitaxel. Studies with interferon and antibodies to epidermal growth factor are being planned. As noted earlier, however, the initial empirical combination trials with cisplatin in ovarian cancer (73) and with doxorubicin in breast cancer (10) have shown that careful attention must be given to the schedule of combinations.

More complete understanding of the mechanisms of resistance will lead to innovative strategies to overcome it. The patterns of cross-resistance between docetaxel and paclitaxel still must be defined. Trials of docetaxel are planned in patients with paclitaxel-resistant breast cancer.

Aggressive development of other taxoids is ongoing. There is one report of a prodrug with aqueous solubility. Whether the presence of the vehicle polyoxyethylated castor oil contributes to paclitaxel's activity is still unclear. Paclitaxel may be only the first of a series of effective taxoid agents. However, clinical enthusiasm must be tempered with hard science to allow careful definition of the optimal doses, schedules, and combinations.

REFERENCES

1. Rowinsky EK, Cazenave LA, Donehower RC. Taxol: A novel investigational antimicrotubule agent. J Natl Cancer Inst 1990;82:1247–1259.
2. Holmes FA, Walters RS, Theriault RL, et al. Phase II trial of taxol, an active drug in the treatment of metastatic breast cancer. J Natl Cancer Inst 1991;83:1797–1805.
3. Ajani JA, Welch SR, Raber MN, et al. Comprehensive criteria for assessing therapy-induced toxicity. Cancer Invest 1990;8:147–159.
4. Reichman BS, Seidman AD, Crown JPA, et al. Paclitaxel and recombinant human granulocyte colony-stimulating factor as initial chemotherapy for metastatic breast cancer. J Clin Oncol 1993;11:1943–1951.
5. Jamis-Dow CA, Klecker RW, Sarosy G, et al. Steady-state plasma concentrations and effects of taxol for a 250 mg/m^2 dose in combination with granulocyte-colony stimulating factor in patients with ovarian cancer. Cancer Chemother Pharmacol 1993;33:48–52.

6. Seidman AD, Crown JPA, Reichman BS, et al. Lack of clinical cross-resistance of taxol with anthracycline in the treatment of metastatic breast cancer (abstract 53). Proc Am Soc Clin Oncol 1993;12:63.
7. Nabholtz JM, Gelmon K, Bontenbal M, et al. Randomized trial of two doses of Taxol in metastatic breast cancer: an interim analysis (abstract 42). Proc Am Soc Clin Oncol 1993;12:61.
8. Bristol-Myers Squibb Taxol Study Group, data presented at Oncology Drug Advisory Committee to the Food and Drug Administration hearings on paclitaxel for metastatic breast cancer, Rockville, MD, December 16, 1993.
9. Holmes FA, Frye D, Valero V, et al. Phase I study of Taxol and doxorubicin with G-CSF in patients without prior chemotherapy for metastatic breast cancer (Abstract 66). Proc Am Soc Clin Oncol 1992;11:60.
10. Holmes FA, Valero V, Walters RS, et al. The M. D. Anderson Cancer Center Experience with Taxol in metastatic breast cancer. Monogr Natl Cancer Inst 1993;15:161–169.
11. Fisherman JS, McCabe M, Noone M, et al. Phase I study of taxol, doxorubicin, plus granulocyte-colony stimulating factor in patients with metastatic breast cancer (abstract). Proceedings of the Second NCI Workshop on Taxol and *Taxus*. Alexandria, VA: National Cancer Institute, September 23–24, 1992.
12. Fisherman JS, McCabe M, Hillig M, et al. Phase I study of Taxol, doxorubicin plus granulocyte colony-stimulating factor (G-CSF) in patients with metastatic breast cancer. Monogr Natl Cancer Inst 1993;15:189–194.
13. O'Shaugnessey JA, Fisherman J, McCabe M, et al. Phase I study of Taxol plus doxorubicin plus granulocyte colony stimulating factor (G-CSF) in patients with metastatic breast cancer (abstract 636). Eur J Cancer 1993;29A(suppl 6):S117.
14. Holmes FA, Newman RA, Madden T, et al. Schedule dependent pharmacokinetics (PK) in a phase I trial of Taxol (T) and doxorubicin (D) as initial chemotherapy for metastatic breast cancer (abstract 489). Ann Oncol 1994;5(suppl 5):197.
15. Berg SL, Cowan KH, Balis FM, et al. Pharmacokinetics of taxol and doxorubicin administered alone and in combination by continuous 72-hour infusion. J Natl Cancer Inst 1994;86:143–145.
16. Sledge GW Jr. Paclitaxel/doxorubicin combinations in breast cancer (abstract). Symposium: Newest Clinical Approaches with Paclitaxel (Taxol). Seventh European Conference on Clinical Oncology and Nursing. Jerusalem, November 15, 1993, p 6.
17. Sledge G, Sparano J, McCaskill-Stevens W, et al. Pilot trial of alternating Taxol and Adriamycin for metastatic breast cancer (abstract 85). Proc Am Soc Clin Oncol 1993;12:71.
18. Sledge GW, Goldstein RN, Sparano J, et al. Phase I trial of Adriamycin (A) + Taxol (T) in metastatic breast cancer (MBC) (abstract 421). Eur J Cancer 1993;29A(suppl 6):S81.
19. Gianni L, Straneo M, Capri G, et al. Optimal dose and sequence finding study of paclitaxel (P) by 3H infusion combined with bolus doxorubicin (D) in untreated metastatic breast cancer patients (pts) (abstract 97). Proc Am Soc Clin Oncol 1994;13:74.
20. Gelmon KA. Phase I/II study of biweekly paclitaxel and cisplatin in advanced ovarian

and breast cancer (abstract). Symposium: Newest Clinical Approaches with Paclitaxel (Taxol). Seventh European Conference on Clinical Oncology and Nursing. Jerusalem, November 15, 1993, p 10.

21. Wasserheit C, Alter R, Speyer J, et al. Phase II trial of paclitaxel and cisplatin (DDP) in women with metastatic breast cancer (abstract 204). Proc Am Soc Clin Oncol 1994; 13:100.

22. Pestalozzi BC, Sotos GA, Choyke PL, et al. Typhlitis resulting from treatment with Taxol and doxorubicin in patients with metastatic breast cancer. Cancer 1993; 71: 1797–1800.

23. Seewaldt V, Cain JM, Greer BE, et al. Bowel complications with Taxol therapy (letter). J Clin Oncol 1993;11:1198.

24. Gotay CC, Korn EL, McCabe MS, et al. Quality-of-life assessment in cancer treatment protocols: Research issues in protocol development. J Natl Cancer Inst 1992;84:575–579.

25. Seidman AD, Reichman S, Crown JPA, et al. Taxol plus recombinant human granulocyte colony-stimulating factor as initial and as salvage chemotherapy for metastatic breast cancer: A preliminary report. Monogr Natl Cancer Inst 1993;15: 171–175.

26. Holmes FA, Valero V, Theriault RL, et al. Phase II trial of Taxol (T) in metastatic breast cancer (MBC) refractory to multiple prior treatments (abstract 178). Proc Am Soc Clin Oncol 1993;12:94.

27. Selby PJ, Chapman JAW, Etazadi-Amoli D, et al. The development of a method for assessing the quality of life of cancer patients. Br J Cancer 1984;50:13–22.

28. Lai GM, Chen YN, Mickley LA, et al. P-glycoprotein expression and schedule dependence of Adriamycin cytotoxicity in human colon carcinoma cell lines. Int J Cancer 1991;49:696–703.

29. Zhan A, Kang Y-K, Regis J, et al. Taxol resistance: in vitro and in vivo studies in breast cancer and lymphomas (abstract 1281). Proc Am Assoc Cancer Res 1993; 34:215.

30. Wilson WH, Berg S, Kang Y-K, et al. Phase I/II study of Taxol 96-hour infusion in refractory lymphoma and breast cancer: Pharmacodynamics and analysis of multi-drug resistance (mdr-1) (abstract 335). Proc Am Soc Clin Oncol 1993;12:134.

31. Wilson WH, Berg SL, Bryan G, et al. Paclitaxel (Taxol) in doxorubicin or mitox-antrone refractory breast cancer: A phase I/II trial of 96-hour infusion. J Clin Oncol 1994;12:1616–1620.

32. Abrams JS, Vena DA, Baltz J, et al. Paclitaxel activity in heavily treated metastatic breast cancer (abstract 494). Ann Oncol 1994;5(Suppl 5):199.

33. Munzone E, Capri G, Demicheli R, et al. Activity of taxol (T) by 3 h infusion in breast cancer patients (pts) with clinical resistance to anthracyclines (A) (abstract 413). Eur J Cancer 1993;29A(suppl 6):S79.

34. Gianni L, Munzone E, Straneo M, Capri G. Paclitaxel in anthracycline-refractory breast cancer. Symposium: Newest Clinical Approaches with Paclitaxel (Taxol). Seventh European Conference on Clinical Oncology and Nursing. Jerusalem, No-vember 15, 1993, p 12.

35. Vermrken JB, Huizing MT, Liefting AJM, et al. High-dose Taxol (HDT) with

G-CSF in patients with advanced breast cancer (ABC) refractory to anthracyclines (abstract 435). Eur J Cancer 1993;29A(suppl 6):S83.

36. Uziely B, Delaflor-Weiss, Lenz HJ, et al. Paclitaxel (Taxol) in refractory breast cancer: response correlates with low levels of MDR1 gene expression (abstract 104). Proc Am Soc Clin Oncol 1994;13:75.

37. Swenerton K, Eisenhauer E, ten Bokkel Huinink W, et al. Taxol in relapsed ovarian cancer: High vs low dose and short vs long infusion. A European-Canadian study coordinated by the NCI Canada Clinical Trials Group (abstract 810). Proc Am Soc Clin Oncol 1993;12:256.

38. Goldberg KB, Goldberg P. NCI's Chabner cautions against 3-hour Taxol infusion, may lower response rate. Cancer Lett 1993;41:1–2.

39. Arbuck SA. Paclitaxel: what schedule? What dose? J Clin Oncol 1994;12:233–235.

40. Lopes NM, Adams EG, Pitts TW, Bhuyan BK. Cell kill kinetics and cell cycle effects of Taxol on human and hamster ovarian cell lines. Cancer Chemother Pharmacol 1993;32:235–242.

41. Huber MN, Murphy WK, Hong WK, Hittelman WN. Characterization of Taxol cytotoxicity against human non-small cell lung cancer (NSCLC) cell lines (abstract 2079). Proc Am Assoc Cancer Res 1993;34:349.

42. Seidman AD, Barrett S, Hudis C, et al. Three-hour Taxol infusion as initial (I) and as salvage (S) chemotherapy of metastatic breast cancer (MBC) (abstract 65). Proc Am Soc Clin Oncol 1994;13:66.

43. Hudis C, Seidman A, Baselga J, et al. Sequential high-dose adjuvant doxorubicin (A), paclitaxel (T), and cyclophosphamide (C) with G-CSF (G) is feasible for women (pts) with resected breast cancer (BC) and $\geq$ 4 (+) lymph nodes (LN) (abstract 65). Proc Am Soc Clin Oncol 1994;13:62.

44. Buzzoni R, Bonadonna G, Valagussa P, Zambetti M. Adjuvant chemotherapy with doxorubicin plus cyclophosphamide, methotrexate, and fluorouracil in the treatment of resectable breast cancer with more than three positive axillary nodes. J Clin Oncol 1991;9:2134–2140.

45. Day RS. Treatment sequencing, asymmetry and uncertainty: Protocol strategies for combination chemotherapy. Cancer Res 1986;46:3876–3885.

46. Norton L, Day R. Potential innovations in scheduling in cancer chemotherapy. In: DeVita VT, Hellman S, Rosenberg SA, eds. Important Advances in Oncology 1991. Philadelphia: Lippincott, 1991:57–73.

47. Schiller JH, Storer B, Tutsch K, et al. Phase I trial of 3-hour infusion of paclitaxel with or without granulocyte colony-stimulating factor in patients with advanced cancer. J Clin Oncol 1994;12:241–248.

48. Hahn SM, Liebmann JE, Cook J, et al. Taxol in combination with doxorubicin or etoposide. Possible antagonism *in vivo*. Cancer 1993;72:2705–2711.

49. Rose WC. Taxol: A review of its preclinical *in vivo* antitumor activity. Anticancer Drugs 1992;149:2459–2465.

50. Hohneker JA, personal communication.

51. Tew KD, Stearns ME. Estramustine–A nitrogen mustard/steroid with antimicrotubule activity. Pharmacol Ther 1989;43:299–319.

52. Woodcock DM, Jefferson S, Linsenmeyer ME, et al. Reversal of the multidrug

resistance phenotype with Cremophor EL, a common vehicle for water-insoluble vitamins and drugs. Cancer Res 1990;50:4599–4603.

53. Lassus M, Scott D, Leyland-Jones B. Allergic reactions (AR) associated with Cremophor (C) containing antineoplastics (ANP) (abstract C-1042). Proc Am Soc Clin Oncol 1985;4:268.

54. Webster L, Linsenmeyer M, Millward M, et al. Measurement of Cremophor EL following Taxol: Plasma levels sufficient to reverse drug exclusion mediated by the multidrug-resistant phenotype. J Natl Cancer Inst 1993;85:1685–1690.

55. Mathew AE, Mejillano MR, Nath JP, et al. Synthesis and evaluation of some water-soluble prodrugs and derivatives of Taxol with antitumor activity. J Med Chem 1992; 35:145–151.

56. Liebmann JE, Hahn SM, Cook JA, et al. Glutathione depletion by L-buthionine sulfoximine antagonizes Taxol cytotoxicity. Cancer Res 1993;53:2066–2070.

57. Choy H, Rodriguez F, Koester S, et al. Investigation of Taxol as a potential radiation sensitizer. Cancer 1993;71:3774–3778.

58. Venook AP, Egorin M, Brown TD, et al. Paclitaxel (Taxol) in patients with liver dysfunction (CALGB 9264) (abstract 350). Proc Am Soc Clin Oncol 1994;13:139.

59. Colin M, Guenard D, Gueritte-Voegelein F, Potier P. Taxol derivatives, their preparation and pharmaceutical compositions containing them. Rhone-Poulenc Sante, U. S. Patent 4814470, granted March 21, 1989 (priority date, July 17, 1986).

60. Piccart MJ. Taxotere: A second generation taxoid compound. ASCO Education Book, 29th Annual Meeting, Orlando, FL.: Bostrom Corporation, 1993:25–32.

61. Choy H, Rodriguez F, Wilcox B, et al. Radiation sensitizing effects of Taxotere (RP 56976) (abstract 2991). Proc Am Assoc Cancer Res 1992;33:500.

62. Fumoleau P, Chevallier B, Kerbrat P, et al. First line chemotherapy with Taxotere (T) in advanced breast cancer (ABC): A phase II study of the EORTC Clinical Screening Group (CSG) (abstract 27). Proc Am Soc Clin Oncol 1993;12:56.

63. Fumoleau P. Current status of Taxotere (docetaxel) as a new treatment in breast cancer. 16th Annual San Antonio Breast Cancer Symposium. San Antonio, TX: November 1993.

64. Trudeau ME, Eisenhauer E, Lofters W, et al. Phase II study of Taxotere as first line chemotherapy for metastatic breast cancer (MBC). A National Cancer Institute of Canada Clinical Trials Groups (NCIC CTG) study (abstract 59). Proc Am Soc Clin Oncol 1993;12:64.

65. Eisenhauer E. Experience with docetaxel in breast cancer. Symposium of the 7th European Conference on Clinical Oncology and Cancer Nursing. Jerusalem, November 14, 1993.

66. Seidman AD, Hudis C, Crown JPA, et al. Phase II evaluation of Taxotere (RP56976, NSC628503) as initial chemotherapy for metastatic breast cancer (abstract 52). Proc Am Soc Clin Oncol 1993;12:63.

67. Ten Bokkel Hunink WW, Van Oosteron AT, Piccart M, et al. Taxotere in advanced breast cancer: A phase II trial of the EORTC Early Clinical Trials Group (abstract 81). Proc Am Soc Clin Oncol 1993;12:70.

68. Valero V, Walters R, Theriault R, et al. Phase II study of Taxotere in refractory metastatic breast cancer (abstract 1636). Proc Am Soc Clin Oncol 1994;13:470.

69. Burris HA, Ravdin PM, Fields SM, et al. Phase II evaluation of Taxotere (RP56976) as chemotherapy for anthracycline-refractory metastatic breast cancer (abstract 6). Br Cancer Res Treat 1993;27:132.

70. Wanders J, Schrijvers D, Bruntsch U, et al. The EORTC-ECTG experience with acute hypersensitivity reaction in Taxotere studies (abstract 94). Proc Am Soc Clin Oncol 1993;12:73.

71. Galindo E, Kavanagh J, Fossella F, et al. Docetaxel (Taxotere) toxicities: Analysis of a single institution experience of 168 patients (623 courses) (abstract 452). Proc Am Soc Clin Oncol 1994;13:164.

72. Schrijvers D, Wanders J, Dirix L, et al. Coping with toxicities of docetaxel (Taxotere). Ann Oncol 1993;4:610–611.

73. Rowinsky EK, Gilbert MR, McGuire WP, et al. Sequences of taxol and cisplatin: A phase I and pharmacologic study. J Clin Oncol 1991;9:1692–1703.

13

Non-Small Cell Lung Cancer

ALEX Y. CHANG

University of Rochester School of Medicine and Dentistry
Rochester, New York

I. INTRODUCTION

Non-small cell lung cancer (NSCLC) comprises about 80% of all bronchogenic neoplasms and is the leading cause of cancer death in both men and women in the United States. It is also one of the major health problems in developing countries. The incidence of NSCLC is 150,000 new cases in the United States in 1993 (1). Most of these patients are not curable by surgery at the time of diagnosis due to advanced stage of disease. Additionally, of the small percentage of patients undergoing curative resection, less than half will remain tumor-free 2 or more years after diagnosis. Thus, most patients with NSCLC will be candidates for systemic therapy at some point.

Although the recent metaanalysis showed modest improvement in median survival by chemotherapy as compared to best supportive care in patients with advanced NSCLC, chemotherapy has not been conclusively demonstrated to provide survival benefit and has not been accepted universally as the treatment choice (2–7). Thus, the main goal of chemotherapy in such patients should be palliation of symptoms. Adverse effects from therapy, however, may supersede any palliation, such that the therapeutic index of any intervention must be carefully assessed. The lack of definite survival benefit and often poor therapeutic index make use of investigational drugs in previously untreated patients both rational and ethical. Ifosfamide, mitomycin-C, cisplatin, vinblastine, and etoposide are the active single agents against NSCLC with response rates of 15% to 20%. Cisplatin- or carboplatin-based combination regimens have commonly been associated with response rates between 10% and 40% (8–10). The median survival time of patients with metastatic NSCLC is between 4 and 8 months, underscoring the urgent need for more effective agents or treatment regimens. Paclitaxel may represent such a compound.

Paclitaxel (NSC-125973) is the first diterpene compound initially approved by the FDA for the treatment of refractory ovarian cancer. It is isolated from the bark of Pacific yew, *Taxus brevifolia*, and has a unique 16-carbon taxene ring (11). Paclitaxel is a microtubule poison. Unlike other antimicrotubule agents such as vinca alkaloids, paclitaxel stabilizes the microtubule assembly and inhibits depolymerization of tubulin dimers, which is an essential process for cell division and other cellular functions (12).

II. PRECLINICAL STUDIES

In preclinical evaluation, paclitaxel was shown to have activity against a variety of tumors, including murine Lewis lung carcinoma and human lung cancer cells, LX-1, implanted in the subrenal capsule of the nude mice (13). These data generated interest in studying paclitaxel in lung cancer patients. The cytotoxicity of paclitaxel is very schedule-dependent. In our laboratory, the cytotoxicity of paclitaxel against A549, human lung adenocarcinoma cells, has been studied (14).

Figure 1 shows that the cytotoxicity of paclitaxel is dependent more on exposure time than on its concentration. In the colony forming assay, higher cell kills of A549 were observed with 0.01 μM of paclitaxel for 96 hr than with 0.1 μM paclitaxel for 24 hr. This is consistent with the improved therapeutic results in p388 leukemia when paclitaxel was given multiple times every 3 hr as compared with other schedules with less frequent treatment.

Rose has studied the interactions between paclitaxel and other cytotoxic agents in the subcutaneously implanted M109 murine lung cancer. In that system, paclitaxel and cisplatin—as compared with paclitaxel alone—significantly delayed tumor growth but did not increase the life span of mice. There was no interaction between paclitaxel and etoposide, doxorubicin, cyclophosphamide, methotrexate, pentamethylmelamine, or bleomycin (15).

III. PHASE I STUDIES

More than 10 phase I studies of paclitaxel were conducted under the auspices of the National Cancer Institute (NCI) (16). After the initial hurdle of hypersensitivity reactions noted in several of these studies was reduced by prolonging the infusion time of paclitaxel and premedicating patients with antihistamines and steroids, a 24-hr IV infusion at 200 to 250 mg/m² was selected for phase II. In a few phase I

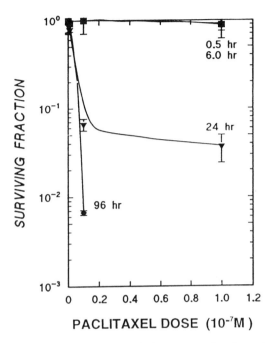

Figure 1   Paclitaxel schedule dependency in lung cancer. In vitro cytotoxicity assay of paclitaxel against A549, adenocarcinoma of the lung. Paclitaxel at high concentration (0.1 μM) for 30 min or 6 hr does not have any cytotoxic effects on A549. Paclitaxel is more effective with 0.01 μM for 96 hr than with 0.1 μM for 24 hr.

reports, patients with NSCLC responded to paclitaxel (16), suggesting a need for phase II studies of paclitaxel in NSCLC.

IV. PHASE II STUDIES

The Eastern Cooperative Oncology Group (ECOG) and M.D. Anderson Cancer Center (MDA) conducted phase II studies of paclitaxel in patients with advanced NSCLC. Each study required patients to have good performance status; normal hematologic, renal, and hepatic functions; measurable diseases; and no prior chemotherapy. The ECOG performed a randomized phase II study of paclitaxel (250 mg/m²), merbarone, and piroxantrone, while MDA conducted a single-arm study of paclitaxel at 200 mg/m². Twenty-five patients entered the ECOG study, with 24 eligible and evaluable; 27 patients were in the MDA trial, with 25 eligible and evaluable. As a single agent, paclitaxel yielded 21% and 24% objective responses in the ECOG and MDA studies, respectively, with an overall response rate of 22.5% (11/49; 95% confidence interval, 12%–37%). The median durations of response were 28 and 27 weeks; the median survivals were 24 and 40 weeks; and the 1-year survival rates were 42% and 37% in the ECOG and MDA studies, respectively. There was one complete responder in the MDA trial. In the ECOG study, four patients lived longer than 2 years (17,18).

The toxicities observed in these studies were not dissimilar. Granulocytopenia was the most common and dose-limiting side effect. Cardiac, neurological, and gastrointestinal (GI) toxicities were infrequent and seldom dose-limiting.

The following conclusions can be drawn from these two studies: (1) Paclitaxel is an active agent against metastatic NSCLC. It is as active as ifosfamide and mitomycin-C and may be more active than cisplatin, carboplatin, vinblastine, and etoposide. (2) The response duration, median survival, and 1-year survival rates are very encouraging. The 1-year survival rate is among the highest reported in the literature, with other phase II trials in similar populations generating 1-year survival rates of 20%. (3) Paclitaxel in the dose and schedule used in these studies is safe in the setting of a community hospital.

More recently, paclitaxel at a dose of 175–250 mg/m^2 has been evaluated as a first-line salvage agent in patients with advanced NSCLC. Modest response (3%–14%) rates were reported (19,20). Paclitaxel combined with other agents active in NSCLC is also under evaluation. Currently, combination regimens include paclitaxel plus carboplatin, paclitaxel plus ifosfamide, paclitaxel plus etoposide plus cisplatin, and paclitaxel plus vinorelbine. Five partial responses have been observed in 23 patients treated with paclitaxel plus carboplatin (135 mg/m^2 by 24-hour intravenous infusion) (21). Leighton et al also reported a 56% response rate in 16 evaluable patients treated with paclitaxel and carboplatin (22). Results of other trials are forthcoming.

V. CONCLUSION: PHASE III STUDIES AND FUTURE DIRECTIONS

Based upon its original experience with paclitaxel, ECOG has started a phase III trial comparing therapy of cisplatin and etoposide with same dose of cisplatin and paclitaxel at either 135 mg/m^2 or 250 mg/m^2 with G-CSF. This study addresses the questions of the dose intensity of paclitaxel in this disease by randomly evaluating two dose levels of paclitaxel as well as the comparative therapeutic index of standard therapy (cisplatin and etoposide) and the new combination paclitaxel and cisplatin.

In addition to dose intensity, there are many questions that remain to be answered with paclitaxel in patients with NSCLC. First, does paclitaxel alone or in combination confer any survival benefit in patients with stage VI NSCLC when compared with best supportive care or to standard chemotherapy? Second, what is the best schedule for paclitaxel administration: 3-hr infusion, 24-hr infusion, or more prolonged infusions? The results from in vitro and preclinical studies suggest that longer exposure time or more frequent treatment has better therapeutic effects. However, clinical data to confirm these observations are not available and suggest a 3-hr and 24-hr schedule lead to similar response rates in patients with refractory ovarian cancer (23). Little information in this regard with NSCLC is available. Third, the mechanism of resistance to paclitaxel of NSCLC is unknown. Tumor cell lines develop resistance to paclitaxel either by increasing the expression of the multidrug resistant (MDR) gene or by microtubule mutation (24). Since a majority of patients with NSCLC are resistant to paclitaxel and most of them do not overexpress MDR, other mechanisms of intrinsic resistance must be explored. Fourth, is there a role for paclitaxel alone or a paclitaxel-based combination in patients with stage III inoperable NSCLC? By analogy from other regimens, one would expect higher response rates to paclitaxel in earlier-stage disease (25). In addition, paclitaxel has radiation-sensitizing properties (26). Radiation and paclitaxel would be a biologically attractive combination in the treatment of stage III inoperable NSCLC. However, our initial in vitro evaluation showed that the interaction between paclitaxel and radiation is complex (14), warranting careful clinical evaluation. The feasibility of using paclitaxel in combination with radiation in treating patients with a locally-advanced non-small cell lung cancer is currently being evaluated (27). Other issues regarding paclitaxel in NSCLC may include the evaluation of therapeutic differences between paclitaxel alone, paclitaxel combined with other agents, and docetaxel.

In summary, paclitaxel is an active agent against advanced NSCLC. Its essential role in the treatment of this disease awaits further studies. Patients should be encouraged to participate in well-designed clinical trials.

REFERENCES

1. Boring CC, Squires TS, Tong T. Cancer statistics, 1993. CA Cancer J Clin 1993; 43:7–26.
2. Idhe DC, Minna JD. Non-small cell lung cancer: II. Treatment. Curr Probl Cancer 1991;15:105–154.
3. Souquest PJ, Boissel JP, Cellerine R, et al. Polychemotherapy in advanced non-small cell lung cancer: a meta-analysis. Lancet 1993;342:19–21.
4. Rapp E, Pater J, Willan A, et al. A comparison of best supportive care to two regimens of combination chemotherapy in the management of advanced non-small cell lung cancer (NSCLC): A report of a Canadian multicenter trial. J Clin Oncol 1988;6:633–641.
5. Williams CJ, Woods R, Page J. Chemotherapy for non-small cell lung cancer: A randomized trial of cisplatin/vindesine vs no chemotherapy. Semin Oncol 1988; 15 (suppl 7):58–61.
6. Ganz PA, Figlin RA, Haskell CM, et al. Supportive care vs supportive care and combination chemotherapy in metastatic lung cancer. Cancer 1989;63:1271–1278.
7. Cormier Y, Bergerson D, LaForge J, et al. Benefit of polychemotherapy in advanced non-small cell bronchogenic carcinoma. Cancer 1982;50:845–849.

8. Bonomi PD, Finkelstein DM, Ruckdeschel JC, et al. Combination chemotherapy versus single agents followed by combination chemotherapy in stage IV non-small cell lung cancer: A study of the Eastern Cooperative Oncology Group. J Clin Oncol 1989;7:1602–1613.

9. Klastersky J, Sculier JP, Lacroix H, et al. A randomized study comparing cisplatin or carboplatin with etoposide in patients with advanced non-small cell lung cancer: European Organization for Research and Treatment of Cancer protocol 07861. J Clin Oncol 1990;8:1556–1562.

10. Rosell R, Abad-Esteve A, Morenno I, et al. A randomized study of two vindesine plus cisplatin-containing regimens with the addition of mitomycin C or ifosfamide in patients with advanced non-small cell lung cancer. Cancer 1990;65:1692–1699.

11. Wani MC, Taylor HL, Wall ME, et al. Plant antitumor agents VI. The isolation and structure of taxol, a novel anti-leukemic and antitumor agent from Taxus brevifolia. J Am Chem Soc 1971;2325–2327.

12. Schiff PB, Fant J, Horwitz SB. Promotion of microtubule assembly in vitro by Taxol. Nature 1979;22:665–667.

13. National Cancer Institute Clinical Brochure: Taxol (NSC-125973). Division of Cancer Treatment, NCI, Bethesda, MD, September 1983:6–12.

14. Chang A, Keng P, Sobel S, Gu CZ. Interaction of radiation and Taxol (abstr). Proc Am Assoc Cancer Res 1993;34:364.

15. Ross WC. Taxol-based combination chemotherapy and other in vivo antitumor studies. Second NCI Workshop on Taxol and Taxus (abstr). Alexandria, VA, National Cancer Institute, 1992.

16. Rowinsky EK, Cazenave LA, Donehower RC. Taxol: A novel investigational anti-microtubule agent. J Natl Cancer Inst 1990;82:1247–1259.

17. Chang AY, Kim K, Glick J, et al. Phase II study of Taxol, merbarone, and piro-xantrone in stage IV non-small cell lung cancer: The Eastern Cooperative Oncology Group results. J Natl Cancer Inst 1993;85:388–394.

18. Murphy WK, Fossella FV, Winn RJ, et al. Phase II study of Taxol in patients with untreated advanced non-small-cell lung cancer. J Natl Cancer Inst 1993;85:384–388.

19. Ruckdeschel J, Wagner H Jr., Williams C, Heise M, Hilstro J. Second-line chemo-therapy for resistant, metastatic, non-small cell lung cancer (NSCLC): The role of Taxol (abstr). Proc Am Soc Clin Oncol 1994;13:357.

20. Murphy WK, Winn RJ, Huber M, et al. Phase II study of Taxol in patients with non-small cell lung cancer who have failed platinum containing chemotherapy (abstr). Proc Am Soc Clin Oncol 1994;13:363.

21. Paul DM, Johnson DH, Hande KR, et al. Carboplatin and Taxol: A well tolerated regimen for advanced non-small cell lung cancer (abstr). Proc Am Soc Clin Oncol 1994;13:352.

22. Leighton J, Comis R, McAleer C, et al. Taxol and carboplatin in combination in stage IV and IIIB non-small cell lung cancer: A phase II trial (abstr). Proc Am Soc Clin Oncol 1994;13:338.

23. Swenerton K, Eisenhauer E, ten Bokkel W, et al. Taxol in relapsed ovarian cancer: High vs low dose and short vs long infusion: A European-Canadian study coordinated

by the NCI Canada Clinical Trials Group (abstr). Proc Am Soc Clin Oncol 1993; 12:256.

24. Horwitz SB, Lothstein L, Manfredi JJ, et al. Taxol: Mechanisms of action and resistance. Ann NY Acad Sci 1986;466:733–744.

25. Johnson DH. Chemotherapy for unresectable non-small cell lung cancer. Semin Oncol 1990;17(suppl 7):20–29.

26. Tishler RB, Geard CR, Hall EJ, et al. Taxol sensitizes human astrocytoma cells to radiation. Can Res 1992;52:3495–3497.

27. Choi H, Akerley W, Safran H, et al. Phase I trial of outpatient weekly paclitaxel and concurrent radiation therapy for advanced non-small cell lung cancer. J Clin Oncol 12:2682–2686.

14

Small Cell Lung Cancer

DAVID S. ETTINGER
Johns Hopkins Oncology Center
Johns Hopkins University School of Medicine
Baltimore, Maryland

I. INTRODUCTION

Small cell lung cancer (SCLC) accounts for approximately 25% of all lung cancers. In the United States in 1993, it is estimated that there will be an estimated 42,500 newly diagnosed cases of SCLC, with 37,250 deaths. Sixty percent of patients with SCLC present with extensive-stage disease, while the other 40% of patients have limited-stage disease. The limited-stage type is defined as disease confined to a hemithorax that can be encompassed in a single radiation therapy port. Some investigators include ipsilateral supraclavicular nodes as well as pleural effusion that is cytologically negative in limited-stage disease. All other patients would then be classified as having extensive-stage disease.

Patients with extensive-stage disease have a median survival, despite treatment, of approximately 10 months, with less than 2% of patients surviving 2 years. In limited-stage disease, patients have a median survival of 16 months with approximately 20% of patients surviving 2 years.

As shown in Table 1, a number of drugs are active as single agents in the treatment of SCLC (1). With so many active drugs, many different effective combination chemotherapeutic regimens have been developed to treat SCLC. Unfortunately, despite these effective therapies, most patients with SCLC will eventually die of their disease.

Table 1 Active Single Agents in SCLC

Drug	Percent approximate response rate
Ifosfamide	50
Teniposide	50
Etoposide	40
Carboplatin	40
Cyclophosphamide	40
Vincristine	35
Methotrexate	35
Doxorubicin	30
Hexamethylmelamine	30
Vinblastine	30
Vindesine	30
Cisplatin	15
CCNU (lomustine)	15

Source: Modified from Ref. 1.

To improve the response rates and duration of responses of the systemic treatment of lung cancer and ultimately increase survival of patients treated, the identification of new drugs with significant activity against lung cancer is needed. The following is a review of the studies evaluating the new drug paclitaxel in the treatment of lung cancer.

Paclitaxel is a novel diterpene plant product isolated from the western yew, *Taxus brevifolia* (2). It exerts its cytotoxic effect by interfering with the structure and function of microtubules (3,4). Paclitaxel in preclinical tumor models, both in vitro and in vivo, has demonstrated significant antitumor activity (5).

In phase I studies where paclitaxel was given as either a 1- or 6-hr infusion, dose-limiting toxicity was either leukopenia or peripheral neuropathy—mainly sensory (6,7). Allergic reactions were frequent with the paclitaxel administration, making it necessary to prolong treatment to 24-hr continuous infusions given every 3 weeks (8). In addition, patients receiving the drug were premedicated with corticosteroids and antihistamines (H_1 and H_2 blockers).

II. THE STUDY

At the time of this writing, there has been one study reported evaluating paclitaxel in the treatment of extensive-stage SCLC (9). In this, the Eastern Cooperative Oncology Group (ECOG) study, patients with extensive-stage SCLC who had not received prior chemotherapy received paclitaxel 250 mg/m^2 administered intravenously over 24 hr every 3 weeks. Because of a limited drug supply at the time this study was activated, patients received a maximum of four doses of paclitaxel as induction therapy. Those patients with progression of their disease after one cycle of therapy or stable disease after two cycles or who achieved only a partial response after four cycles of paclitaxel received salvage chemotherapy consisting of etoposide 120 mg/m^2 intravenously over 45 min on days 1, 2, and 3 and cisplatin 60 mg/m^2 intravenously as a short infusion on day 1. Cycles were repeated every 3 weeks. Prophylactic whole brain irradiation was to be given to patients who achieved a complete response (Fig. 1).

Table 2 details the characteristics of the evaluable SCLC patients in the study; none of them showed a complete response. Of the total, 11 patients (34%) had a partial response while 6 patients had stable disease. It is of interest that in 3 of the 6 patients who had stable disease, there was a greater than 50% shrinkage of tumor; however, there were no 4-week follow-up measurements, partly because the patients received salvage chemotherapy 3 weeks after their last dose of paclitaxel. Therefore, three patients were not considered as having had a partial response since, by definition, such a response must last at least 4 weeks. The median survival time for all evaluable patients was 43 weeks (Fig. 2). The major toxicity was leukopenia; the other toxicities are specified in Table 2.

III. CONCLUSION

Paclitaxel, in the one reported study evaluating its activity in patients with extensive-stage SCLC, was found to be active. The overall response rate was only 34% in the ECOG study. However, if the three SCLC patients who had a 50%

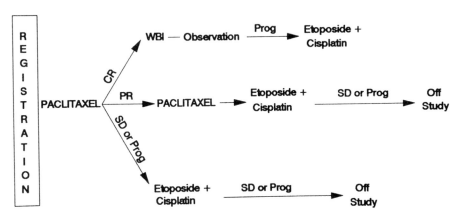

Figure 1 Schema of study.

Table 2 ECOG SCLC Study—Patient and
Disease Characteristics

Characteristics	No. of patients
Entered	36
Evaluable for toxicity	34
Evaluable for response	32
Sex	
Male	21
Female	13
Age	
Median	63 yr
Range	40–78 yr
Initial performance status	
0	9
1	19
2	6
Sites of distant metastases	
Ipsilateral lung	22
Contralateral lung	3
Mediastinum	24
Pleura	7
Scalene lymph node	7
Liver	22
Bone marrow	9
Bone	7
Subcutaneous	1
Other	10
Response	
Complete	0
Partial	11 (34%)
Stable	6 (19%)
Progression	15 (47%)
Toxicity	
Leukopenia	19 (56%)
Pulmonary	3 (9%)
Hepatic	2 (6%)
Cardiac	1 (3%)
Thrombocytopenia	1 (3%)
Stomatitis	1 (3%)
Allergic reaction	1 (3%)

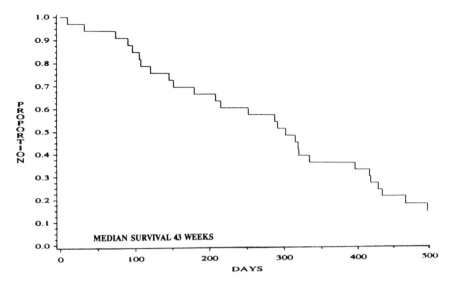

Figure 2 Survival of patients receiving paclitaxel.

shrinkage of tumor but were considered as having stable disease where included as responding, the overall response rate would be 44%. The North Central Cancer Treatment Group (NCCTG) has also conducted a study similar to the ECOG study to confirm the activity of paclitaxel (250 mg/m^2 over 24 hrs and granulocyte colony-stimulating factor (G-CSF) 5 μg/kg days 2 to 15 every 3 weeks) in treating patients with extensive stage SCLC (11). In their study, the number of cycles of paclitaxel was not limited to four, as it was in the ECOG study. Patients experiencing disease progression were crossed over to an etoposide–cisplatin combination. At the time of their initial report, 37 of 43 patients were evaluable for response. There were 27 males and 16 females; median age was 66. Of the 37 total evaluable patients, there were no CRs and 15 PRs (objective response rate, 40.5%). However, if both evaluable and measurable patients are considered, there were 15 PRs and 10 additional responses in patients with nonmeasurable disease (major response rate, 68 percent). The median time to progression was 98 days. Of the 12 patients crossed over to etoposide–cisplatin, there were 1 CR, 3 PRs, and 2 other regressions among nonmeasurable patients. This study corroborates the impressive single agent activity of paclitaxel in extensive stage SCLC.

There are a number of potential combination chemotherapeutic regimens to be evaluated in patients with SCLC. These include paclitaxel combined with the following: (1) etoposide, (2) cisplatin, (3) topotecan, and (4) etoposide plus cisplatin.

Paclitaxel has been shown to cause radiosensitization in a human grade 3 astrocytoma cell line (10). The drug selectively blocks cells in the G_2 and M phases, which are the most radiosensitive phases of the cell cycle. Studies using either low-dose paclitaxel given frequently or higher doses of the drug administered intermittently along with radiation therapy in the treatment of lung cancer have been proposed.

REFERENCES

1. Feld R, Ginsberg RJ, Payne DG. Treatment of small cell lung cancer. In: Roth RA, Ruckdeschel JC, Weisenburger JH, eds. Thoracic Oncology. Philadelphia, Saunders, 1989;229–262.
2. Wani MC, Taylor HL, Wall ME, et al. Plant antitumor agents: VI. The isolation and structure of Taxol, a novel antileukemic and antitumor agent from *Taxus brevifolia*. J Am Chem Soc 1971;93:2325–2327.
3. Schiff PB, Fant J, Horwitz SB. Promotion of microtubule assembly in vitro by Taxol. Nature 1979;277:665–667.
4. Parness J, Horwitz SB. Taxol binds to polymerized tubulins in vitro. J Cell Biol 1981;91:479–487.
5. Clinical brochure: Taxol (NSC-125973). Bethesda, MD, National Cancer Institute, 1983.
6. Donehower RC, Rowinsky EK, Grochow LB, et al. Phase I trial of Taxol in patients with advanced cancer. Cancer Treat Rep 1987;71:1171–1177.
7. Wiernik PH, Schwartz EL, Strauman JJ, et al. Phase I clinical and pharmacokinetic study of Taxol. Cancer Res 1987;47:2486–2493.
8. Wiernik PH, Schwartz EL, Einzig A, et al. Phase I trial of Taxol given as a 24-hour infusion every 21 days: Responses observed in metastatic melanoma. J Clin Oncol 1987;5:1232–1239.
9. Ettinger DS, Finkelstein DM, Sarma R, Johnson DH. Phase II study of Taxol in patients with extensive-stage small cell lung cancer (SCLC): An Eastern Cooperative Oncology Group Study. Proc Am Soc Clin Oncol 1993;12:329.
10. Tischler RB, Schiff PB, Geard CR, Hall EJ. Taxol: A novel radiation sensitizer. Int J Radiat Oncol Biol Phys 1992;22:613–617.
11. Kirschling RJ, Jung SH, Jett JR. A Phase II trial of taxol and G-CSF in previously untreated patients with extensive stage small cell lung cancer. Proc Am Soc Clin Oncol 1994;13:326.

15

Head and Neck Malignancies

ARLENE A. FORASTIERE
Johns Hopkins Oncology Center
Johns Hopkins University School of Medicine
Baltimore, Maryland

I. INTRODUCTION

Malignancies of the head and neck represent approximately 5% of invasive cancers diagnosed annually in the United States. The currently accepted treatment of newly diagnosed patients with local/regional confined disease is surgery and/or radiotherapy. Chemotherapy, when followed by radiotherapy, has a role in the initial management of patients with advanced cancer of the larynx who desire preservation of natural speech (1). For all others, chemotherapy is reserved for palliation of metastatic or recurrent disease after failure of curative attempts with surgery and radiotherapy. Using these accepted guidelines for employing chemotherapy and local treatment modalities, survival data for patients diagnosed between 1960 and 1988, as depicted in Table 1, have shown no significant change (2). These poor survival rates have driven clinical research efforts to identify new compounds with activity against squamous cancers of the head and neck and salivary gland tumors.

Over the last decade, the combination of cisplatin and 5-fluorouracil (5-FU) has become the most frequently used chemotherapy regimen for treatment of all stages of head and neck cancer. The overall response rate in newly diagnosed patients given 2 to 4 cycles of induction chemotherapy prior to surgery or radiotherapy is approximately 85%, with a 35% to 40% clinical complete response rate. Unfortunately, this approach has not resulted in a survival advantage. In contrast, only

Table 1 Survival Trends

Primary site	Five-year relative survival (%) by year of diagnosis		
	1960–1963	1970–1973	1983–1988
Oral cavity + pharynx			
White patients	45	43	54
Black patients	—	—	32
Larynx			
White patients	53	62	67
Black patients	—	—	53

32% of patients with recurrent disease treated for palliation respond to cisplatin plus 5-FU and complete response is unusual. Although the 32% response rate to the combination is significantly higher than that observed for either cisplatin, 5-FU, or methotrexate used as single agents, median survival is not different—approximately 6 months—for all patients regardless of palliative treatment (3,4).

Thus, a major challenge for the next decade of clinical research trials in head and neck cancer is the identification of a regimen that is superior to cisplatin plus 5-FU in order to improve survival rates when used for palliation or as initial curative combined-modality treatment. Paclitaxel is the first new compound since the discovery of cisplatin which has promise for altering current response rates and survival statistics.

In 1990, the National Cancer Institute initiated phase II trials in multiple solid tumors, including head and neck cancer. These trials used a 24-hr continuous infusion schedule and the maximum tolerated dose from phase I trials (5).

II. TRIALS IN PATIENTS WITH RECURRENT DISEASE

One phase II trial of paclitaxel in patients with metastatic or recurrent disease has been completed. Confirmatory single-agent paclitaxel studies and combination regimens are currently in phase II testing.

The Eastern Cooperative Oncology Group (ECOG) evaluated a 24-hr infusion schedule of paclitaxel, 250 mg/m^2, administered every 3 weeks, along with granulocyte colony stimulating factor (G-CSF) support (6). Patients had either local/regional recurrent or metastatic disease or were newly diagnosed with locally advanced incurable disease. Thirty-four patients were registered on the study, 32 with recurrent/metastatic disease and 2 newly diagnosed. Four patients had received prior adjuvant cisplatin-based chemotherapy at least 12 months before study entry; all others were chemotherapy-naive. Of these 34, one never received paclitaxel and 3 were ineligible. There were 2 early deaths (sepsis, myocardial infarction) during cycle 1. In a preliminary analysis, response was observed in 12 patients: 2 complete, 10 partial, 10 stable, 6 progressions. Including the 2 nonassessable patients (early deaths), the complete and partial response rate was 40% (Table 2). Responses were observed in both previously irradiated sites of disease and distant metastases.

In all, 33 patients and 138 courses were evaluable for toxicity. The toxicity was very similar to that reported in other trials evaluating this dose and schedule of paclitaxel. Grade III to IV neutropenia lasting an average of 2 days occurred in 30 patients (91%). Peripheral neuropathy occurred in 13 patients (39%; grade I, 7; Grade II, 3; Grade III, 3) and mild to moderate myalgias/arthralgias in 13 patients (39%). Those developing grade II neuropathy were able to continue treatment at a reduced dose of paclitaxel, 135 mg/m^2, without progression of their neuropathy. Patients with grade III neuropathy had paclitaxel discontinued, after which functional impairments reversed. Stomatitis, nausea, and vomiting were infrequent; alopecia was universal.

These results indicate that paclitaxel is an active new agent for the treatment of squamous cell carcinoma of the head and neck. In patients with recurrent disease and an excellent performance status, the response rate to the 250 mg/m^2 dose administered as a 24-hr infusion was 40%. The primary toxicity was severe neutropenia lasting an average of 2 days.

The current ECOG trial is shown in Figure 1. This is a randomized phase II trial evaluating high- (200 mg/m^2) and low- (135 mg/m^2) dose paclitaxel in combination with cisplatin (75 mg/m^2). In addition, G-CSF is employed in the high-dose arm.

Table 2 Results of the Eastern Cooperative Oncology Group Phase II Trial

Treatment:	*Paclitaxel* 250 mg/m^2 as a 24-hr continuous infusion *G-CSF* 5 μg/kg/day SC daily, starting day 3		
Response:	complete	2	7%
	partial	10	33%
	stable	10	33%
	progression	6	20%
	nonassessable	2	7%
	Total	30	100%

Abbreviations: G-CSF, granulocyte–colony stimulating factor; SC, subcutaneous.

290

Forastiere

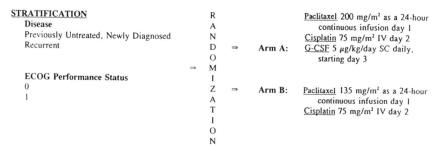

Figure 1   Schema of ECOG protocol 1393: A randomized phase II evaluation of high-dose paclitaxel plus G-CSF plus cisplatin and low-dose paclitaxel plus cisplatin in advanced head and neck cancer.

The sequencing of the two agents and doses selected for each arm was based on the phase I studies conducted by Rowinsky and colleagues (7,8), which established the maximum tolerable doses for paclitaxel (24-hr infusion) combined with cisplatin, with and without G-CSF support.

III. ISSUES IN THE DEVELOPMENT OF PACLITAXEL

A. Optimal Infusion Schedule

A number of important questions must be addressed in the development of paclitaxel in head and neck cancer (Table 3). One of the most pressing is determining the optimal infusion schedule. Initial studies sponsored by the National Cancer Institute utilized a 24-hr continuous infusion because of the high incidence of hypersensitivity reactions associated with shorter infusion times (9). With the development of effective prophylactic regimens (dexamethasone, diphenhydramine, and H_2 blockers), shorter infusions of 1 to 3 hr are being evaluated. The pharmacokinetics and pharmacodynamics of shorter infusions are quite different from 24-hr or longer infusion schedules (10). Because of the unique

Table 3   Issues in the Development of Paclitaxel

- Optimal schedule
- Dose-response effects
- Efficacy and toxicity of combination regimens
- Potential for radiation enhancement

mechanism of action of paclitaxel, causing a phase-specific (G_2/M) block in the cell cycle, one would expect longer infusions to achieve greater cell kill. Thus, studies in progress in head and neck cancer run the gamut from 3-hr weekly dosing to 35-day prolonged continuous infusion.

B. Dose-Response Effects

In addition to the scheduling issue, there is the question of dose response. Are high-dose more effective than low-dose regimens? The ECOG is attempting to look at this in their current head and neck cancer trial. Phase III trials in ovary, breast, and lung cancer that specifically address this question are also in progress.

C. Combination Regimens

The logical development of a new drug with antitumor activity is to combine it with other agents effective in the treatment of that particular tumor type. Thus, a number of phase I and phase II trials are in progress in head and neck cancer evaluating paclitaxel in combination with one other cytotoxic drug. These include cisplatin, carboplatin, methotrexate, and ifosfamide (Table 4). In all combination trials, the sequencing of paclitaxel with other agents may have profound effects on paclitaxel, pharmacokinetics, toxicity, and efficacy. This appears to be true for cisplatin (7), doxorubicin (11), and alkylating agents (i.e., cyclophosphamide) (12). Thus, drug sequencing will need to be carefully evaluated as new combination regimens are explored.

Table 4   Paclitaxel Trials in Progress in Head and Neck Cancer

Phase I
P 24-hr CI + carboplatin
P 24-hr CI + methotrexate
Phase II
P 135 mg/m^2 24-hr CI
P 250 mg/m^2 24-hr CI + G-CSF
P 170 mg/m^2 24-hr CI + Ifosfamide + G-CSF
P 200 mg/m^2 24-hr CI + cisplatin 75 mg/m^2 + G-CSF[a]
P 135 mg/m^2 24-hr CI + cisplatin 75 mg/m^{2a}
P 175 mg/m^2 24-hr CI[a]
P 175 mg/m^2 3-hr infusion[a]
Phase III
P 175 mg/m^2 vs methotrexate 40 mg/m^2/wk

[a]Randomized phase II trial design.
Abbreviations: CI, continuous infusion; P, paclitaxel; G-CSF, granulocyte colony stimulating factor.

D. Radiosensitizing Effects

In vitro studies with various cell lines indicate that paclitaxel is a cell-cycle-selective radiosensitizer (13–15). This effect is dependent on the concentration of paclitaxel and the fraction of cells in the G_2 and M phases of the cell cycle. Phase I trials evaluating various infusion schedules of paclitaxel are in progress (Table 5). Pharmacokinetic monitoring and measurement of paclitaxel concentrations in tumor are part of some of these studies.

The availability of a true radiosensitizer that also has antitumor activity and does not have mucositis as a primary toxicity opens up a whole new arena of clinical and laboratory investigation for head and neck cancer. Several cytotoxics (mitomycin, 5-FU, bleomycin) have been shown to improve disease-free and overall survival when used concomitantly with radiotherapy in patients with advanced head and neck cancer (16–19). However, because of often severe mucocutaneous toxicity occurring within the radiation port, this approach has never gained wide acceptance. Concomitant chemoradiation as initial curative therapy is of great interest because of the potential for improved local/regional control. Multicenter randomized controlled trials are in progress evaluating cisplatin plus 5-FU or cisplatin alone and concomitant radiotherapy with or without surgical salvage for (1) locally advanced unresectable squamous cancers of the head and neck; (2) stage III and IV resectable laryngeal cancer; and (3) stage III and IV cancer of the nasopharynx (20). These pivotal studies may change the current practice of head and neck oncology. It is reasonable to expect that the next generation of chemoradiation studies will include paclitaxel.

IV. CONCLUSION: FUTURE DIRECTIONS

In summary, paclitaxel has antitumor activity against squamous cell cancer of the head and neck. In addition, it will likely prove to be a very effective radiosensitizer. Studies are in progress evaluating multiple infusion schedules and doses of

Table 5 Phase I Trials in Progress of
Paclitaxel and Radiotherapy in Head and Neck
Cancer—Schedule of Paclitaxel

35-day CI[a]
96-hr CI every 3 weeks
24-hr CI every 3 weeks
3-hr infusion per week + cisplatin each week
3-hr infusion per week + carboplatin each week

---

[a]CI, continuous infusion.

paclitaxel used singly, in combination with other active drugs, and with radiotherapy. Future studies in patients with recurrent disease will include comparative trials of paclitaxel-based combinations versus/Cisplatin plus 5-FU. For newly diagnosed patients, strategies to improve survival include induction or neoadjuvant chemotherapy, post-operative adjuvant chemotherapy, and concomitant chemoradiation. As the current phase I and II studies of paclitaxel with other agents and radiotherapy are completed, a logical next step will be to incorporate these regimens into combined-modality treatments.

Paclitaxel will also have to be evaluated in other tumor types, specifically salivary gland cancers—adenoid cystic, mucoepidermoid, and adenocarcinoma. Such trials are planned within the cooperative groups. Over the next decade, investigators will strive to learn how to utilize this drug most effectively to palliate and cure patients with head and neck cancer. Carefully designed clinical trials with laboratory correlates will be necessary to achieve this.

REFERENCES

1. Department of Veterans Affairs Laryngeal Study Group. Induction chemotherapy plus radiation compared with surgery plus radiation in patients with advanced laryngeal cancer. N Engl J Med 1991;324:1685–1690.
2. Boring CC, Squires TS, Tong T. Cancer statistics, 1993. CA Cancer J Clin 1993;43: 7–26.
3. Forastiere AA, Metch B, Schuller DE, et al. Randomized comparison of cisplatin plus fluorouracil and carboplatin plus fluorouracil versus methotrexate in advanced squamous-cell carcinoma of the head and neck: A Southwest Oncology Group Study. J Clin Oncol 1992;10:1245–1251.
4. Jacobs C, Lyman G, Velez-Garcia E, et al. A phase III randomized study comparing cisplatin and fluorouracil as single agents and in combination for advanced squamous cell carcinoma of the head and neck. J Clin Oncol 1992;10:257–263.
5. Rowinsky EK, Onetto N, Canetta RM, Arbuck SG. Taxol: The first of the taxanes, an important new class of antitumor agents. Semin Oncol 1992;19:646–662.
6. Forastiere AA, Neuberg D, Taylor SG IV, et al. Phase II Evaluation of Taxol in advanced head and neck Cancer: An Eastern Cooperative Oncology Group Trial. Proceedings of the Second National Cancer Institute Meeting on Taxol and *Taxus*. Monogr Natl Cancer Inst 1993;15:181–184.
7. Rowinsky EK, Gilbert MR, McGuire WP, et al. Sequences of Taxol and Cisplatin: A phase I and pharmacologic study. J Clin Oncol 1991;9:1692–1703.
8. Rowinsky EK, Chaudhry V, Forastiere AA, et al. A phase I and pharmacologic study of paclitaxel and cisplatin with granulocyte colony-stimulating factor: Neuromuscular toxicity is dose-limiting. J Clin Oncol 1993;11:2010–2020.
9. Rowinsky EK, Cazenave LA, Donehower RC. Taxol: A novel investigational antimicrotubule agent. J Natl Cancer Inst 1990;82:1247–1259.
10. Huizing MT, Keung ACF, Rosing H, et al. Pharmacokinetics of paclitaxel and

metabolites in a randomized comparative study of platinum-pretreated ovarian cancer patients. J Clin Oncol 1993;11:2127–2135.

11. Sledge GW, Robert N, Goldstein LJ, et al. Phase I trial of Adriamycin + Taxol in metastatic breast cancer. Eur J Cancer 1993;29A(suppl 6):S81.

12. Kennedy MJ, Armstrong D, Donehower R, et al. The hematologic toxicity of the Taxol/Cytoxan doublet is sequence-dependent. Proc Am J Clin Oncol 1994;13:137.

13. Tishler RB, Schiff PB, Geard CR, Hall EJ. Taxol: A novel radiation sensitizer. Int J Radiat Oncol Biol Phys 1992;22:613–617.

14. Tishler RB, Geard CR, Hall EJ, Schiff PB. Taxol sensitizes human astrocytoma cells to radiation. Cancer Res 1992;52:3495–3497.

15. Choy H, Rodriquez FF, Koester S, et al. Investigation of Taxol as a potential radiation sensitizer. Cancer 1993;71:3774–3778.

16. Lo TCM, Wiley AL Jr, Ansfield FJ, et al. Combined radiation and 5-fluorouracil for advanced squamous cell carcinoma of the oral cavity and oropharynx: A randomized study. AJR 1976;126:229–235.

17. Weissberg JB, Son YH, Papac RJ, et al. Randomized clinical trial of mitomycin C as an adjunct to radiotherapy in head and neck cancer. Int J Radiat Oncol Biol Phys 1989; 17:3–9.

18. Shanta V, Krishnamurthi S. Combined bleomycin and radiotherapy in oral cancer. Clin Radiol 1980;31:617–620.

19. Fu KK, Phillips TL, Silverger IJ, et al. Combined radiotherapy and chemotherapy with bleomycin and methotrexate for advanced inoperable head and neck cancer: Update of a Northern California Oncology Group randomized trial. J Clin Oncol 1987;5:1410–1418.

20. Forastiere AA. Cisplatin and radiotherapy in the management of locally advanced head and neck cancer. Int J Radiat Oncol Biol Phys 1993;27:465–470.

16

Hematological Malignancies

BRUCE D. CHESON and WYNDHAM H. WILSON
National Cancer Institute
National Institutes of Health
Bethesda, Maryland

I. INTRODUCTION

Over the past few decades, significant advances have been made in the therapy of many of the hematological malignancies. The incorporation of doxorubicin into combinations of other drugs led to a number of chemotherapy regimens such as CHOP (cyclophosphamide, doxorubicin, vincristine, prednisone), which resulted in the cure of 30% to 40% of patients with intermediate and high-grade non-Hodgkin's lymphomas (NHL) (1). 2'-Deoxycoformycin (pentostatin) and 2'-chloro-deoxyadenosine (cladribine) achieve durable complete remissions in approximately 60% to 80% of patients with hairy cell leukemia (2,3). Fludarabine achieves responses in more than 50% of refractory patients with chronic lymphocytic leukemia (CLL), of which almost 15% are complete, with responses in more than 80% of previously untreated patients, of which 30% to 40% are complete (4).

Unfortunately, the rate of progress appears to be diminishing. Recent studies suggest that newer multiagent regimens such as m-BACOD (methotrexate, bleomycin, doxorubicin, cyclophosphamide, vincristine, dexamethasone), ProMACE/CytaBOM (Prednisone, doxorubicin, cyclophosphamide and etoposide followed by cytarabine, bleomycin, vincristine, and methotrexate), or MACOP-B (methotrexate, doxorubicin, cyclophosphamide, vincristine, prednisone, and bleomycin) have not improved on the results achievable with CHOP (5,6). Limited progress has been made in patients with indolent lymphomas; neither adding doxorubicin to combination programs nor the use of more intensive multimodality regimens has provided a meaningful improvement in survival compared to less intensive alkylator-based therapy (7). Similarly, multiagent chemotherapy regimens have not improved on the results achievable with melphalan and prednisone in patients with multiple myeloma (8). In addition, since the combination of cytarabine and an anthracycline was introduced as induction chemotherapy for adult patients with acute myeloid leukemia (AML) or acute lymphoblastic leukemias (ALL), further modification of induction, consolidation, or maintenance regimens has provided only modest improvements in outcome (9,10).

A number of approaches are being evaluated to improve the available treatments for patients with hematological malignancies. These include the development of new cytotoxic agents, modifications of the schedule of administration of currently available drugs (i.e., continuous intravenous infusion), increasing the dose intensity of cytotoxic agents, requiring hematopoietic growth factor and/or stem cell support, the

Table 1 Active Clinical Trials of Paclitaxel in Hematological Malignancies[a]

Disease	NCI protocol no.	Group/ institution	Phase	Dose (mg/m^2) schedule
AML	T92-0235	M. D. Anderson	I	80–200/24hr q1wk × 3
Lymphoma	T92-0017	NCI	I/II	40–80/d over 96hr q21d
Lymphoma	T92-0125	UCLA, COH, USC, Cedars	II	250/24hr q22d
Myeloma/ Waldenström's	T92-0204	M. D. Anderson	II	135–225/3hr q4wk
Myeloma	E1A93	ECOG	II	250/24hr q21d
AML	EST-P-A490	ECOG	II	315/24hr
ALL	T92-0222	M. D. Anderson	II	250/24hr
CLL	T92-0245	M. D. Anderson	II	175–275/24hr q21–28d
Leukemia[a]	CCG-0903	CCG	I	250–430/24hr q21d
Leukemia[b]	T92-0110	St. Jude	I	315/24hr q21d
Lymphoma	SWOG-9246	SWOG	II	175/24hr q21d
Lymphoma[c]	T92-0199	U. of Colorado	I	135–725/24hr

[a]Studies current as of October 15, 1993.
[b]Pediatric.
[c]Autologous bone marrow transplantation regimen.
Abbreviations: AML, acute myeloid leukemia; ALL, acute lymphoblastic leukemia; CLL, chronic lymphocytic leukemia; CCG, Children's Cancer Group; NCI, National Cancer Institute; ECOG, Eastern Cooperative Oncology Group; UCLA, University of California at Los Angeles; COH, City of Hope National Medical Center; USC, University of Southern California.

use of agents to reverse acquired drug resistance (e.g., cyclosporine, verapamil, R-verapamil), and the development of new biological therapies.

A substantial portion of the drug development programs of both the National Cancer Institute (NCI) and the pharmaceutical industry have focused on evaluating new analogs of currently available, active drugs. This practice has been relatively unsuccessful in identifying agents that achieve a substantial improvement in efficacy for the hematological malignancies compared with the parent compound. Many of the major therapeutic advances made in the past few years have resulted from agents with unique mechanisms of action.

One class of agents that has stimulated considerable recent attention is the taxanes, notably paclitaxel and docetaxel. Wani et al.(11) first isolated a crude extract of paclitaxel from the bark of the pacific yew tree, *Taxus brevifolia*, and demonstrated that it was cytotoxic to a wide range of murine tumors, including L1210, P388, and P145 leukemias. Although the taxanes have exhibited impressive antitumor activity against a range of solid tumors, particularly ovarian carcinoma and breast cancer (described elsewhere in this volume), there are as yet only limited data on the efficacy of these agents in patients with hematological malignancies. One explanation for the lack of experience in these disorders with paclitaxel, in particular, was that the availability of this agent for clinical trials was initially quite limited. Once the drug supply issue was resolved, active clinical development of this agent began. In this chapter we review the rationale for the use of paclitaxel in hematological malignancies and the current and planned clinical trials (Table 1).

II. ACUTE AND CHRONIC LEUKEMIA

During the early evaluation of paclitaxel as a potential antineoplastic agent, the drug was noted to exhibit cross-resistance with doxorubicin in a doxorubicin-resistant P388 leukemia cell line (12). This early observation led Fuchs and Johnson (13) to further characterize the mechanism of action of this new agent. They inoculated P388 leukemia cells intraperitoneally into mice, following this in 7 days by the administration of paclitaxel. Ascites fluid was sampled prior to drug treatment and at regular intervals following administration of paclitaxel, the smears were examined, and the mitotic index was quantified. At doses of paclitaxel that were well tolerated by the mice, mitotic abnormalities of the P388 cells were observed. These alterations included disrupted and abnormal mitotic figures and a transient increase in the mitotic index, although paclitaxel was less efficient than other spindle poisons in inducing mitotic arrest. There was also a time-dependent increase in cell size of unclear significance. Their conclusion was that the mechanism of action of paclitaxel was as a mitotic spindle poison.

Rowinsky et al. (14) further evaluated the effect of paclitaxel on microtubules of leukemic cell lines. They assessed whether such changes could be used as a predictor of drug sensitivity. The cell lines used included the HL-60 promyelocytic cell line, a K562 myeloblastic cell line, and a Daudi lymphoblastic cell line. The effects of paclitaxel on microtubules were evaluated with an indirect immunofluorescent assay with antitubulin antibody; flow cytometry was used to evaluate the effects on cell cycle; and a clonogenic assay of drug sensitivity was used to assess drug sensitivity. The various paclitaxel-treated cell lines were then compared with untreated leukemic cell lines. At clinically achievable doses (0.1–10.0 μM) for 2, 4 or 22 hours, paclitaxel induced a time-dependent formation of microtubular bundles or mitotic aster formations, depending on the particular cell line. The reversibility of this effect was also cell line–dependent. Microtubule bundling occurred in cells in G_1 or G_2/M. Persistent microtubule bundle formation was strongly correlated with cytotoxicity, whereas reversible bundling was present in the resistant cell lines.

Recent data also suggest that one mechanism by which paclitaxel may result in leukemic cell death is by activation of apoptosis. Bhalla et al. (15) exposed HL-60 and KG-1 leukemia cells to clinically achievable concentrations of paclitaxel and noted morphological changes and oligonucleosome-sized DNA fragmentation, consistent with programmed cell death, as well as inhibition of clonogenic survival. A possible effect on oncogene expression was noted with decreased expression of *bcl*-2 and c-*myc* but without an influence on c-*jun*. Whereas high levels of *bcl*-2 may lead to paclitaxel resistance in human leukemic cells by inhibiting apoptosis without influencing the drug's antimicrotubule effects, overexpression of p-glycoprotein interferes with both paclitaxel-induced apoptosis and antimicrotubule activity (16). Whether these mechanisms are clinically relevant remains to be determined.

The rationale for subsequent clinical trials of paclitaxel in hematological malignancies was based on a number of factors: the cytotoxicity of paclitaxel against in vitro leukemic cell lines and in vivo models (11,13–17), the dose-limiting myelosuppression of the drug, and the fact that other drugs that interfere with microtubules (e.g., vincristine) may have activity in leukemia. The first clinical trial of paclitaxel in acute leukemia was reported by Rowinsky et al. (18), who conducted a phase I study of this agent in 17 patients with acute leukemia, including 13 with acute myeloid leukemia (AML), 2 with acute lymphoblastic leukemia (ALL), and 2 with biphenotypic acute leukemia, one of whom had the Philadelphia chromosome but was *bcr*-negative. All patients had failed extensive prior chemotherapy. The dose of paclitaxel began at 200 mg/m^2 as a 24 hr infusion and was increased in a stepwise fashion to 250 mg/m^2, 315 mg/m^2, and 390 mg/m^2. Patients were premedicated with dexamethasone, diphenhydramine, and ranitidine to prevent a possible hypersensitivity reaction. Twenty-eight courses were evaluable for toxicity. Although mucositis was relatively uncommon in the clinical trials in solid tumors, using lower doses of paclitaxel, severe mucositis was the dose-limiting nonhematological toxicity at these doses; at the highest dose level, grade IV mucositis (alimentation not possible) occurred during three courses, with grade III mucositis (liquid alimentation only) during two courses. Other side effects included peripheral neuropathy, characterized by a glove-stocking loss of pain, temperature and vibratory sensation; arthralgias; myalgias; nausea and vomiting; and diarrhea. One patient experienced an acute pulmonary reaction thought to be related to the polyoxyethylated castor oil vehicle. The maximum tolerated dose (MTD) was determined to be 390 mg/m^2, and the recommended phase II dose was 315 mg/m^2. The mean peak plasma concentrations achieved at all dose levels were in the range required to induce in vitro microtubule bundle formation. Clinical responses to paclitaxel were limited; there were no complete remissions. Transient reductions in leukemic blasts were noted in 13 courses administered to 9 patients, although leukemia cells persisted in the blood and bone marrow. Complete clearing of blasts from the peripheral blood and bone marrow occurred at a dose of 315 mg/m^2 in one patient and in two courses administered to two patients at 390 mg/m^2. Tumor lysis was observed in the responders, with a white blood cell nadir occurring between days 3 and 8. Nevertheless, the leukemia returned within 2 weeks, 2.5 weeks, and 4 weeks. A partial remission was also noted following one course, although the duration of this response was not provided. Of interest was the observation that microtubule bundle formation occurred ex vivo in the leukemia blasts from eight patients who exhibited clinical responsiveness, but this effect was not detected in the cells from four patients who were totally refractory to the therapy.

III. MALIGNANT LYMPHOMA

Like other hematological malignancies, lymphomas are responsive to a broad range of chemotherapy drug classes, including alkylating agents, anthracycline and related drugs, plant alkyloids, epipodophyllotoxins, and antimetabolites (19,20). Despite this wide variety of chemotherapy agents, cure rates of have not appreciably improved since the development of MOPP (mechlorethamine, vincristine, procarbazine, and prednisone) or ABVD (doxorubicin, bleomycin, vinblastine, dacarbazine) for Hodgkin's disease (21–23) and CHOP for intermediate and high-grade NHL (1,5). Thus, there is a need for new agents which are non-cross-resistant and/or synergistic with drugs currently in use.

Paclitaxel, the first taxane to be clinically used in lymphomas, was considered potentially promising as a new antilymphoma agent because of its broad in vivo and clinical antitumor activity and its unique interactions with tubulin (14,24,25). The sensitivity of lymphomas to vinca alkyloids suggests that tubulin is an important intracellular target, and preliminary in vitro evidence suggests that cells that develop vincristine resistance may develop collateral paclitaxel sensitivity (24).

The efficacy and toxicity of paclitaxel in lymphomas is being studied in four phase I/II clinical trials using a variety of paclitaxel doses and schedules and targeting both chemotherapy-sensitive and -resistant patient populations (Table 1). Two phase II studies in progress are evaluating paclitaxel at a standard dose (175 mg/m^2) without myeloid growth factor support and at a higher dose (250 mg/m^2) with granulocyte colony stimulating factor (G-CSF) in patients with relapsed Hodgkin's disease and NHL. Patients eligible for these trials are not heavily pretreated (≤ 2 prior regimens) so as to assess the activity of paclitaxel in patients who are potentially still sensitive to chemotherapy. A third study is evaluating the toxicity of high-dose paclitaxel as part of a preparative regimen for autologous bone marrow transplantation in patients with relapsed Hodgkin's disease, NHL, and solid tumors. In this trial, the dose of paclitaxel is escalated with fixed high doses of cyclophosphamide and cisplatin.

Although paclitaxel is delivered as a 24-hr infusion in each of these studies, the optimal schedule of administration has yet to be defined. However, there is ample in vitro evidence suggesting that the cytotoxicity of paclitaxel may be schedule-dependent. In both ovarian and colon cancer cell lines, increasing the time of exposure of tumor cells to paclitaxel markedly increases cytotoxicity (14,26). Studies by Lopes et al. (27) suggest that paclitaxel is a phase-specific drug that is more cytotoxic to cells in mitosis. They observed that, like other phase-specific agents, the dose-survival pattern of paclitaxel reaches a plateau at a specific drug concentration, and that cells are more sensitive to increases in exposure time than to doses above this plateau. Longer drug exposure times may also partially overcome multidrug resistance (mdr-1), a mechanism of resistance to paclitaxel that has been identified in vitro (28). Lai et al. (29) demonstrated that tumor cells in culture that express the mdr-1 phenotype display relatively less resistance when exposed to prolonged exposures of low concentrations of the natural product class of drugs, such as doxorubicin and vincristine, as compared with brief, high-concentration exposure. Zhan et al (29) reported similar findings for paclitaxel. Thus, longer exposure times may increase the intracellular concentration of paclitaxel in tumor cells expressing mdr-1, thereby potentially increasing cytotoxicity.

Based on these observations, Wilson et al. (31) performed a phase I study of a 96-hr continuous infusion of paclitaxel including 12 patients with lymphoma or solid tumors. Paclitaxel was escalated from a dose of 120 mg/m^2 to 160 mg/m^2 (total dose over 96 hr) with a cycle length of 21 days. A MTD of 140 mg/m^2 was identified, with grade III mucositis and grade IV granulocytopenia as the dose-limiting toxicities at 160 mg/m^2. Pharmacokinetic measurement of serum paclitaxel concentration in seven patients treated at the MTD revealed a steady-state concentration of 0.06 ± 0.003 μM, a concentration that is cytotoxic in vitro. A total of 25 assessable patients with a variety of histologies of lymphoma were treated on a subsequent phase II study (32); 4 patients each with mycosis fungoides and Hodgkin's disease and 17 patients with NHL. The median age of the patient group was 49 years (range 22–72); they had a median performance status of 2 (range 1-3, ECOG scale), and 72% were male. Most patients had received extensive prior therapy in order to assess whether paclitaxel was non–cross resistant with agents commonly used for the treatment of lymphomas, particularly doxorubicin, vincristine, and cyclophosphamide. The patient group had received a median of 4 (range 1–5) previous combination chemotherapy regimens, including a median of 9 (range 4–12) drugs. All patients had previously received doxorubicin and vincristine. Sixty-eight percent of patients had failed to achieve a complete response with their initial chemotherapy regimen and 92% had received EPOCH (infusion etoposide, vincristine, and doxorubicin, with cyclophosphamide and prednisone) chemotherapy in the salvage setting (33). Most patients had advanced disease with stage IV in 68% and stages II or III in the remaining 32%. In general, this schedule of administration of paclitaxel was well tolerated without the use of myeloid growth factors.

An assessment of the toxicity of paclitaxel by prolonged infusion was conducted in 20 patients who received 114 cycles without growth factor support; 9 (45%) of these had a lymphoma, the remainder were primarily women with breast cancer. Granulocyte nadirs of 100 to $500/mm^3$ and $<100/mm^3$ occurred in 25% and 11% of all cycles, respectively. However, fever and neutropenia were observed in only 6% of all cycles and in 17% of cycles in which grade IV neutropenia occurred. Platelet counts below $50,000/mm^3$ were observed in 11% of all cycles; grade II or worse mucositis (painful ulcers or erythema but able to eat) was noted in 6% of cycles. Eighty-eight percent (41.3 ± 8 mg/m^2/week) of the projected dose intensity (46.7 mg/m^2 week) of paclitaxel was administered over all cycles, with a mean cycle length of 21.5 days.

The response rate of these heavily pretreated patients with lymphomas in this trial was disappointing. None of the four patients with mycosis fungoides responded, and only one of four patients with Hodgkin's disease achieved a partial response. Of interest, however, was that the sole responder with Hodgkin's disease had failed standard chemotherapy, including EPOCH salvage, but achieved an excellent partial response with paclitaxel. This response demonstrated non–cross resistance between paclitaxel and conventional agents. Of 17 patients with an intermediate-grade NHL, 4 responded (1 complete response, 3 partial responses); these responses were of brief duration. Most patients exhibited no response to paclitaxel and rapidly progressed after the first or second cycle.

In a second trial, paclitaxel was administered at a starting dose of 200 mg/m^2 over 3 h to 19 patients with NHL. Two complete remissions and 4 partial remissions were achieved of 12 patients with a diffuse large cell lymphoma, one partial remission was reported of 5 patients with a low grade histology, and one partial remission of 2 patients with mantle cell lymphoma (34). However, with additional accrual to 52 evaluable patients, the overall response rate has decreased to 25% with responses being more frequent in less heavily pre-treated cases (A. Younes, personal communication).

Although the clinical experience with paclitaxel in lymphomas is limited, these trials suggest that there may be significant cross-resistance between paclitaxel and the other natural products in the treatment of lymphomas. It is possible that paclitaxel may be more effective in less heavily pretreated patients, and such trials are nearing completion; however, the high incidence of disease progression within the first two cycles of therapy with paclitaxel suggests a high degree of drug resistance, which may also be present in less heavily pretreated patients. Indeed, if paclitaxel is cross-resistant with standard agents in the majority of patients with lymphomas, as this trial suggests, it is highly unlikely that this drug will improve the cure rate of these diseases. However, experience with paclitaxel in less heavily pretreated patients, further investigation of the optimal dose and schedule, and further studies of the mechanisms of drug resistance (e.g., mdr-1) are needed to accurately assess the value of paclitaxel in lymphomas. Ultimately, if paclitaxel is to have an impact on the treatment of lymphomas, it will have to be integrated into combinations with other agents. Potentially, integration of paclitaxel into combination regimens may be difficult, because experimental evidence suggests the possibility of antagonism between paclitaxel and other natural products such as doxorubicin and vincristine.

IV. MULTIPLE MYELOMA

The number of active agents to treat multiple myeloma is limited to alkylating agents, nitrosoureas, and corticosteroids. Therefore, a drug with a unique mechanism of action is of interest for study in this disease. Recently published in vitro data suggest that paclitaxel should be an active agent for the treatment of multiple myeloma. Bleiler et al. (35) incubated an IL-6–responsive human myeloma cell line (AF10) with paclitaxel. Such treatment induced stable intracellular microtubule bundles, resulting in arrested growth in the G_2/M phases of the cell cycle. This agent also induced DNA fragmentation characteristic of cellular apoptosis. Coculture of cells with interleukin-6 (IL-6) had no effect. Doxorubicin-resistant cells, which overexpress the multidrug resistance phenotype (mdr-1), were resistant to the effects of paclitaxel.

Despite the apparent in vitro activity of paclitaxel against human myeloma cell lines, the limited available preliminary data suggest that the clinical activity of paclitaxel in even previously untreated patients with myeloma is limited. Dimopoulos et al (36) reported 22 previously untreated patients; the first 10 received 125 mg/m^2 (5) or 150 mg/m^2 (5) over 24 h. An additional 12 patients received 135 mg/m^2 as a 3 h infusion. A decrease in the myeloma protein of more than 50% was noted in only 5 patients lasting 2+ to 8+ months.

V. CONCLUSION

Paclitaxel is a unique antineoplastic agent with substantial activity against a variety of human solid tumors. The evaluation of this agent in hematological malignancies is still early (Table 1). However, the results to date have been disappointing in lymphomas and multiple myeloma. For those patients with lymphoma, this might be explained by the extensive prior therapy they had received. On the other hand, the patients with multiple myeloma had not received prior chemotherapy, yet, in the preliminary observations, the drug exhibited limited activity.

Although combinations of paclitaxel with other cytotoxic agents are in development in solid tumors (e.g., cyclophosphamide, cisplatin, doxorubicin), this approach is not yet appropriate in the hematological disorders until such time as this agent has demonstrated substantial activity. The explanation for this limited activity is unclear. It may be that different doses and schedules must be tested in these disorders. More likely it represents differences in mechanisms of cellular drug resistance. Ultimately, significant progress in the treatment of these diseases will require a better understanding of their biology, leading to therapeutic strategies based on a strong scientific rationale.

REFERENCES

1. Coltman CA Jr, Dahlberg S, Jones SE, et al. CHOP is curative in thirty percent of patients with large cell lymphoma: A twelve-year Southwest Oncology Group follow-up. In: Update on treatment for diffuse large cell lymphoma. (Skarin A.T., ed) Park Row Pub, New York 1985, p.71.
2. Grever M, Kopecky K, Head D, et al. A randomized comparison of deoxycoformycin (DCF) versus alpha-2a interferon (IFN) in previously untreated patients with hairy cell leukemia (HCL): An NCI-sponsored intergroup study (SWOG, ECOG, CALGB, NCIC CTG). Proc Am Soc Clin Oncol 1992;11:264.
3. Piro LD, Saven A, Ellison D, Beutler E. Prolonged complete remissions following 2-chlorodeoxyadenosine (2-CdA) in hairy cell leukemia (HCL). Proc Am Soc Clin Oncol 1992;11:259.
4. Keating MJ, O'Brien S, Kantarjian H, et al. Long-term follow-up of patients with chronic lymphocytic leukemia treated with fludarabine as a single agent. Blood 1993; 81:2878.
5. Fisher RI, Gaynor E, Dahlberg S, et al. Comparison of a standard regimen (CHOP) with three intensive chemotherapy regimens for advanced non-Hodgkin's lymphoma. N Engl J Med 1993;328:1002.
6. Gordon LI, Harrington D, Andersen J, et al. Comparison of a second-generation combination chemotherapeutic regimen (m-BACOD) with a standard regimen (CHOP) for advanced diffuse non-Hodgkin's lymphoma. N Engl J Med 1992; 327:1342.

7. Dana BW, Dahlberg S, Nathwani BN, et al. Long-term follow-up of patients with low-grade malignant lymphomas treated with doxorubicin-based chemotherapy or chemo-immunotherapy. J Clin Oncol 1993;11:644.
8. Blade J, San Miguel JF, Alcala A, et al. Alternating combination VCMP/VBAP chemotherapy versus melphalan/prednisone in the treatment of multiple myeloma: A randomized multicentric study of 487 patients. J Clin Oncol 1993;11:1165.
9. Mayer RJ, Davis RB, Schiffer CA, et al. Intensive post-remission therapy in adults with acute myeloid leukemia. N Engl J Med 1994;331:896.
10. Hoelzer D, Thiel E, Loffler H, et al. Prognostic factors in a multicenter study for treatment of acute lymphoblastic leukemia in adults. Blood 1988;71:123.
11. Wani MC, Taylor HL, Wall ME, et al. Plant antitumor agents: VI. The isolation and structure of Taxol, a novel antileukemic and antitumor agent isolated from *Taxus brevifolia*. J Am Chem Soc 1971;94:2325.
12. Johnson RK, Chitnis MP, Goldin A. Characteristics of resistance and cross-resistance in vivo of a subline of P388 leukemia resistant to adriamycin. Pharmacologist 1976; 18:173.
13. Fuchs DA, Johnson RK. Cytologic evidence that Taxol, an antineoplastic agent from *Taxus brevifolia*, acts as a mitotic spindle poison. Cancer Treat Rep 1978;62:1219.
14. Rowinsky EK, Donehower RC, Jones RJ, Tucker RW. Microtubule changes and cytotoxicity in leukemic cell lines treated with taxol. Cancer Res 1988;48:4093.
15. Bhalla K, Ibrado AM, Tourkina E, et al. Taxol induces internucleosomal DNA fragmentation associated with programmed cell death in human myeloid leukemia cells. Leukemia 1993;7:563.
16. Ponnathpur V, Tang C, Reed JC, et al. Mechanisms of resistance to taxol induced apoptosis in human leukemic cells. Blood 82(suppl.): 255a (abstr 1007), 1993.
17. Clinical Brochure: Taxol (NSC-125973). Bethesda, MD, National Cancer Institute, 1990.
18. Rowinsky EK, Burke PJ, Karp JE, et al. Phase I and pharmacodynamic study of Taxol in refractory acute leukemias. Cancer Res 1989;49:4640.
19. Coltman C Jr. Adriamycin in the treatment of lymphomas: Southwest Oncology Group Studies. Cancer Chemother Rep 1975;36:375.
20. Cheson BD: New chemotherapeutic agents for non-Hodgkin's lymphomas. Hematol Oncol Clin North Am 1991;5:1027.
21. DeVita VT Jr, Serpick AA, Carbone PP. Combination chemotherapy in the treatment of advanced Hodgkin's disease. Ann Intern Med 1970;73:881.
22. Bonadonna G, Valagussa P, Santoro A. Alternating non-cross-resistant combination chemotherapy or MOPP in stage IV Hodgkin's disease. Ann Intern Med 1986; 104:739.
23. Canellos GP, Anderson JR, Propert KJ, et al. Chemotherapy of advanced Hodgkin's disease with MOPP, ABVD, or MOPP alternating with ABVD. N Engl J Med 1992; 327:1478.
24. Schiff PB, Fant J, Horwitz SB. Promotion of microtubule assembly in vitro by Taxol. Nature 1979;77:665.
25. Arbuck SG, Canetta R, Onetto N, Christian MC. Current dosage and schedule issues in the development of paclitaxel. Semin Oncol 1993;20:31.

26. Rowinsky EK, Donehower R, Tucker RW. Microtubule changes and cytotoxicity produced by Taxol in human ovarian cell lines. Proc Am Assoc Cancer Res 1987; 28:423.

27. Lopes NM, Adams EG, Pitts TW, Bhuyan BK. Cell kill kinetics and cell cycle effects of Taxol on human and hamster ovarian cell lines. Cancer Chemother Pharmacol 1993;32:235.

28. Jachez B, Nordmann R, Loor F. Restoration of Taxol sensitivity of multidrug-resistant cells by the cyclosporine SDZ PSC833 and the cyclopeptide SDZ 280-446. J Natl Cancer Inst 1993;85:478.

29. Lai G-M, Chen Y-N, Mickley LA, et al. P-glycoprotein expression and schedule dependence of Adriamycin cytotoxicity in human colon carcinoma cell lines. Int J Cancer 1991;49:696.

30. Zhan Z, Kang Y-K, Regis et al. Taxol resistant *in vitro* and *in vivo* studies in breast cancer and lymphoma. Proc Amer Assoc Cancer Res 1993;34:215.

31. Wilson WH, Berg S, Kang Y-K, et al. Phase I/II study of Taxol 96-hour infusion in refractory lymphoma and breast cancer: Pharmacodynamics and analysis of multi-drug resistance (mdr-1). Proc Am Soc Clin Oncol 1993;12:134.

32. Wilson WH, Chabner BA, Bryant G, et al.: A phase II study of paclitaxel in relapsed non-Hodgkin's lymphomas. J Clin Oncol (in press).

33. Wilson WH, Bryant G, Bates S, et al. EPOCH chemotherapy: Toxicity and efficacy in relapsed and refractory non-Hodgkin's lymphoma. J Clin Oncol 1993;11:1573.

34. Younes A, Sarris A, McLaughlin P, et al. Phase II trial of Taxol given as a 3-hour infusion every 3 weeks in relapsed non-Hodgkin's Lymphoma (NHL) Proc Am Soc Clin Oncol 1994;13 (abstr 1267):374, 1994.

35. Bleiler JK, Tang C, Lutzky J, et al. Taxol induced apoptosis in human myeloma cells. Blood. In press.

36. Dimopoulos M, Arbuck S, Weber D, et al. Primary paclitaxel (Taxol) therapy for previously untreated multiple myeloma. Proc Am Soc Clin Oncol 1994;13:409 (abstr 1394).

17

The Pediatric Experience

STEVEN D. WEITMAN
Medical College of Wisconsin
Milwaukee, Wisconsin

MARY V. RELLING
St. Jude Children's Research Hospital
and College of Pharmacy
University of Tennessee
Memphis, Tennessee

CRAIG A. HURWITZ
Maine Medical Center
Portland, Maine
and University of Vermont College of Medicine
Burlington, Vermont

I. INTRODUCTION

Survival rates from various childhood cancers have improved over the past decade. This progress is predominantly the result of better supportive care measures and more intensive administration of available agents. Clinical pediatric oncology trials during this period, however, have been hampered by the lack of new chemotherapeutic agents.

Observations from adult clinical and preclinical studies suggest that a new drug with a unique mechanism of action is effective against adult epithelial ovarian cancer (1–4), breast cancer (4,5), lung cancer (4,6,7), melanoma (8–10), and acute leukemia (11). Paclitaxel, an antimicrotubular agent, is now being investigated for its potential usefulness in pediatric clinical oncology. Although conventional preclinical screening of paclitaxel showed it to have differential cytotoxicity against several human tumor cell lines, no pediatric tumor cell lines are currently used in the conventional preclinical drug screen (12,13). Thus, knowledge that useful advances in pediatric medicine may not parallel results found in adults has led to a cautious yet optimistic testing of the potential benefits of paclitaxel against pediatric malignant diseases.

Paclitaxel is a plant product isolated from the bark (or associated fungus) of the Pacific yew tree *Taxus brevifolia* (14). Plant products remain an important source of medical drugs. However, extensive screening of various plant compounds has identified few clinically active anticancer agents. To date, only vinca alkaloids, derived from leaf extracts of the periwinkle plant (15), and epipodophyllotoxins, extracted from mandrake roots (16), have been shown to have clinical efficacy in the treatment of childhood cancer. After completion of the ongoing phase I and II pediatric clinical testing, paclitaxel will, it is hoped, join the list of natural products with wide clinical utility against pediatric malignancies.

II. PEDIATRIC EXPERIENCE WITH PACLITAXEL

A. Phase I Clinical Studies

Children, relative to adults, more often have cancers for which potentially curative therapy exists; they are infrequently eligible for phase I studies in adequate numbers to successfully evaluate new agents. Thus, childhood phase I studies are not usually performed until the maximum tolerated dose (MTD) of a new drug has been established in adults. Unlike the situation in adults, therefore, experience with paclitaxel in pediatrics is limited and incomplete.

To date, three pediatric phase I studies have acquired enough information to allow some preliminary observations. The Pediatric Oncology Group (POG) recently completed their phase I trial of paclitaxel in children with refractory solid tumors (17). In this trial, a total of 31 heavily pretreated patients (median age: 13; range: 2–22) received paclitaxel by 24-hr continuous infusion over five dosage levels before the dose-limiting toxicity (DLT) was determined. The MTD of paclitaxel in this study of children with solid tumors was 350 mg/m^2 when delivered as a 24-hr continuous infusion. This dose is approximately 100 mg/m^2 greater than the MTD established in similar phase I studies in adults (18).

Major toxicities in this study are summarized in Table 1. Significant myelosuppression (absolute neutrophil count [ANC] <500/mm^3) was documented at all dosage levels but was of short duration and was not related to the dose level or to repeated courses. As in adult studies, the onset of neutropenia usually occurred within 1 week of treatment and reached a nadir 3 to 4 days later (1,8,18–20). No patient remained neutropenic for >7 days, and, as noted by McGuire in adults (1), paclitaxel administration was associated with a neutropenic fever that required hospitalization in fewer than one-third of the courses delivered.

Thrombocytopenia (platelet count ≤100,000/mm^3) was documented in less than half of the courses of paclitaxel administered and generally occurred coincident with the neutrophil nadir. No child had grade 4 thrombocytopenia (platelet

Table 1 Toxicities Observed During the POG Phase I Study of Paclitaxel

Toxicity	Dose (mg/m^2)				
	200	240	290	350	420
No. patients treated at each dose level	3	3	6	7	12
Neurotoxicity					
Paresthesias	0%	0%	17%	29%	50%
Diffuse myalgias	0%	0%	17%	14%	25%
Fine motor deficit	0%	0%	0%	0%	8%
Seizure	0%	0%	0%	0%	8%
Neutropenia (ANC <500/mm^3)	100%	33%	100%	86%	83%
Hypersensitivity	33%	0%	0%	14%	0%
Mucositis	0%	0%	33%	14%	0%

count <25,000/mm^3), and no renal, electrolyte, liver, or coagulation abnormalities resulted, nor did any patient complain of nausea during the 24-hr infusion.

Neuropathy was dose-limiting in this phase I study of paclitaxel in children with solid tumors and occurred at a dose of 420 mg/m^2. At this dose, one patient developed significant motor weakness following the paclitaxel infusion and a second patient had a generalized seizure within 24 hr of completion of the drug. Two instances of generalized seizure activity have previously been reported. One occurred during the paclitaxel infusion, the other after drug administration in a patient with a history of seizures secondary to brain metastases (1,21). In our study, the seizure followed infusion of the drug. Interestingly, the child was receiving intravenous meperidine at the time the seizure occurred. Meperidine typically causes seizures in patients with significant renal dysfunction (22), but it is possible that paclitaxel potentiated the neurotoxic effect of meperidine in this patient. As paclitaxel is combined with other neurotoxic chemotherapeutic agents like cisplatin in pediatric and adult trials, attention to an increased incidence of significant neurotoxicity will have to be considered (23). In fact, one recent adult study used granulocyte colony stimulating factor (G-CSF) to protect against neutropenia in a phase I trial of paclitaxel and cisplatin (24). A higher MTD was reached, but significant neuromuscular toxicity became dose-limiting.

High grade neurotoxicity was observed in one patient in a phase I trial of paclitaxel administered on a 4-day fractionated infusion schedule to children with recurrent solid tumors (25). This toxicity was observed when paclitaxel was administered at a dose of 120 mg/m^2 daily for four days.

Neuropathy has not been identified as a major toxicity in the ongoing Children's Cancer Group (CCG) phase I study of paclitaxel administered as a continuous 24 hour infusion every 3 weeks to children with refractory leukemia (26). The MTD for this study is 430 mg/m², compared with a MTD of 390 mg/m² in adults with leukemia (11). Dose limiting toxicities on this schedule included stomatitis, diarrhea and hyperbilirubinemia. Accrual continues with an amended schedule of administration of paclitaxel every 2 weeks.

The greater dose tolerance to paclitaxel in children compared to adults is not surprising, in that the MTD determined by phase I trials is often higher in children than in adults (27). Wide variations in drug distribution and elimination via renal excretion and hepatic metabolism exist between children and adults (28,29). Although some examples of children tolerating higher dosages are at least partly due to increased clearance of the anticancer drug, paclitaxel clearance was not higher in children compared to adults with solid tumors (8,30). Whether clearance in children with leukemia will be higher than in adults with leukemia is not known.

B. Paclitaxel Pharmacokinetics in Pediatrics

The toxicity and pharmacokinetic disposition of paclitaxel delivered as a continuous 24-hr infusion were evaluated in children treated on the POG and CCG studies described above (17,26,30). Prior to paclitaxel infusion, patients received dexamethasone and diphenhydramine intravenously as prophylaxis against the known hypersensitivity reactions associated with paclitaxel infusions. A histamine H_2 blocker was also used in the CCG leukemia trial. Extensive plasma samples were obtained during and following infusion of the drug. Paclitaxel plasma concentrations were measured using high-performance liquid chromatography with ultraviolet (UV) detection in both studies.

Unfortunately, no data are available on the urinary excretion of paclitaxel, metabolite formation, drug interactions (i.e., cisplatin, cimetidine), or serum protein binding of drug in the pediatric population. In addition, while adult and animal studies suggest that minimal concentrations of paclitaxel are achieved in cerebrospinal fluid (or neural tissue) following systemic drug administration (11,31), no data exist to address this issue in children.

In the POG study of children with solid tumors, pharmacokinetic data were available on 30 patients at five dose levels (200–420 mg/m²) of paclitaxel (30). The data from this pediatric study suggested that paclitaxel tissue distribution/binding involved a saturable process that resulted in high predicted estimates of paclitaxel concentrations early during infusion, when standard linear equations were used. A two-compartment model with saturable tissue distribution/binding is consistent with these findings. Studies (phase I) in adults usually employed a first-order (linear) two-compartment model to describe the disposition of paclitaxel. However, recent studies using shorter infusion times (3 hr) suggest that a nonlinear process may also be involved (32).

End-of-infusion or peak paclitaxel concentrations have previously been reported in adult studies that delivered paclitaxel as a 24-hr continuous infusion (Table 2). In the POG solid tumor trial, median paclitaxel concentrations generally increased with increasing dosages (200 mg/m^2→1.08 μM; 240 mg/m^2→0.62 μM; 290 mg/m^2→1.47 μM; 350 mg/m^2→2.32 μM; 420 mg/m^2→3.15 μM), but there was considerable interpatient variability within each dosage level. The paclitaxel concentrations found in this study tended to correspond to those observed in the adult trials (Fig. 1).

In the POG phase I trial, patients who developed neurotoxicity had areas under the plasma concentration × time curve (AUC) for paclitaxel above the median (>62 μM × hr/ml). Adult studies have not correlated pharmacokinetic parameters following 24-hr continuous administration with paclitaxel toxicity. However, a phase I study of paclitaxel using a 6-hr infusion in adults did correlate AUC with myelosuppression (AUC >25 μg × hr/ml) and peripheral neuropathy (AUC >25 μg × hr/ml) (21).

The CCG phase I and pharmacokinetic trial of paclitaxel in children with refractory leukemia is currently under way (26). Paclitaxel pharmacokinetics have been studied in seventeen patients treated at doses that have ranged from 250 mg/m^2 to 500 mg/m^2. The post-infusion AUC data were fit to a two-compartment open model. The terminal half-life for elimination was 9.58 hr, with total body clearance and volume of distribution at steady state being 318 ml/min/m^2 and 81 L/m^2, respectively (Table 2). Since the doses used in this study are approximately twofold greater than those in comparable adult trials that used 24-hr continuous infusions, direct comparison is difficult. However, one adult phase I trial treated patients with doses in the range achieved in this pediatric study and found similar values for clearance (337–393 ml/min/m^2) and volume of distribution (65–182 L/m^2) (8). These clearances are somewhat higher than the median observed in the POG phase I trial, which was 135 ml/min/m^2 (30). Thus the preliminary estimates of clearance from the CCG study in children with leukemia appear to be higher than those from the POG study (26,30).

Future phase I and II studies should continue to evaluate paclitaxel pharmacokinetics in the pediatric population. Since cisplatin has already been shown to decrease paclitaxel clearance in adult trials (23), studies evaluating potential drug-drug interactions during combination chemotherapy are especially pertinent. These studies may also determine whether a critical systemic exposure correlates with tumor response to paclitaxel.

C. Preliminary Evidence of Activity in Pediatric Solid Tumors

Phase II studies to examine the efficacy of paclitaxel against childhood cancers are ongoing. However, there are hints from the recently completed phase I trial in children with refractory solid tumors that this drug will play a significant role in future pediatric chemotherapeutic regimens. Table 3 summarizes the objective

Table 2 24-Hr Paclitaxel Infusion-Pharmacokinetic Studies

	Dose (mg/m²)	Cpeak (μM)[a]	T½ (hr)[b]	Cl (ml/min/m²)[c]	Vd (L/m²)[d]	Comments
Adult—single-agent studies						
Rowinsky et al., 1989 (11)	250	1.57				No CSF paclitaxel penetration
	315	2.93				
	390	3.50				
Wiernik et al., 1987 (8)	200	0.56	3	348	65	Cpeak and Vd correlated with dose
	250	0.88	3	337	110	
	275	0.94	4	393	182	
Horikoshi et al., 1993 (39)	50	0.10	10	375	213	
	100	0.47	24	187	193	
	150	0.63	22	248	188	
	200	0.75	13	230	149	
Tamura et al., 1993 (40)	50	0.10	3	554	117	Cpeak and AUC[e] correlated with dose
	75	0.22	19	247	267	
	105	0.21	25	386	394	
	135	0.48	17	246	164	
	180	0.69	14	288	169	

						Paclitaxel Cl ↓ C → T compared to T → C
Adult—multiagent studies						
Rowinsky et al., 1991	110	0.21		503		
(T-paclitaxel/C-cisplatin) (23)	135	0.35		400		
	170	0.61		246		
	200	0.83		238		
Pediatric—single-agent studies						
Hurwitz et al., 1993 (17)	200	1.08				
	240	0.62				
	290	1.47				
	350	2.32				
	420	3.15				
Seibel et al., 1994 (26)	250–500		10	318	81	
Sonmichsen et al., 1994 (30)	200–420			135	51	Saturable tissue distribution

[a]Peak plasma concentrations of Paclitaxel
[b]Half-life for elimination
[c]Clearance
[d]Volume of distribution
[e]Area under the plasma concentration time curve

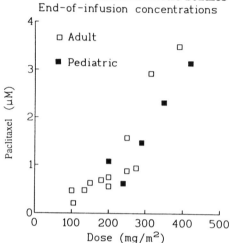

Figure 1 The average paclitaxel plasma end-of-infusion concentrations following 24-hr continuous intravenous administration from adult and pediatric patients with refractory malignancies (8,11,17,38,39).

Table 3 Responses to Paclitaxel Observed During the POG Phase I Study of Children with Solid Tumors

Diagnosis	Dose (mg/m²)	Response
Alveolar soft sarcoma	240	Partial response
Ewing sarcoma	240	Stable disease
Osteosarcoma	290	Stable disease
Hepatocellular carcinoma	290	Partial response
Intrathoracic chordoma	350	Stable disease
Osteosarcoma	350	Stable response
Synovial sarcoma	350	Stable response
Ewing sarcoma	420	Stable response
Pontine glioma	420	Stable response
Synovial sarcoma	420	Stable response
Papillary serous carcinoma	420	Complete response
Ewing sarcoma	420	Minimal response

clinical responses to paclitaxel observed with the POG study. Antitumor responses to paclitaxel as a single agent were observed at all but the lowest dose level. Eight patients had stable disease during the treatment period. One patient treated at a dose of 420 mg/m^2 had a minimal response and two other patients had partial responses: one at a dose of 240 mg/m^2 and another at a dose of 290 mg/m^2 (Fig. 2). A fourth patient treated at 420 mg/m^2 had a complete response of 8 months duration for an overall response rate of 13%. The average antitumor response rate of new agents in phase I trails is, in general, thought to be approximately 2.9% (33). A response rate that is greater than 4 times this average response rate to a single agent is encouraging, and phase II single agent trials are under way.

III. PLANNED AND ONGOING CLINICAL PEDIATRIC STUDIES

Traditional phase II and drug combination studies of paclitaxel have not been completed in children. Therefore, the spectrum of activity of this new agent against common pediatric tumors—including soft tissue and bone sarcomas, neuroblastoma, Wilms' tumor, germ cell tumors, brain tumors, or hepatoblastomas and hepatocellular carcinomas—is unknown.

The completion of phase II studies of paclitaxel in children is important for several reasons. First, phase I trials do not clearly predict eventual clinical activity. Second, estimates of response to paclitaxel for specific tumors will be useful in planning subsequent trials of efficacy. The POG phase II study of paclitaxel in children with solid tumors is currently under way, but response data for specific tumor types are not yet available.

In certain pediatric tumors where response rate is high but cure is rare, phase II "window" studies may be useful as front-line therapy. Disseminated neuroblastoma is such a tumor. Importantly, paclitaxel inhibits neurite growth and induces microtubule bundles in neurons and Schwann cells in dorsal root ganglion cultures (18,34,35). These effects predict that neurotoxicity would be a major side effect of paclitaxel, but they also lead to the logical conclusion that disseminated neuroblastoma takes a high priority in the phase II testing of this drug. The POG has designed such a protocol to specifically determine the response rate of paclitaxel in children with previously untreated disseminated neuroblastoma. Paclitaxel will be delivered to children with stage IV neuroblastoma as a single agent. Following evaluation of response, traditional therapy will be administered. Such studies will allow accurate assessment of the efficacy of paclitaxel against this tumor and no doubt will affect the development of future phase III trials.

IV. COMBINATION CHEMOTHERAPY TRIALS WITH PACLITAXEL

The MTD for drugs used in combination is not usually the MTD of each single drug. In fact, there are probably a range of safely tolerated MTD combinations.

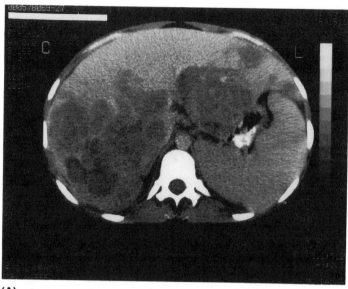

(A)

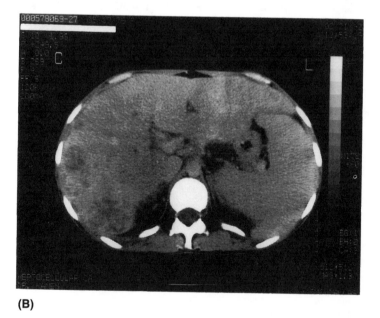

(B)

Figure 2 Partial response (liver) to paclitaxel in a 16-year-old with metastatic hepato-cellular carcinoma: (**A**) computered tomography (CT) scan of liver prior to paclitaxel (290 mg/m²) administration; (**B**) CT scan of liver after second course of paclitaxel therapy

Therefore, it is reasonable to attempt to define the MTD for drug combinations in phase I trials more precisely (36).

Because of the variety of objective antitumor responses noted in heavily pretreated children when paclitaxel is used as a single agent (Table 3), the POG is planning to initiate two phase I studies that will combine paclitaxel with agents having known activity. The first trial will seek to establish an MTD for the drug ifosfamide followed by paclitaxel; the second POG trial will use the drug carboplatin followed by paclitaxel. Ifosfamide and carboplatin were selected because of the known efficacy of these agents in solid tumors and because of the nonoverlapping nonhematological side-effects of each as compared with paclitaxel (with the possible exception of neuropathy associated with platinum-based compounds) (24).

A previously reported adult phase I study that combined paclitaxel and cyclophosphamide found no sequence-dependent difference in toxicity (37). A recent study by Rowinsky et al. (23), however, indicated that neutropenia, the predominant toxicity, was significantly worse when cisplatin preceded paclitaxel. Further, in vitro studies have shown that the sequence of paclitaxel followed by cisplatin 24 hr later resulted in the greatest degree of cytotoxicity of L1210 cells (38). The mechanism proposed for this sequence-dependent cytotoxicity was paclitaxel-induced downregulation of DNA excision repair with subsequent slowing of platinum-DNA adduct repair. Pediatric clinical phase I trials (such as those described above) that combine paclitaxel and known active agents in a rational sequence based on prior in vivo and in vitro data should provide useful information on the effects of cumulative treatment in these patients as well as preliminary antitumor information.

REFERENCES

1. McGuire WP, Rowinsky EK, Rosenshein NB, et al. A unique antineoplastic agent with significant activity in advanced ovarian epithelial neoplasms. Ann Intern Med 1989;111:273–279.
2. Einzig AI, Wiernik PH, Sasloff J, et al. Phase II study and long-term follow-up of patients treated with taxol for advanced ovarian adenocarcinoma. J Clin Oncol 1992; 10:1748–1753.
3. Runowicz CD, Wiernik PH, Einzig AI, et al. Taxol in ovarian cancer. Cancer 1993; 71:1591–1596.
4. Rowinsky EK, Onetto N, Canetta RM, Arbuck SG. Taxol: the first of the taxanes, an important new class of antitumor agents. Semin Oncol 1992;19:646–662.
5. Holmes FA, Walters RS, Theriault RL, et al. Phase II trial of taxol, an active drug in the treatment of metastatic breast cancer. J Natl Cancer Inst 1991;83:1797–1805.
6. Murphy WK, Fossella FV, Winn RJ, et al. Phase II study of taxol in patients with untreated advanced non-small-lung cancer. J Natl Cancer Inst 1993;85:384–388.
7. Chang AY, Kim K, Glick J, et al. Phase II study of taxol, merbarone, and piroxantrone in stage IV non-small-cell lung cancer: The Eastern Cooperative Oncology Group Results. J Natl Cancer Inst 1993;85:388–394.

8. Wiernik PH, Schwartz EL, Einzig A, et al. Phase I trial of taxol given as a 24-hour infusion every 21 days: Responses observed in metastatic melanoma. J Clin Oncol 1987;5:1232–1239.
9. Legha SS, Ring S, Papadopoulos N, et al. A phase II trial of taxol in metastatic melanoma. Cancer 1990;65:2478–2481.
10. Einzig AI, Hochster H, Wiernik PH, et al. A phase II study of taxol in patients with malignant melanoma. Invest New Drugs 1991;9:59–64.
11. Rowinsky EK, Burke PJ, Karp JE, et al. Phase I and pharmacodynamic study of taxol in refractory acute leukemias. Cancer Res 1989;49:4640–4647.
12. DeVita VT. Principles of chemotherapy. In: DeVita VT, Hellman S, Rosenberg SA, eds. Cancer Principles and Practice of Oncology. Vol 1. 4th ed. Philadelphia: Lippincott, 1993:276–292.
13. Skehan P, Storeng R, Scudiero D, et al. New colorimetric cytotoxicity assay for anticancer-drug screening. J Natl Cancer Inst 1990;82:1107–1112.
14. Wani MC, Taylor HL, Wall ME, et al. Plant antitumor agents: VI. The isolation and structure of taxol, a novel antileukemic and antitumor agent from *Taxus brevifolia*. J Am Chem Soc 1971;93:2325–2327.
15. Creasy WA. Plant alkaloids. In: Becker FA, ed. Cancer: A Comprehensive Treatise. Vol 5. New York: Plenum Press, 1977:379–425.
16. Issell BF, Crooke ST. Etoposide (VP 16-213). Cancer Treat Rev 1979;6:107–124.
17. Hurwitz CA, Relling MV, Weitman SD, et al. Phase I trial of taxol in children with refractory solid tumors: A Pediatric Oncology Group study. J Clin Oncol 1993;11:2329.
18. Rowinsky EK, Cazenave LA, Donehower RC. Taxol: A novel investigational antimicrotubule agent. J Natl Cancer Inst 1990;82:1247–1259.
19. Donehower RC, Rowinsky EK, Grochow LB, et al. Phase I trial of taxol in patients with advanced cancer. Cancer Treat Rep 1987;71:1171–1177.
20. Wiernik PH, Schwartz EL, Strauman JJ, et al. Phase I clinical and pharmacokinetic study of taxol. Cancer Res 1987;47:2486–2493.
21. Brown T, Havlin K, Weiss G, et al. A phase I trial of taxol given by a 6-hour intravenous infusion. J Clin Oncol 1991;9:1261–1267.
22. Kaiko RF, Foley KM, Grabinski PY, et al. Central nervous system excitatory effects of meperidine in cancer patients. Ann Neurol 1983;13:180–185.
23. Rowinsky EK, Gilbert MR, McGuire WP, et al. Sequences of taxol and cisplatin: A phase I and pharmacologic study. J Clin Oncol 1991;9:1692–1703.
24. Rowinsky EK, Chaudhry V, Forastiere AA, et al. Phase I and pharmacologic study of paclitaxel and cisplatin with granulocyte colony-stimulating factor: Neuromuscular toxicity is dose-limiting. J Clin Oncol 1993;11:2010–2020.
25. Don Francesco A, Deb G, Sio L, et al. Phase I trial of a Q4D taxol regimen in pediatric patients with recurrent solid tumors. Proc Am Soc Clin Oncol 1994;13:426.
26. Seibel N, Ames M, Ivy P, et al. Phase I and pharmacokinetic trial of paclitaxel: A Children's Cancer Group Study. Proc Am Soc Clin Oncol 1994;13:324.
27. Marsoni S, Ungerleider RS, Hurson SB, et al. Tolerance to antineoplastic agents in children and adults. Cancer Treat Rep 1985;69:1263–1269.
28. Evans WE, Relling MV, Rodman JH, Crom WR. Anticancer therapy as a pediatric pharmacodynamic paradigm. Dev Pharmacol Ther 1989;13:85–95.

29. Evans WE, Petros WP, Relling MV, et al. Clinical pharmacology of cancer chemo-therapy in children. Pediatr Clin North Am 1989;36:1199–1230.

30. Sonnichsen D, Hurwitz C, Pratt C, et al. Saturable Pharmacokinetics and paclitaxel pharmacodynamics in children with solid tumors. J Clin Oncol 1994;12:532–538.

31. Lesser GJ, Grossman SA, Eller S, Rowinsky EK. Distribution of ^{3}H-taxol in the nervous system (NS) and organs of rats. Proc Am Soc Clin Oncol 1993;12:160.

32. Kearns C, Gianni L, Vigano L, et al. Non-linear pharmacokinetics of taxol in humans. Proc Am Soc Clin Oncol 1993;12:341.

33. Estey E, Hoth D, Simon R, Marsoni S, et al. Therapeutic response in phase I trials of anti-neoplastic agents. Cancer Treat Rep 1986;70:1105–1115.

34. Letourneau PC, Ressler AH. Inhibition of neurite initiation and growth by taxol. J Cell Biol 1984;98:1355–1362.

35. Letourneau PC, Shattuck TA, Ressler AH. Branching of sensory and sympathetic neurites in vitro is inhibited by treatment with taxol. J Neurosci 1986;6:1912–1917.

36. Korn EL, Simon R. Using the tolerable-dose diagram in the design of phase I combination chemotherapy trials. J Clin Oncol 1993;11:794–801.

37. Kennedy MJ, Donehower RC, Sartorius SE, et al. Sequences of taxol and cyclophos-phamide: A phase I and pharmacologic study in doxorubicin resistant metastatic breast cancer. Proc Am Soc Clin Oncol 1993;12:165.

38. Citardi M, Rowinsky EK, Schaefer KL, Donehower RC. Sequence-dependent cytotoxicity between cisplatin and the antimicrotubule agents taxol and vincristine. Proc Am Assoc Cancer Res 1990;31:410.

39. Horikoshi N, Ogawa M, Inoue K, et al. Pharmacokinetics of a 24 hour infusion of taxol. Proc Am Soc Clin Oncol 1993;12:146.

40. Tamura T, Sasaki Y, Shinkai T, et al. Phase I and pharmacokinetic study of taxol by a 24-hour intravenous infusion. Proc Am Soc Clin Oncol 1993;12:143.

18

Melanoma

AVI I. EINZIG and PETER H. WIERNIK

Montefiore Medical Center
and Albert Einstein Cancer Center
Albert Einstein College of Medicine
Bronx, New York

I. INTRODUCTION

The worldwide increase in the incidence of melanoma is unsurpassed by any other neoplasm with the exception of lung cancer in women. Even with disease that is apparently localized to the skin at the time of diagnosis, up to 30% of patients will develop systemic metastases and the majority of these will die (1). The development of systemic agents to treat melanoma is, therefore, of paramount importance.

After surgical treatment for primary or regional disease, the most frequent distant sites for first recurrence are the skin, subcutaneous tissues, and distant lymph nodes. The median survival of patients with skin, subcutaneous tissue, and distant lymph node metastases is 7 months, but there is wide variability in survival for this group of patients. The second most common site for the first relapse is the lung, and patients with lung involvement have a median survival of 11 months.

Systemic therapy for melanoma, both as adjuvant therapy and for treatment of disseminated (stage IV) disease, remains unsatisfactory. Few chemotherapeutic agents have demonstrated antitumor activity against metastatic melanoma. In a review of phase II trials supported by the National Cancer Institute (NCI), only 2 of 30 drugs that were tested demonstrated a response rate greater than 10% (with 80% confidence limits) in melanoma patients (2). The best-studied single agents for the treatment of melanoma, dacarbazine (DTIC) and nitrosoureas, have objective response rates between 10% to 20%; complete responses are uncommon. Responses are observed most frequently in patients with skin, subcutaneous tissue, lymph node, and lung metastases—sites that are associated with longer median survival (3–5). The median duration of response to DTIC is 5 to 6 months (6). Complete responses were observed in about 5% of 580 patients entered into phase II trials, and most of these complete responses occurred in subcutaneous and lymph node metastases. Overall, about 2% of patients treated with DTIC sustain long-term complete responses.

The nitrosoureas are a second group of agents with defined activity against melanoma. Response rates are generally between 10% and 20%, with response sites similar to those with DTIC (skin, subcutaneous tissues, lymph nodes, lung) (7–8).

Cisplatin and carboplatin have measurable although generally limited activity against melanoma, with short durations of response.

Numerous combinations of drugs have failed to show convincing superiority over DTIC alone.

II. BIOLOGICAL THERAPY

There is evidence that the immune system can influence the pathogenesis of melanoma. Several biological agents have been tested in patients with metastatic melanoma and have demonstrated antitumor activity. Interferon-alpha is an active agent in the treatment of metastatic melanoma (9). Objective response rates average 15%; most responses have been partial and short-lived and occur mainly in skin, subcutaneous tissue, lymph node, and lung. Complete responses have been observed in only 5% of treated patients, but occasional durable complete responses have been observed (10).

Clinical trials of high-dose bolus injections of interleukin-2 (IL-2), with or without the addition of lymphokine-activated killer (LAK) cells, have demonstrated response rates of 10% to 25% in patients with metastatic melanoma, using several doses and schedules of administration (11–13). Partial responses are typically of short duration, but durable complete responses have been observed in a small proportion of patients.

A. Paclitaxel: Preclinical and Phase I Results in Metastatic Melanoma

Preclinical studies of paclitaxel demonstrated significant antitumor activity against murine B16 melanoma (14), while Slichenmyer and Von Hoff reported activity against melanoma in a human tumor stem cell assay equivalent to activity against breast- and ovarian cancer–derived cells (15).

In a phase I clinical trial of paclitaxel as a 6-hr continuous infusion, Wiernik et al. (16) treated one patient with metastatic melanoma at a dose of 15 mg/m^2; there was no clinical response. However, the patient's melanoma cells obtained from a pleural effusion were sensitive to paclitaxel in vitro. In a phase I trial of paclitaxel given as a 24-hr infusion (17), partial responses were noted in 4 of 12 patients with metastatic melanoma. Responses were observed at 200mg/m^2 and 250 mg/m^2. One of these patients had received prior chemotherapy and radiation therapy, one had received immunotherapy with bacille Calmette-Guérin, and two patients had not received prior therapy. Sites of responses were satellite skin lesions, lymph nodes, a vulvar mass, neck masses, a chest mass, and a liver mass. Response durations were 13 weeks, 16 weeks, 16 weeks, and 22+ weeks.

B. Phase II Results

Based on the activity of paclitaxel in melanoma in this phase I study, 34 patients were entered onto an ECOG phase II study (18). Patients had documented metastatic melanoma and received paclitaxel 250 mg/m^2 as a 24-hr continuous infusion with the standard premedication regimen. None of the patients had received prior chemotherapy; 10 patients had received prior immunotherapy. 4 of 28 (14%) evaluable patients demonstrated objective responses, including 3 complete responses and 1 partial response. Two of the complete responders have remained in complete remission, off all therapy, for over 4 years. One of these patients, who presented with inguinal adenopathy, had a CR after 14 courses and received a total of 37 courses at 250 mg/m^2. A second patient who initially had pelvic and inguinal adenopathy demonstrated a complete response, received a total of 23 courses, and required a dosage reduction to 180 mg/m^2 due to peripheral neuropathy. A third patient who had complete regression of clinical and axillary nodes received a total of 10 cycles of therapy but relapsed with meningeal carcinomatosis. There was also a partial response (of 5 months duration) in a patient with skin lesions and lymph nodes.

Additional evidence of the activity of paclitaxel occurred in four patients. Two patients had mixed responses with significant regression of multiple skin lesions but with development of new skin lesions, while the other lesions continued to respond (2 months duration). One patient had a minor response of skin lesions for 2 months. One patient had a 37% reduction of a lung mass after the initial course of treatment, but an acute hypersensitivity reaction at the initiation of the second course precluded continuation of treatment. The bulk of tumor or sites of metastatic disease may have had an impact on responses in patients receiving paclitaxel. Responses in this study were seen primarily in patients whose measurable disease was limited to regional lymph nodes, skin lesions, and subcutaneous nodules. There were 10 patients who had metastatic disease to the liver and no responses were observed in these individuals.

Grade 4 neutropenia was observed in 23 patients but was characterized by rapid recovery. Ten patients required antibiotic therapy for febrile episodes during neutropenia. Six patients developed grade 3 peripheral neuropathy. Other toxicities were not significant.

In another phase II study conducted at M. D. Anderson Cancer Center (19), paclitaxel was administered as a continuous intravenous infusion over 24 hr at 3-week intervals, with the standard premedication regimen. All patients were previously untreated with chemotherapy. Two patients had previously received radiation therapy and one had prior treatment with interferon. All 25 patients entered onto this study were evaluable for response. Three patients (12%) achieved a partial response for durations of 8, 12 and 17 months; responses were seen in subcutaneous lesions. In addition, four patients had objective responses which were minor responses. These responses were seen in the liver, lung, and subcutaneous nodules, with duration of response from 6 to 11 months.

In the M.D. Anderson study, paclitaxel was generally well tolerated. No significant hypersensitivity reactions were observed. The dose-limiting toxicity was myelosuppression, predominately in the form of neutropenia. Although the duration of neutropenia was brief, 14 patients developed neutropenic fever after the first course of paclitaxel, required hospitalization for intravenous antibiotics, and had a dose reduction in subsequent courses of paclitaxel to 200 mg/m^2. The nonhematological side effects included alopecia in all patients and arthralgias and peripheral neuropathy in the majority of patients. None of these adverse effects required a dose reduction and there was no evidence of cumulative toxicity.

The results of this study confirmed that paclitaxel has a definite albeit low level of activity against malignant melanoma (Tables 1 and 2). However, the observation of relatively prolonged duration of response was uncharacteristic of other active drugs used in the treatment of melanoma.

Table 1 Melanoma Patients Treated with Paclitaxel[a]

	No. treated	CR	PR	MR	SD	PD	NE
Albert Einstein—phase I	1	0	0	0	0	1	0
Albert Einstein—phase I	12	0	4	1	1	3	0
ECOG—phase II	34	3	1	2	2	20	6[b]
M. D. Anderson—phase II	25	0	3	4	4	14	0
Albert Einstein (paclitaxel + G-CSF)	10	0	2	0	2	6	0

[a]Total of 66 evaluable patients with CR + PR = 12, 18% resposne.
[b]Four patients had anaphylactoid reactions to the first dose and were taken off study.
Abbreviations: CR, complete response; PR, partial response; MR, minor response—reduction in size by >25% but <50%; SD, stable disease; PD, progressive disease; NE, not evaluable.

Table 2 Clinical Response in Melanoma Patients

Investigator (Ref)	Measurable response	Response	Duration
Albert Einstein	Neck mass, liver, chest mass	PR	13 weeks
phase I (17)	Vulvar mass, lymph nodes	PR	22+ weeks
	Satellite skin lesions	PR	16 weeks
	Neck mass, lymph nodes	PR	16 weeks
	Lymph nodes	MR	12 weeks
ECOG phase II	Lymph nodes	CR	4+ years
(18)	Lymph nodes	CR	4+ years
	Lymph nodes	CR	11 weeks
	Lung nodules, skin lesions, groin mass	PR	5 months
	Lung nodules	MR	2 months
	Skin lesions	MR	2 months
M. D. Anderson	Skin lesions, lung, liver	PR	12 months
phase II (19)	Skin lesion, lung	PR	17 months
	Hilar mass	PR	8 months
	Liver, skin lesions	MR	6 months
	Lymph nodes, lung	MR	7 months
	Hilar nodes, skin lesions	MR	11 months
	Skin lesions	MR	11 months

III. CONCLUSION

The course of metastatic melanoma remains largely unperturbed by the multitude of available systemic agents. In terms of new agents, what is sought are drugs of novel structure and/or mechanism of action. New compounds should have meaningful single-agent response rates, which have traditionally been defined to be in the range of 15% to 20%.

How does one interpret the paclitaxel results in these trials? Paclitaxel was initially identified as showing activity in phase I trials, although there was evidence suggested by preclinical tumor screens. Paclitaxel satisfied the criterion of being novel both in structure and mechanism of action. The phase II studies satisfy the criteria of optimal phase II study design: chemotherapy-naive patients with measurable disease treated with the highest dose of paclitaxel without growth-factor support.

In both phase II trials, the observed response rate was below the target rate of 15% to 20%, but confidence limits are wide because of small sample sizes and results compare favorably with other single-agent responses in metastatic melanoma. Sites of responses are similar to those of other agents, the majority of responses appearing in subcutaneous lesions; responses are more favorable than those of other agents in visceral sites (lung, liver). Durations of response are longer than in other single-agent studies and unique in documenting two complete responses that have continued for over 4 years. It is not yet known whether this activity will be translated into cure for some patients or an improved median survival for responders. The schedule of administration and dosage of paclitaxel are being tested in other diseases (3-hr infusion versus 24-hr infusion and reduced toxicity with growth factor), and this could be pursued in melanoma.

In a phase I study of paclitaxel and G-CSF, 10 patients with metastatic melanoma were treated and two patients have had partial responses at 250 mg/m^2 and 350 mg/m^2. A dose-response relationship has not been clearly established for paclitaxel. Combining paclitaxel with other active agents (interferon, IL-2, cis-platin, DTIC) appears warranted. A trial is under way testing docetaxel, a semi-synthetic analogue of paclitaxel in patients with metastatic melanoma, and preliminary results show activity.

REFERENCES

1. Karjalainen S, Hakulinen T. Survival and prognostic factors of patients with skin melanomas. Cancer 1988;62:2274.
2. Marsoni S, Hoth D, Simon R. Clinical drug development: An analysis of phase II trials, 1970–1985. Cancer Treat Rep 1987;71:71.
3. Comis RL. DTIC in malignant melanomas: A perspective. Cancer Treat Rep 1976; 64:1123.
4. Luce JK. Chemotherapy of malignant melanomas. Cancer 1972;30:1604.
5. Costanza ME, Nathanson L, Schoenfeld D, et al. Results with methyl-CCNU and DTIC in metastatic melanoma. Cancer 1977;40:1010.
6. Hill GJ II, Krementz ET, Hill HZ. Dimethyl triazeno imidazole carboxamide and combination therapy for melanoma: Late results after complete response to chemotherapy. Cancer 1984;53:1299.
7. Ramirez G, Wilson W, Graze T, Hill G. Phase II evaluation of 1,3-bis (2-chloroethyl)-1-nitrosourea in patients with solid tumors. Cancer Chemother Rep 1972;56:787.
8. DeVita VT, Carbone PP, Owens AH Jr, et al. Clinical trials with 1,3-bis (2-chloroethyl)-1-nitrosourea. Cancer Res 1965;25:1876.
9. Kirkwood JM, Ernstoff M. Potential application of the interferons in oncology: Lessons drawn from studies of human melanoma. Semin Oncol 1986;13:48.
10. Creagan ET, Ahman DL, Frytak S, et al. Recombinant leukocyte α interferon (r IFN-alpha 2A) in the treatment of disseminated malignant melanoma: Analysis of complete and long-term responding patients. Cancer 1986;58:2576.
11. Rosenberg SA, Lotee MT, Muul LM, et al. A progress report on the treatment of 157 patients with advanced cancer using lymphokine-activated killer cells and inter-leukin-2 or high-dose interleukin-2 alone. N Engl J Med 1987;316:889.
12. Dutcher J, Gaynor E, Bold DH, et al. Phase II study of high dose intravenous continuous infusion (IVCI) interleukin-2 (IL2) and lymphokine activated killer (LAK) cells in patients with metastatic melanoma (abstr). Proc Am Soc Clin Oncol 1987;98:2827.

13. Dutcher JP, Creekmore S, Weiss GR, et al. A phase II study of interleukin-2 and lymphokine-activated killer cells in patients with malignant melanoma. J Clin Oncol 1989;7:477.
14. Clinical Brochure: Taxol (NSC-125973). Bethesda, MD, National Cancer Institute, 1990.
15. Slichenmyer WJ, Von Hoff D. Taxol: A new and effective anticancer drug. Anti-Cancer Drugs 1991;2:519–530.
16. Wiernik PH, Schwartz EL, Strauman JJ, et al. Phase I clinical and pharmacokinetic study of Taxol. Cancer Res 1987;47:2486–2493.
17. Wiernik PH, Schwartz EL, Einzig A, et al. Phase I trial of Taxol given as a 24-hour infusion every 21 days: Responses observed in metastatic melanoma. J Clin Oncol 1987;5:1232–1239.
18. Einzig AI, Hochster H, Wiernik PH, et al. A phase II study of Taxol in patients with malignant melanoma. Invest New Drugs 1991;9:59–64.
19. Legha SS, Ring S, Papadopoulos N, et al. Taxol: A Phase II study in patients with metastatic melanoma. Cancer 1990;65:2478–2481.

19

Clinical Activity in Other Tumors

FRANCO M. MUGGIA

University of Southern California School of Medicine
and USC/Norris Comprehensive Cancer Center
Los Angeles, California

I. INTRODUCTION

Exploratory phase II studies of paclitaxel in a wide range of tumors beyond ovarian, breast, lung, and head and neck cancers have for the most part not been published in detailed form. In addition, except for the above tumors and malignant melanoma (see Chap. 18), many tumor sites have not had confirmatory studies to verify the initial level of activity. In particular, this situation pertains to disease sites that are relatively uncommon and for those that have initially negative preliminary data. In this review we utilize both published sources and personal communications from clinical trials that have been completed but not yet published. Because of the tentative nature of this source of material, a firm interpretation is not possible.

This chapter represents also a broad overview of paclitaxel's potential spectrum of activity beyond the initial tumor types covered in earlier chapters. Therefore, a survey of currently ongoing clinical trials is included. Table 1 describes the number of clinical trials completed and ongoing in relation to a specific cancer. Unless specified, all trials have been performed with the 24-hr schedule of paclitaxel given every 3 weeks. Occasional reference to clinical trials with docetaxel, on the other hand, relate to a 1-hr infusion schedule unless otherwise specified.

Table 1 Published and Ongoing Trials with Paclitaxel in Miscellaneous Tumors

Disease sites	No. published (Ref.)	No. ongoing (group)
I. Gastrointestinal cancer		
Esophagus	1 (1,2)	
Stomach	1 (4)	
Colorectal	1 (7)	
Pancreas	1 (9)	
Liver	0	1 (Ohio State)
II. Gynecological cancer		
Cervix	1 (11)	1 (GOG)
Endometrium	0	1 (GOG)
Trophoblast	0	0
III. Urological cancer		
Bladder	1 (13)	1[a] (MDA)
Kidney	1 (14)	0
Prostate	1 (14a)	1[b] (Fox Chase)
Testis	1 (16,17)	1 (Indiana U)
IV. Hematologic malignancies (exclusive of lymphoma)		
Leukemia	2 (18,20,21)	2 (MDA, POG[c])
Multiple myeloma	1 (6)	1 (ECOG)
V. Miscellaneous		
Sarcoma	0	2 (MDA, SWOG)
Kaposi's sarcoma	1 (23)	1 (NCI)
Mesothelioma	1 (24)	2 (CALGB, EORTC)
Glioma/CNS	1 (3,12,25)	2 (CU, UCSF)
Endocrine/Carcinoid	0	1 (Mayo Clinic)

[a]In combination with cisplatin and methotrexate.
[b]In combination with estramustine phosphate.
[c]In combination with ifosfamide.
Abbreviations: GOG, Gynecologic Oncology Group; MDA, M. D. Anderson Cancer Center; MSK, Memorial Sloan-Kettering Cancer Center; POG, Pediatric Oncology Group; ECOG, Eastern Cooperative Oncology Group; CU, Columbia University; UCSF, University of California, San Francisco; SWOG, Southwest Oncology Group; CALGB, Cancer and Acute Leukemia Group B; EORTC, European Organization for Research and Treatment of Cancer; NCI, National Cancer Institute.

II. GASTROINTESTINAL CANCER

A. Esophageal Cancer

With paclitaxel's activity in head and neck cancers (see Chap. 15) and in lung cancers (see Chaps. 13 and 14) and its radiosensitizing potential, there has been mounting interest in testing paclitaxel in esophageal cancer. Ongoing studies have not yet been fully published. Results from a joint study conducted at Memorial Sloan Kettering and at M. D. Anderson Cancer Centers were recently summarized by Kelsen et al. at the Paclitaxel (Taxol) ECCO 7 Satellite Symposium in Jerusalem on November 15, 1993 (1), and at the American Society of Clinical Oncology in May 1994 (2). The starting dose was 250 mg/m^2, with escalation to 280 mg/m^2 if tolerable myelosuppression was present in the preceding cycle. Thirteen patients with squamous cancer have been entered; 3 of 12 evaluable (25%) have had partial responses (PR). Of 30 with adenocarcinomas entered and evaluable, 10 (33%) have had PR. Median duration of response has been 16.5 weeks (range 4 to 45+ weeks). Eleven patients required hospitalization for febrile neutropenia, but no treatment-related deaths occurred. With this demonstrable activity, combinations with cisplatin and other drugs will undoubtedly be pursued. Also, paclitaxel with radiation is ongoing at the Johns Hopkins Oncology Center (3).

B. Gastric Cancer

In this tumor site, again, ongoing studies have not yet been published except in abstract form (4). A dose of 250 mg/m^2 over 24 hr was employed, and only one PR had been recorded out of 20 evaluable patients in the preliminary report by the Eastern Cooperative Oncology Group (ECOG). A full report is awaited, particularly since 24% activity has been preliminarily reported with docetaxel by the Early Clinical Trials Group (5).

C. Colonic Cancer

This tumor site is notoriously chemoresistant to most chemotherapeutic agents except fluoropyrimidines. In part, this has been explained by the frequent over-expression of the MDR1 phenotype that would be expected to be associated with intrinsic resistance to paclitaxel (6). One study has been completed by ECOG in previously untreated patients, and no response was noted in 19 patients (7). Of interest, a liposomal preparation was found to restore sensitivity to paclitaxel in preclinical models (8).

D. Pancreatic Cancer

The Southwest Oncology Group (SWOG) has just completed a phase II study in this disease. Forty patients who had received no prior chemotherapy or radiotherapy were entered, and only a preliminary analysis of the data in 20 patients is available in abstract form. Disease progression had already been documented in 13 patients, but 4 others had received at least four courses of therapy with stable disease (9). Docetaxel has shown activity in this disease, with objective responses noted among 18 patients entered in a trial by the Institut Gustave-Roussy, Villejuif, France (10).

E. Hepatocellular Cancer

Results of ongoing studies are awaited.

III. GYNECOLOGICAL (OTHER THAN OVARIAN)

A. Cervical Cancer

The Gynecologic Oncology Group (GOG) conducted a phase II study in patients with recurrent or metastatic squamous cell carcinoma without prior treatment exposure. Among 30 patients, 3 responses were observed (11). This degree of activity, while somewhat disappointing, did encourage entry of 12 additional patients to provide more narrow confidence intervals of response rates; these results are not yet available. Another study is awaiting activation by the GOG in previously chemotherapy-naive patients with non-squamous cervical cancer. Interest in cervical cancer is also spurred by the radiosensitizing properties of paclitaxel, although work on one cervical carcinoma cell line did not show enhancement of radiation response by 5 and 10 nM of paclitaxel (12).

B. Endometrial Adenocarcinoma

This GOG study utilized a paclitaxel dose of 250 mg/m^2 over 24 hr with granulocyte colony stimulating factor (G-CSF) used routinely beginning 1 day after completion of the infusion. Patients entered into this study received no prior treatment. Results have not yet been published, but activity comparing favorably to that of other active drugs has been documented, with 3 complete responses (CR) and 11 PR being recorded out of 36 patients (H. Ball, study chair, personal communication). The GOG is actively developing additional phase II and III protocols to pursue this important lead.

No trials have been performed in resistant *gestational trophoblastic tumors*, but interest has been generated because of reports of activity in germ cell tumors (see below).

IV. UROLOGICAL CANCER

A. Bladder Cancer

A study by ECOG indicates activity for paclitaxel in this tumor type (13). The dose studied was 250 mg/m^2 over 24 hr, and 26 patients unexposed to prior chemotherapy or radiation with advanced transitional urothelial cancer were entered. A total of 5 clinical CR and 6 PR were documented, with 9 of these responses lasting for 6 months or more. Such activity has been followed up at M. D. Anderson by integrating it in a primary combination with cisplatin and methotrexate (A. A. Zukiwski, personal communication).

B. Kidney Cancer

No response was noted in a phase II trial of paclitaxel given at a dose of 250 mg/m^2 in a 24-hr infusion to 18 patients with cytotoxic, untreated, measurable renal cell cancer (14). This study appears quite definitive in view of its inclusion of 9 patients who had actually undergone nephrectomy and only 3 with prior immunotherapy.

C. Prostate Cancer

A study performed by ECOG revealed minimal activity in hormonally refractory disease. All 23 patients had bidimensionally measurable disease; 1 patient was considered nonevaluable because of death on day 4. One patient had a complete response of lymphadenopathy and a drop in PSA from 66 to 11. Eleven others were considered to have stable and 10 progressive disease; the median survival was 5 months (14a). In spite of this minimal activity, interest in testing paclitaxel against prostate cancer continues because of in vitro studies indicating enhanced effects with paclitaxel and estramustine phosphate (Emcyt) combinations (15). Clinical trials with this combination are ongoing at the Fox Chase Cancer Center (G. R. Hudes, personal communication).

D. Testicular and Other Germ Cell Cancers

Trials in platinum-resistant germ cell tumors have been ongoing in major centers dealing with this disease. Of 6 patients evaluated so far in the M. D. Anderson trial, 2 have achieved PR after failure of two cisplatin-based programs (16). Activity has also been seen in a yet to be published trial at Indiana University and at Memorial Sloan-Kettering Cancer Center (17). The latter study indicates 5 PR and 3 CR out of 31 patients with platinum-refractory germ cell tumors treated with paclitaxel 250 mg/m^2 in 24-hr infusions (17) and including dose escalations to 275 mg/m^2 in 10 and to 300 mg/m^2 in 5.

V. LEUKEMIAS AND MULTIPLE MYELOMA

A. Leukemia

A phase I study by Rowinsky and coworkers in refractory adult acute leukemia observed some antitumor activity as reflected by decrease in blasts and, in two instances, transient total clearance of blasts (18,19). These patients received from 250 to 390 mg/m^2 over 24 hr, and this observation led to a recommended dose of

315 mg/m^2 by 24-hr infusion every 2 to 3 weeks for subsequent phase II trials. Mucositis was the dose-limiting toxicity in this study. Other observations included indirect immunofluorescence staining of tubulin following incubation of patients' blasts with paclitaxel ex vivo. The ability to form microtubular bundles in these leukemic blasts correlated with the antitumor activity observed. Subsequent clinical trials have been ongoing within either large institutions (M. D. Anderson Cancer Center, Houston, Texas), or pediatric cooperative groups. Only pharmacological and toxicological results on 19 patients entered by the Children's Cancer Group are available in abstract form. In these children, doses were escalated to 500 mg/m^2 and the recommended dose for subsequent study will be 430 mg/m^2 as a 24-hr infusion (20). On the other hand, a group from New York Medical College has employed 24-hr infusions of 0.75 mg/m^2/min every 4 days × 3 in 19 adults with refractory adult leukemias. Four aplastic marrows but no complete remissions were noted. However, cumulative doses of 405 mg/m^2/cycle were tolerable, with mucositis as the dose-limiting toxicity (21).

B. Multiple Myeloma

Trials of paclitaxel in this disease ar ongoing within ECOG and at the M. D. Anderson Cancer Center (6). Results from the latter have appeared in a recent abstract and indicate responses in untreated patients, both in 24-hr (2 PR/10) and 3-hr schedules (3 PR/12); duration of responses was 2+ to 8+ months (6). In vitro studies have demonstrated that MDR1-mediated resistance to paclitaxel in human myeloma cell lines may be reversed by a large number of resistance modifiers (22).

VI. MISCELLANEOUS TUMORS (SARCOMA, MESOTHELIOMA, GLIOMA, ENDOCRINE TUMORS)

A. Sarcomas

Adult soft tissue sarcomas with metastatic disease and no prior chemotherapy have been entered in a phase II study by the Southwest Oncology Group, but an analysis is not yet forthcoming. Another trial is ongoing at M. D. Anderson. Interest in this tumor type is further fueled by the 17% response rate noted in a phase II study of docetaxel by the Soft Tissue and Bone Sarcoma Group of the EORTC (5). Three patients with HIV-associated Kaposi's sarcoma have been treated at the National Cancer Institute with 96-hr infusions of paclitaxel, with 2 achieving a response (23). This group shifted to study 3-hr infusions to avoid myelosuppression; one PR has been achieved, with five other patients also still on treatment.

B. Mesothelioma

No experience in this tumor type has been published in full form, but trials are ongoing within the Cancer and Leukemia Group B (CALGB) and the European

Organization for Research and Treatment of Cancer (EORTC). Preliminary data of the CALGB indicate 2 PR out of 15 patients receiving 250 mg/m² as 24-hr infusions (24).

C. Gliomas

Activity has been noted against some glioma human and rodent cell lines (29), and paclitaxel has been shown to enhance the cytotoxicity of radiation in one of these (12). Accordingly, trials in combination with radiation have been planned by P. Schiff (Columbia University, New York) and by M. Prados (University of California, San Francisco). Four patients received a 96-hr infusion for three cycles preceding radiotherapy for gliomas. No responses were noted, but pharmacological studies indicate lower paclitaxel steady-state concentrations than in patients with lymphoma or breast cancer (25). Phase II studies to determine its antitumor activity as a single agent are ongoing at the University of California, San Francisco, and at the M. D. Anderson Cancer Center. Pharmacological studies by Huizing and colleagues and by Beijnen (26,27) in patients dosed with paclitaxel 175 mg/m² over 3 hr prior to surgery indicate that the blood-brain barrier is sufficiently disrupted in central nervous system tumors to allow 100-fold or greater uptake of paclitaxel relative to normal brain tissue.

D. Endocrine Tumors

No information is available to date on the effect of paclitaxel on tumors of the endocrine organs, carcinoids, and neuroendocrine tumors. A trial on carcinoid tumors is currently ongoing at the Mayo Clinic (C. Moertel, personal communication).

VII. CONCLUSIONS

The spectrum of activity of paclitaxel has not been fully established. Not only are most of the studies still of a preliminary nature, but no studies in combination with other drugs or with radiation have yet been carried out in most tumor types. Moreover, studies testing shorter or longer infusion schedules must also be performed. Guiding principles outlined below are likely to influence future developments.

Overexpression of MDR1 by tumors may predict for intrinsic resistance and may explain the lack of responsiveness of colonic and renal cell cancers. Prior treatment may alter the sensitivity of tumors by induction of MDR1, and this must be considered in interpreting data from these trials. Also, MDR1 may be important in factors influencing drug distribution, such as the blood-brain barrier. Nevertheless, pharmacological studies indicate good penetrance into central nervous system tumors. On the other hand, cerebrospinal fluid levels have been determined to be very low.

In combination chemotherapy, sequencing has proven to be crucial. In addition, combinations with doxorubicin, for example, have been complicated by increasing mucosal toxicity. For many tumor types reviewed, however, combinations with cisplatin may prove desirable to explore. In this context, the preliminary data in esophageal and bladder cancers are promising and may lead to improved therapeutic strategies. Future studies incorporating radiation therapy are also eagerly awaited. As the exploration of cisplatin more than a decade ago led to substantial therapeutic gains in a number of previously refractory diseases (29), the use of paclitaxel may be predicted to evolve in the ensuing years for many of the conditions covered in this chapter.

REFERENCES

1. Kelsen D, Ajani J, Ilson D. Phase II trial of paclitaxel in esophageal cancer. Paclitaxel (Taxol) ECCO 7 Satellite Symposium, Jerusalem, Nov 15, 1993.
2. Ajani JA, Ilson D, Daugherty K, et al. Activity of Taxol in patients with squamous cell carcinoma and adenocarcinoma of the esophagus. J Natl Cancer Inst 1994;86:1086–1091.
3. Donehower R. Overview of studies with paclitaxel. 8th NCI-EORTC Symposium on New Drugs in Cancer Therapy. Amsterdam, March 15–18, 1994.
4. Einzig AI, Wiernik PH, Lipsitz S, Benson AB III. Phase II trial of Taxol in patients with adenocarcinoma of the upper gastrointestinal tract (UGIT): The Eastern Cooperative Oncology Group (ECOG) results. Proc ASCO 1993;12:194.
5. Verweij J. Recent clinical developments and future directions with docetaxel. 8th NCI-EORTC Symposium on New Drugs in Cancer Therapy. Amsterdam, March 15–18, 1994.
6. Dimopoulos M, Arbuck S, Weber D, et al. Primary paclitaxel (Taxol) therapy for previously untreated multiple myeloma (abstr 1394). Proc ASCO 1994;13:409.
7. Arbuck SG, Christian MC, Fisherman JC, et al. Clinical development of Taxol. Natl Cancer Inst Monogr 1993;15:11–24.
8. Straubinger RM, Sharma A, Murray M, Mayhew E. Novel Taxol formulations: Taxol-containing liposomes. Natl Cancer Inst Monogr 1993;15:69–78.
9. Brown T, Tangen C, Fleming T, Macdonald J. A phase II trial of Taxol and granulocyte colony stimulating factor (G-CSF) in patients with adenocarcinoma of the pancreas (abstr 592). Proc ASCO 1993;12:200.
10. DeForni A, Rougier P, Adenis A, et al. Phase II study of Taxotere (RP 56976, docetaxel) in locally advanced and/or metastatic pancreatic cancer. 8th NCI-EORTC Symposium on New Drugs in Cancer Therapy. Amsterdam, March 15–18, 1994.
11. Rowinsky EK, Onetto N, Canetta RM. Taxol: The first of the taxanes, an important new class of antitumor agents. Semin Oncol 1992;19:646–662.
12. Geard CR, Jones JM, Schiff PB. Taxol and radiation. Natl Cancer Inst Monogr 1993; 15:89–94.
13. Roth BJ, Dreicer R, Einhorn LH, et al. Significant activity of paclitaxel in advanced transitional cell carcinoma of the urothelium: A phase II trial of Eastern Cooperative Oncology Group. J Clin Oncol 1994;12:2264–2270.

14. Einzig AJ, Gorowski E, Sasloff J, Wiernik PH. Phase II trial of Taxol in patients with renal cell carcinoma (abstr 884). Proc Am Assoc Cancer Res 1988;29:222.

14a. Roth BJ, Yeap BY, Wilding G, et al. Taxol in advanced, hormone-refractory carcinoma of the prostate: A Phase II trial of the Eastern Cooperative Oncology Group. Cancer 1993;72:2457–2460.

15. Tew KD, Sheridan VR, Speicher LA. Determinant factors in estramustine cytotoxicity and resistance. Cell Pharmacol 1993;1(suppl 1):S53–S58.

16. Nazario A, Amato R, Hutchinson L, et al. Preliminary results of Taxol in patients with refractory or second relapse non-seminomatous germ cell tumors of the testis (abstr 1387). Proc Am Assoc Cancer Res 1994;35:232.

17. Motzer R, Bajorin DF, Schwartz LH, et al. Phase II trial of paclitaxel shows antitumor activity in patients with previously treated germ cell tumors. J Clin Oncol 1994;12: 2277–2283.

18. Rowinsky EK, Burke PJ, Karp JE. Phase I study of Taxol in refractory adult acute leukemia. Cancer Res 1989;49:4640–4647.

19. Rowinsky EK. Clinical pharmacology of Taxol. Natl Cancer Inst Monogr 1993;15: 25–38.

20. Seibel N, Ames M, Ivy P, et al. Phase I and pharmacologic study of paclitaxel in refractory pediatric leukemia: A Children's Cancer Group study (abstr 1068). Proc ASCO 1994;13:324.

21. Feldman E, Seiter K, Helson L, et al. Phase I evaluation of a short infusion of every 4 day schedule of Taxol in refractory acute leukemia (abstr 1022). Proc ASCO 1994; 13:311.

22. Horwitz SB, Cohen D, Rao S, et al. Taxol: Mechanisms of action and resistance. Natl Cancer Inst Monogr 1993;15:55–62.

23. Saville MW, Lietzau J, Wilson W, et al. A trial of paclitaxel (Taxol) in patients with HIV-associated Kaposi's sarcoma (KS) (abstr 20). Proc ASCO 1994;13:54.

24. Vogelzang NJ, Herndon J, Clamon GH, et al. Paclitaxel (Taxol) for malignant mesothelioma: A phase II study of the Cancer and Leukemia Group B (CALGB 9234) (abstr 1382). Proc ASCO 1994;13:405.

25. Fetell MR, Grossman SA, Balmaceda, et al. Clinical and pharmacologic study of pre-irradiation Taxol administered as a 96 hour infusion in adults with newly diagnosed glioblastoma multiforme (abstr 504). Proc ASCO 1994;13:179.

26. Huizing MT, Keung ACF, Rosing H, et al. Pharmacokinetics of paclitaxel and metabolites in a randomized comparative study in platinum pretreated ovarian cancer patients. J Clin Oncol 1993;11:2127–2135.

27. Beijnen JH. Pharmacology of paclitaxel. 8th NCI-EORTC Symposium on New Drugs in Cancer Therapy. Amsterdam, Mar 15–18, 1994.

28. Cahan MA, Walter KA, Colvin OM, Brem H. Cytotoxicity of Taxol in vitro against human and rat malignant brain tumors. Cancer Chemother Pharmacol 1994;33: 441–444.

29. Muggia FM. Future of cancer chemotherapy with cisplatin. Semin Oncol 1989; 16(suppl):123–128.

Index

About the Editors

WILLIAM P. MCGUIRE is Professor of Medicine in the Division of Hematology/ Oncology of the Department of Medicine at Emory University, Atlanta, Georgia. The author or coauthor of over 180 book chapters, professional papers, and abstracts, he is a member of the American Society of Clinical Oncology, the International Association for the Study of Lung Cancer, the Gynecologic Oncology Group, and the International Gynecological Cancer Society, among other organizations, and he serves on the editorial boards of several journals, including *Gynecologic Oncology* and *Physician Data Query*. Dr. McGuire, a diplomate of the American Board of Internal Medicine, received the M.D. degree (1971) from Baylor Medical College, Houston, Texas.

ERIC K. ROWINSKY is Associate Professor of Oncology in the Division of Pharmacology and Therapeutics at Johns Hopkins Oncology Center and Staff Oncologist at Johns Hopkins Hospital, Baltimore, Maryland. A Fellow of the American College of Physicians and a member of the American Society of Clinical Oncology and the American Association for Cancer Research, among other organizations, he is the author or coauthor of more than 150 book chapters, professional papers, and abstracts and serves on the editorial boards of several journals, including the *Journal of Cancer Research and Clinical Oncology* and *Clinical Cancer Research*. Dr. Rowinsky received the M.D. degree (1981) from Vanderbilt University School of Medicine, Nashville, Tennessee. He is a diplomate of the American Board of Internal Medicine.